Respiratory Physiology II

Publisher's Note

The *International Review of Physiology* remains a major force in the education of established scientists and advanced students of physiology throughout the world. It continues to present accurate, timely, and thorough reviews of key topics by distinguished authors charged with the responsibility of selecting and critically analyzing new facts and concepts important to the progress of physiology from the mass of information in their respective fields.

Following the successful format established by the earlier volumes in this series, new volumes of the *International Review of Physiology* will concentrate on current developments in neurophysiology and cardiovascular, respiratory, gastrointestinal, liver, endocrine, kidney and urinary tract, environmental, and reproductive physiology. New volumes on a given subject generally appear at two-year intervals, or according to the demand created by new developments in the field. The scope of the series is flexible, however, so that future volumes may cover areas not included earlier.

University Park Press is honored to continue publication of the *International Review of Physiology* under its sole sponsorship beginning with Volume 9. The following is a list of volumes published and currently in preparation for the series:

Volume 1: **CARDIOVASCULAR PHYSIOLOGY** (A. C. Guyton and C. E. Jones)
Volume 2: **RESPIRATORY PHYSIOLOGY** (J. G. Widdicombe)
Volume 3: **NEUROPHYSIOLOGY** (C. C. Hunt)
Volume 4: **GASTROINTESTINAL PHYSIOLOGY** (E. D. Jacobson and L. L. Shanbour)
Volume 5: **ENDOCRINE PHYSIOLOGY** (S. M. McCann)
Volume 6: **KIDNEY AND URINARY TRACT PHYSIOLOGY** (K. Thurau)
Volume 7: **ENVIRONMENTAL PHYSIOLOGY** (D. Robertshaw)
Volume 8: **REPRODUCTIVE PHYSIOLOGY** (R. O. Greep)
Volume 9: **CARDIOVASCULAR PHYSIOLOGY II** (A. C. Guyton and A. W. Cowley, Jr.)
Volume 10: **NEUROPHYSIOLOGY II** (R. Porter)
Volume 11: **KIDNEY AND URINARY TRACT PHYSIOLOGY II** (K. Thurau)
Volume 12: **GASTROINTESTINAL PHYSIOLOGY II** (R. K. Crane)
Volume 13: **REPRODUCTIVE PHYSIOLOGY II** (R. O. Greep)
Volume 14: **RESPIRATORY PHYSIOLOGY II** (J. G. Widdicombe)

(Series numbers for the following volumes will be assigned in order of publication)
ENDOCRINE PHYSIOLOGY II (S. M. McCann)
ENVIRONMENTAL PHYSIOLOGY II (D. Robertshaw)

Consultant Editor: Arthur C. Guyton, M.D., Department of Physiology and Biophysics, University of Mississippi Medical Center

INTERNATIONAL REVIEW
OF PHYSIOLOGY

Volume 14

Respiratory
Physiology II

Edited by

John G. Widdicombe, M.D., Ph.D., F.R.C.P.

Department of Physiology
St. Georges Hospital Medical School
Tooting, London, England

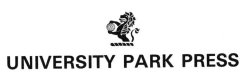

UNIVERSITY PARK PRESS

Baltimore • London • Tokyo

UNIVERSITY PARK PRESS
International Publishers in Science and Medicine
Chamber of Commerce Building
Baltimore, Maryland 21202

Copyright © 1977 by University Park Press

Typeset by The Composing Room of Michigan, Inc.

Manufactured in the United States of America by Universal Lithographers, Inc.,
and The Optic Bindery Incorporated

Library of Congress Cataloging in Publication Data
Main entry under title:

Respiratory physiology II.
  (International review of physiology; v. 14)
  Includes bibliographical references and index.
  1. Respiration. I. Widdicombe, J. G.
II. Series. [DNLM: 1. Respiration—Periodicals.
W1 IN834F v. 14 etc.]
QP1.P62 vol. 14 [QP121] 599'.01'8s [599'.01'2]
ISBN 0-8391-1063-4   77-823

Consultant Editor's Note

In 1974 the first series of the *International Review of Physiology* appeared. This new review was launched in response to unfulfilled needs in the field of physiological science, most importantly the need for an in-depth review written especially for teachers and students of physiology throughout the world. It was not without trepidation that this publishing venture was begun, but its early success seems to assure its future. Therefore, we need to repeat here the philosophy, the goals, and the concept of the *International Review of Physiology*.

The *International Review of Physiology* has the same goals as all other reviews for accuracy, timeliness, and completeness, but it also has policies that we hope and believe engender still other important qualities often missing in reviews, the qualities of critical evaluation, integration, and instructiveness. To achieve these goals, the format allows publication of approximately 2,500 pages per series, divided into eight subspecialty volumes, each organized by experts in their respective fields. This extensiveness of coverage allows consideration of each subject in great depth. And, to make the review as timely as possible, a new series of all eight volumes is published approximately every two years, giving a cycle time that will keep the articles current.

Yet, perhaps the greatest hope that this new review will achieve its goals lies in its editorial policies. A simple but firm request is made to each author that he utilize his expertise and his judgment to sift from the mass of biennial publications those new facts and concepts that are important to the progress of physiology; that he make a conscious effort not to write a review consisting of an annotated list of references; and that the important material that he does choose be presented in thoughtful and logical exposition, complete enough to convey full understanding, as well as woven into context with previously established physiological principles. Hopefully, these processes will continue to bring to the reader each two years a treatise that he will use not merely as a reference in his own personal field but also as an exercise in refreshing and modernizing his whole store of physiological knowledge.

A. C. Guyton

Contents

Preface ix

1
Structure of the Lungs 1
W. M. Thurlbeck

2
Gas Mixing and Distribution in the Lung 37
L. A. Engel and P. T. Macklem

3
Pulmonary Gas Exchange 83
J. B. West

4
Respiratory Function of Hemoglobin 107
H. Bartels and R. Baumann

5
Pulmonary Circulation and Fluid Balance 135
J. M. B. Hughes

6
Control of the Breathing Pattern 185
G. W. Bradley

7
**Comparative Physiology of Respiration: Functional Analysis
of Gas Exchange Organs in Vertebrates** 219
J. Piiper and P. Scheid

8
Control of Breathing in Diseases of the Respiratory System 255
F. Paleček

9

Defense Mechanisms of the Respiratory Tract and Lungs 291
J. G. Widdicombe

Index 317

Preface

The second edition of *Respiratory Physiology* contains chapters that fill some of the more obvious gaps in the first edition; other contributions bring up to date rapidly expanding aspects of respiratory physiology previously dealt with. This edition might be said to resemble the postnatal development of the lung (Thurlbeck, Chapter 1), in that there is a combination of recruitment of new areas and expansion of those already functioning. Over the past decade one striking development concerning respiratory physiology has been its increasing correlation with lung structure, including morphology and ultrastructure. This partnership between two of the basic medical disciplines, sometimes academic competitors, is displayed in many of the chapters of this edition. Several of the chapters also describe or touch on the applications of physiology in experimental or human respiratory disease. This is no new trend; however, it is one of increasing significance and value as the results of basic research accumulate.

I am grateful to all the authors not only for their valuable and expert contributions, but also for their apparently willing acceptance of editorial constraints and procedures. I am also grateful to Margaret Conroy, who has felicitously organized the administrative juggling of the nine chapters without mishap.

Respiratory Physiology II

International Review of Physiology
Respiratory Physiology II, Volume 14
Edited by John G. Widdicombe
Copyright 1977   University Park Press   Baltimore

1
Structure
of the Lungs

W. M. THURLBECK

University of Manitoba, Faculty of Medicine, Winnipeg, Canada

CONTINUING MYSTERY OF THE CLARA CELL   2

POSTNATAL LUNG GROWTH   4
  Nature of Lung Growth   4
    Animals   4
    Human Lung   12
  Growth of Other Structures in Lungs   15
    Airways   15
    Vascular System   15
  Alterations in Postnatal Lung Growth   16
    Resection of Lung Tissue   16
    Diminution of Lung Volume   17
    Growth Hormone   17
    Hypoxia and Hypobaric Conditions   18
    Hyperoxia   18

LUNG EXPANSION   18
  Alveolar Expansion   19
  Lung Inflation Primarily by Alveolar
    Enlargement and Stretching   20
  Lung Inflation by Alveolar Recruitment or Unfolding   23
  Effects of Lung Inflation on Capillary Bed   26
  Expansion of Airways   27

LUNG AND ITS NERVES   28
  Airways and Nonadrenergic Inhibitory Nervous System   28
  Nerves in Alveoli and Airway Epithelium   29

This chapter is chiefly concerned with three topics that have become of major interest since the last edition of this book (1)—postnatal lung growth, the manner in which the lung expands, and the nerve supply of the lung. Admittedly, much of the information concerning the latter two topics predates the previous edition of this book, but the issues are of considerable current interest and there have been some notable recent contributions. In addition, some recent data concerning the Clara cell are reviewed; this topic was reviewed in more detail in the previous edition.

CONTINUING MYSTERY OF THE CLARA CELL

Clara cells are distinctive cells which are most obvious in the distal conducting airways of rats, mice, and rabbits. They are nonciliated cells which line the airways and have characteristic tongue-shaped protections into the airway lumen. The function of the Clara cell has been a source of lively controversy. In the previous edition of this book, the evidence concerning the cellular source of pulmonary surfactant was reviewed in detail. It was concluded that the type II alveolar cells (granular pneumonocytes) probably secreted surfactant and that, although the Clara cells were an unlikely source of surfactant, they might contribute to the "hypophase" upon which surfactant lies. Three recent papers have supported the notion that the Clara cells may be the chief source of surfactant. Etherton et al. (2) have recently expanded their initial observations (3) that tritiated palmitate labeled Clara cells much more heavily than it did type II cells 0.5 and 1.5 min after injection. At 60 min, more grains were found over type II cells, suggesting that surfactant was secreted by Clara cells and phagocytosed by type II cells. Their most recent paper (2) has reaffirmed the preferential labeling of Clara cells for palmitate; it also indicated that the secretion of Clara cells was of apocrine type and that the tips of the tongue-shaped processes were secreted into the lumen of the airways. Smith et al. (4) also claimed that apocrine secretion occurred in Clara cells. They observed that the apical cap of the Clara cells commonly projected from the rest of the cell. They noted that the cytoplasm of this part of the cell was often less dense than the rest of the cell and was sharply demarcated from it. The apical cap contained large quantities of endoplasmic reticulum. They observed "islands of cytoplasm," lying apparently free in the bronchiolar lumen, that were identical in appearance to the apical caps in some instances; organelles were lacking in the islands in other instances. These findings were more prominent in adult rats acutely exposed to hypoxia, and they interpreted the observations to indicate an attempt on the part of the Clara cells to increase the amount of available surfactant. When chlorphentermine was administered to rats, hyperplasia of Clara cells was observed, and the amount of phospholipid in the alveolar spaces was increased. Lamelated electron-dense inclusions, thought to be phospholipid, appeared in the Clara cells. The authors concluded "that the Clara cell secretes the phospholipid pulmonary surfactant."

The critical concept reviewed in both of the papers is the notion of apocrine secretion by the Clara cell. The papers ignore the membrane-bound granules within the Clara cells, usually thought to be secretory granules. The evidence for apocrine secretion is less than convincing. Wang et al. (5) attempted to affect Clara cell secretion with the use of adrenaline and pilocarpine, but were unable to convince themselves of the presence of true apocrine secretion in Clara cells. A variety of blebs and apical caps was apparent in Clara cells in these experiments, but similar changes were seen in other cells and these were interpreted as nonspecific changes of cell damage.

Petrik and Collet (6) have observed the incorporation of tritiated leucine, choline, acetate, and galactose into Clara cells of mice. They found that labeled choline was not incorporated into Clara cells, but was incorporated into type II cells. Because choline is such an important constituent of surfactant, it thus seems unlikely that surfactant is secreted by the Clara cells. They also noted that labeled leucine (used as an estimate of protein synthesis), galactose (carbohydrate metabolism), and acetate rapidly appeared in the cell cytoplasm in smooth and rough endoplasmic reticulum. Subsequently, the substances were found in the Golgi apparatus and then in the secretory granules. At 4 hr after injection of tritiated leucine and galactose, labeling was found in the "acellular layer located on the free surface of bronchiolar cells, usually considered an extracellular surfactant." These observations suggest the synthesis of complex molecules within the cell, packaging in the Golgi apparatus, and then secretion into the lumen as secretory granules. However, the material appears to be different from the usual surface-active material which is rich in choline. These authors also suggested that the material secreted by the Clara cell was the hypophase. However, the small number of granules compared to the large volume of hypophase suggests that this explanation may not necessarily be the correct one. It is also true that no one has observed the granules passing through the cell membrane. It is known that airways behave functionally as if they are lined by surface-active material (7), and osmiophilic material, similar to that seen in alveoli, has been found in small airways (8). The composition of this material, however, is unknown. It could be that there is more than one surface-active material in the lung and that both Clara cells and type II cells secrete their own surface-active products. It still seems unlikely that the Clara cell is the major source of surfactant in the lung. We (9) are widely quoted as supporting the hypothesis that the Clara cell secretes surfactant: our observation was that the Clara cells were rich in choline-containing phospholipids, tightly bound to protein, whereas type II cells contained choline-rich phospholipid weakly bound or not bound to protein. Because the current evidence is that surfactant is only loosely linked to its apoprotein, this suggests that the positive staining in the Clara cell probably corresponds to the large amount of endoplasmic reticulum present in these cells. At the time we wrote, "if ... (the view) ... that the surfactant is not a lipoprotein is correct then the type II alveolar cell should still be regarded as the prime source of surfactant. The function of the secretion of the Clara cell would then be obscure." This statement still appears to be correct.

POSTNATAL LUNG GROWTH

While birth may only be a minor milestone in the development of some organs, it is a major functional event for the lungs when they begin to exchange gas. It is also a major morphological event, because alveoli are absent in many species at birth and in most species the majority of alveoli develop in the postnatal period. Thus, in the lung, as in many other organs, there is a qualitative as well as a quantitative change. Because of the unique expansile character of the lung, some have considered that the lung could grow mainly, or only, by expansion. A simple observation indicates the nature of growth of the lung. At birth the human lung weighs about 60 g, whereas an adult lung weighs about 700 g. This 10- to 12-fold increase in lung weight compares to the 15- to 25-fold increase in body weight. Postnatal growth of the lung should not be viewed as fundamentally different from growth in other organs. In general terms, an organ can grow and enlarge in one or both of two ways—it may grow by cellular multiplication or by cell enlargement. The increase in weight that occurs argues for a major role in cell multiplication. Increase in weight of an organ can also be brought about by another mechanism, best exemplified in the brain—that of secretion and accumulation of material within and between cells. In the brain, myelination is a major event, but in most other organs, including the lung, synthesis of scleroproteins adds significantly to organ mass. The cells within an organ may be laid down in units, such as the nephron, so that, theoretically, organs can grow by multiplying the units or by enlarging the units.

In the next section, the manner in which the lung grows and how it differs from other organs is considered. Naturally, the process is better studied in experimental animals than in man, so the data for animals is discussed first and then results in man are compared to this information.

Nature of Lung Growth

Animals Cell multiplication and enlargement in the whole rat and its organs are illustrated in Figures 1 and 2. In Figure 1 it is apparent that there is rapid increase in DNA in all organs, reflecting rapid cellular multiplication, in fetal and early life. The patterns differ in the various organs, and cellular multiplication in lung and kidney ceased at about 2 weeks of age. In the other organs, significant cellular multiplication continued for a further 3–4 weeks. Figure 2 expresses the amount of protein per nucleus in the various organs and is thus an expression of cell size. It is apparent, when taken in conjunction with Figure 1, that kidney and lung grow primarily by cellular multiplication for the first 2 weeks of life and by cellular enlargement until 9–10 weeks of age.

In addition, the lung expands more in volume than it does in weight. Figure 3 illustrates the relative proportion that tissue forms of the lung; it is apparent that the relative amount of tissue decreases steadily during fetal life and that this process continues through much of postnatal life. Thus, in general terms, the lung grows more in volume than it does in weight. This is not brought about

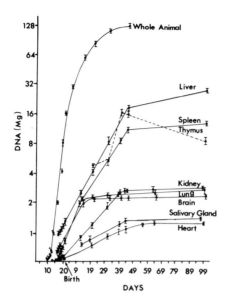

Figure 1. The increase in deoxyribose nucleic acid (DNA) with increasing age is compared in several organs in the rat. The rate of cellular multiplication varies between organs, but the lung and brain behave similarly. In the lung, cellular multiplication has largely ceased by age 14 days. Reprinted with permission of Dev. Biol. 12:451 (1965).

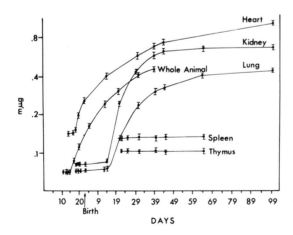

Figure 2. The amount of protein per nucleus (ordinate in $m\mu g$ or ng) is compared in a variety of organs and in the whole rat. In the lung, cell size remains approximately constant to 2 weeks of age and then increases to about 9 weeks of age. Cell size of the spleen and thymus remains unchanged. Reprinted with permission of Dev. Biol. 12:451 (1965).

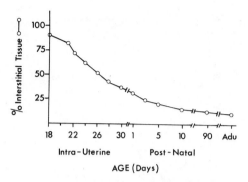

Figure 3. When the percentage of the lung that is tissue (interstitial tissue) is plotted against age in the rabbit, there is a decrease throughout intrauterine life that continues into the postnatal period and lasts until at least 3 months of age. Reprinted with permission of Am. Rev. Respir. Dis. 111:803 (1975).

only by simple expansion of the lung; it is accompanied by a radical restructuring of the lung. This process is best illustrated by comparing histological slides from animals of different ages (Figure 4). Rats and mice have been studied most thoroughly, but it is probable that rabbits and dogs show similar features. At birth, the peripheral lung units are simple structures with relatively smooth walls; their length considerably exceeds their diameter (Figure 5). Thus, these units differ in shape from the smallest lung units in the adult (alveoli) and are also much larger. They do not correspond to adult structures, and they are often referred to as "primary saccules" (10, 11). Three phases of growth in the rat lung have been described, and perhaps a fourth should be added. In the 1st day of life, little cellular multiplication occurs so that phase is one of simple expansion (12). From days 2–4, there is both cellular multiplication and lung expansion. In rats, lung volume increases less than body weight, so that the ratio of lung volume to body weight decreases (10); but in mice lung weight-body weight ratios remain essentially unchanged during this period (12). In the rabbit, lung volume changes little in the 1st day of life (13). Not only is the primary saccule different in shape from any adult structure, but there is a double capillary network in its wall. A double capillary network must necessarily occur at some stage. Each developing airway in the fetus has its own capillary network. The airways keep the capillary bed as they branch and develop respiratory epithelium. As airway and lung development proceeds, adjacent airways approach each other and then become apposed. At this stage, the original capillary networks still persist, forming a double network between airways. Where the airway does not abut on the wall of any other, such as at lobular septa or vessels, the capillary layer is single. Progressive fusion of the capillary layers occurs during postnatal development. The wall of the saccule is relatively thick and characteristically contains cells which have been referred to as "primary interstitial cells" or "fibroblasts." These cells contain large numbers of lipid vacuoles

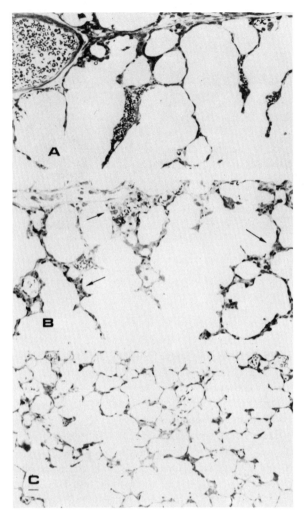

Figure 4. The development of the mouse lung. *A*, photomicrograph at 1 day of age. The respiratory portion of the lung is formed by primary saccules and no alveoli can be recognized. *B*, photomicrograph at 5 days of age. Septal crests produce poorly formed alveoli. The interstitium is thick and contains many "fibroblasts" or primitive interstitial cells. *C*, at 7 days of age, alveoli are deeper and more obvious. The interstitium is almost of adult type (1μ-thick epon section, × 150). Reprinted with permission of Pathobiology Annual, 1975. Appleton-Century-Crofts, New York, p. 1.

and glycogen granules. They also contain much rough endoplasmic reticulum, and collagen and elastic fibers are seen close to them (14). These cells are thought to be responsible for synthesis of elastic tissue and collagen, and they may also be progenitor cells that can differentiate into fibroblasts, muscle cells, or endothelium. The other noteworthy feature in the primary saccule is the

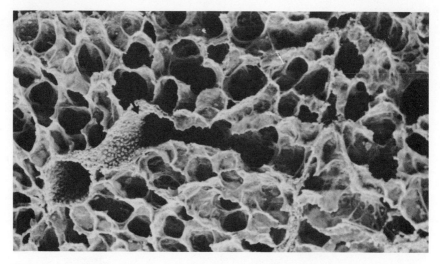

Figure 5. A scanning electronmicrograph shows a simple primary saccule in a 1-day-old mouse. The primary saccule arises from a terminal bronchiole, indicated by the *arrow*. (X 184). Reprinted with permission of Am. Rev. Respir. Dis. 111:803 (1975).

presence of low ridges, disposed primarily transversely (Figure 6). A thin elastic fiber is found at the margins of the ridges which represent the site of the development of the "secondary crests" which are characteristic of the next phase of development (Figure 7). This has been referred to as "the phase of tissue proliferation," although it might be more dramatically described as the phase of restructuring of the lung. It lasts from day 4 to days 10–14 and results in the rapid development of alveoli (Figures 8–11) brought about by subdivision of the primary saccules by secondary crests to form definitive alveoli. These secondary crests are characterized by an elastic fiber in their margins, numerous interstitial cells, and a single capillary layer. Cells in the crest label 1.4 times as frequently as do cells in other parts of the saccule wall (15). Elastic tissue may play a central role in alveolar development, but it should be noted that collagen fibers are also invariably associated with the elastic fibers at the mouths of alveoli. The margin of each crest that forms the mouth of alveoli contains an elastic fiber, and the appearance of elastic fibers in the newborn has been compared to that of a fishnet (16, 17). Some authors compare alveolar development to the events that would occur if a balloon with a very pliant wall were inflated in a container formed by a semirigid mesh. The balloon would protrude through the mesh, forming smaller spaces that would correspond to alveoli in the developing lung. Alveolar multiplication produces a dramatic increase in the surface area of the lung. Figure 12 plots alveolar surface area against lung volume. The stage of the restructuring of the lung is indicated by the middle (*solid*) line. During this phase, the surface area increases disproportionately to the lung volume—to the 1.6 power. Were the lung to expand by simple expansion, the change would approximate the 2/3 power of lung volume.

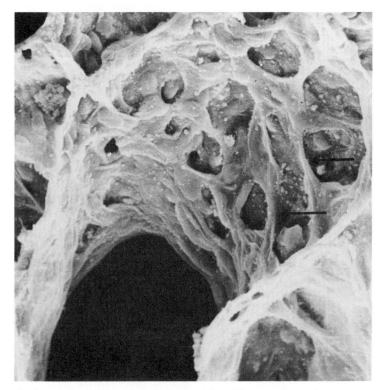

Figure 6. A scanning electronmicrograph of a 1-day-old mouse shows the transverse ridges (*arrows*) in which elastic fibers lie in the walls of a primary saccule × 980. Reprinted with permission of Am. Rev. Respir. Dis. 111:803 (1975).

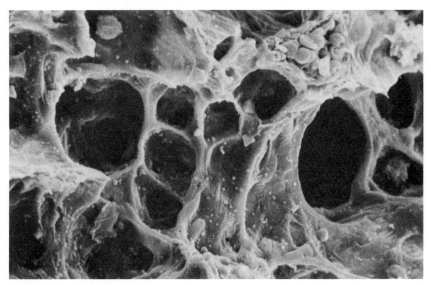

Figure 7. The secondary crests are now more prominent in this 3-day-old mouse. Elastic and collagen fibers lie at the free margin of each ridge. (Scanning electron micrograph × 920.) Reprinted with permission of Rev. Respir. Dis. 111:803 (1975).

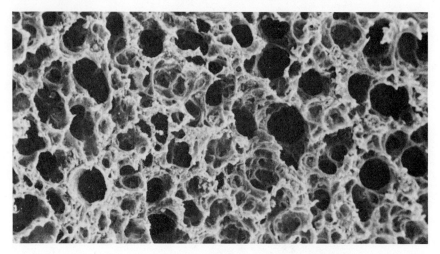

Figure 8. The development of alveoli in the lung of a mouse 4 days of age; the development of the secondary crests is well shown.

The final phase is described as "the phase of equilibrated growth." It is indicated by the final line in Figure 12. During this stage, the lung grows primarily by expansion and by cell enlargement, rather than by cellular multiplication. The surface area increases to the 0.71 power of the increase in lung volume, suggesting that the lung is growing almost entirely by expansion. The interstitium of the lung matures, so that the primary interstitial cells disappear and the secondary crests lengthen. Only a single capillary layer can be found in the walls of the airspaces. A notable feature after day 14 is the dramatic increase

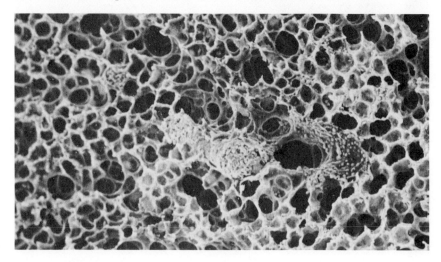

Figure 9. The development of alveoli in a 6-day-old mouse, showing subdivision into well demarcated alveoli.

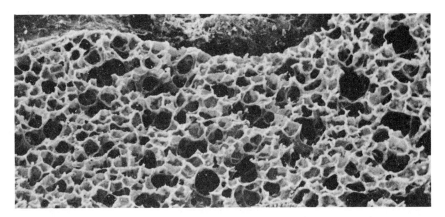

Figure 10. The development of alveoli in the lung of a 2-week-old mouse; alveoli are well developed and any change after this stage is due to dilatation.

in the number of pores of Kohn that can be seen in the mouse. Although these are present occasionally in the newborn (Figure 6), they are only easily recognizable after about day 14. There is some question about whether or not the phase of equilibrated growth can be divided into two parts—one in which growth is primarily by expansion, but during which alveoli are still being formed, and one in which no alveoli are added. It is not certain at exactly what age alveoli cease to multiply in various species, but it appears likely that most alveoli are present by the age of 2 weeks in rats and mice and 12 weeks in rabbits (18).

Growth of other parts of the lung, such as airways and blood vessels, has not been studied in the same detail as has parenchymal growth. Bronchial length

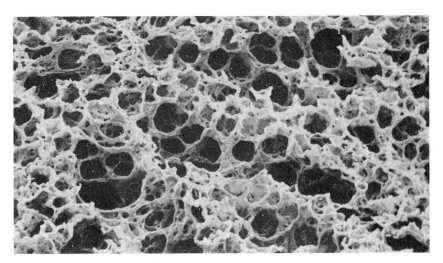

Figure 11. The development of alveoli in the lung of an adult mouse. Note the marked increase in the number of pores of Kohn seen in the adult animal.

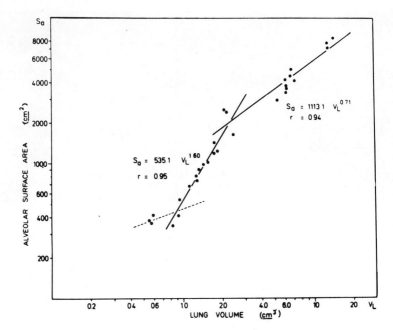

Figure 12. Alveolar surface area plotted against lung volume. The relationship appears to follow three phases. The *broken line* indicates the first 4 days of life and the first *solid line* indicates days 4–21. Note that in the second phase the surface area increased more than lung volume, indicating disproportionate increase of alveolar surface area, which represents alveolar multiplication. In the final phase, from days 21–131 (*solid line, right*), surface area increases approximately to the 2/3 power of lung volume, suggesting enlargement primarily by expansion. Reprinted with permission of Anat. Rec. 178:711 (1974).

increases by approximately the cube root of the increase of lung volume in cats (19), suggesting isotropic growth in this species. In rats, airway volume increases less than lung volume (10). It is also not clear whether proximal and distal airways increase to the same extent; in dogs it has been suggested that distal airways increase approximately 10 times in length, whereas proximal airways increase only about 3 times (20).

Human Lung In contrast to animal lungs, relatively little is known about alveolar growth and cell multiplication in the human lung, whereas rather more is known about growth of other structures, such as airways and blood vessels. As is the case in animal lungs, the amount of air per unit of tissue increases in the lungs in the postnatal period. As was mentioned earlier, at birth lungs weigh about 60 g compared to the adult value of about 700 g, an 11- to 12-fold increase. Lung volume (tissue plus air at total lung capacity) is about 200–250 ml at birth, compared to 5–6 liters in adult life, a 25-fold increase. Stigol et al. (21) found that the human lung contains approximately 3 ml of air/g of tissue at full inflation at birth and, at about 6 years of age, the adult value of about 6 ml of air/g of tissue was reached.

The human lung must go through similar phases of growth and development as was described for animals. It is still not certain whether alveoli are present at birth in the human and, if so, how many are present. The weight of evidence, however, supports the presence of alveoli at birth, which means that the phases of tissue proliferation and restructuring of the lung start in utero in most instances, rather than at birth as in animals. However, many observers have noted the lack of development of the lung of newborn infants and the resemblance of their lungs to those of newborn animals (19, 20). Both objective (22) and subjective (23) observations have suggested that the terminal airspaces are larger in newborn children than in older children, suggesting that either alveoli are absent or are very poorly developed at birth. As long ago as 1928, Willson (23) asked, "By what process do these large airspaces in the very young child develop into a number of smaller airspaces in a child of 13 years? Can it be by any other process than invagination of the respiratory air passages?" Thus, the estimates of the number of alveoli at birth in the human have varied from none (24, 25), few (17 million (26) and 20 million (22)), or many (71 million (27)). In general, these authors accepted the adult complement of alveoli to be 300 million or more. Hieronymi found 70 million alveoli at birth but considered the adult number to be 110 million (28, 29). These differences of opinion probably result from several different causes. It is not generally recognized how hard it is to define and recognize an alveolus in the neonatal period. Because considerable alveolar multiplication occurs after birth, all stages of alveolar development are present, and it may become arbitrary what structure is regarded as an alveolus and what is not. Less well appreciated is the wide variation between observers that may be found when the same observers examine the same slides. In our own laboratory, we have encountered consistent differences of 10–20% between different observers despite the fact that careful attempts were made to use uniform criteria. Discussions with other observers have suggested that this is usual. It is likely that biological variations may be more important, and it is not unusual to find striking differences on subjective observation of the lungs of infants of the same gestation or postnatal age. A further variable is the method of preparation of the lung. The appearance of the lung is entirely different when the lungs are fully distended by fixative before sectioning compared to the appearance of the undistended lungs. Some have interpreted this to mean that alveoli are formed by distension (13), but it is more likely that there is much collapse in uninflated lungs and that alveoli are very hard to find. Most pathologists, however, would agree that it is an unusual full term infant in whom alveoli cannot be recognized at postmortem examination. There is also a technical but less interesting reason why alveolar counting has significant limitations in the growth period. This has been discussed at length elsewhere (18).

There is even more controversy about the time at which alveolar multiplication ceases. Most observers believe that alveolar multiplication is more active in the immediate postnatal period. Hieronymi (28, 29) found what he considered to be the adult number of alveoli (110 million) at the end of the first year of life.

He also observed that the alveolar surface area per unit of volume grew faster between birth and 3 months, indicating that this was the peak phase of alveolar multiplication. Boyden (30) also observed that the most rapid phase of alveolar multiplication was in the first 2 months of life, followed by a period of slower multiplication until 4 years of age. A subjective description suggests that alveolar multiplication continues until at least 7 years of age (23). Dunnill (22) has produced the classic and most widely accepted data. He noted a 5-fold increase in the number of alveoli in the first year of life (from 24 million to 129 million). Alveolar multiplication was slower thereafter. A child 4 years old had 260 million alveoli, and a child 8 years old had 280 million alveoli. He considered the total number of alveoli in the adult to be about 300 million and, therefore, deduced that alveolar multiplication slowed between 1 and 4 years and ceased at about 8 years. Others have found very similar numbers to those of Dunnill and concluded that alveolar multiplication ceased between 5 and 11 years of age (31). Emery and Mithal (32) used an indirect method of assessing alveolar number which suggested that the number of alveoli quadrupled from birth to the end of the first year of life and increased a further 2.5 times by the age of 12–13 years. An important observation of theirs was the large variation in alveolar number between children of the same age. Emery and Wilcock (33) and Naka-mura et al. (34) have suggested that alveolar multiplication may occur through-out childhood. Our initial observation was related to adults (35). We found that the normal range of alveoli in adults varied from 200–600 million; this suggested that the conclusions that have been drawn from Dunnill's data are not neces-sarily correct. For example, the 8-year-old child with 280 million alveoli may have been destined to have 500 million alveoli. From our data it could be reasoned that only half of the alveoli were added before age 8 years. Alterna-tively, it could be reasoned that the 4-year-old child with 250 million alveoli had reached the adult complement and, therefore, alveolar multiplication had ceased at this age. We subsequently counted alveoli in a group of children and found a wide variation (27). Our data were, however, roughly comparable to those of Dunnill (22) and Davies and Reid (31) and indicated, like those of all other observers, that alveolar multiplication is probably most rapid in infancy. How-ever, the exact age of cessation of alveolar multiplication must be regarded as uncertain at the present time. It may even be that alveolar multiplication and lung regeneration can occur in adolescence and even adult life. Bates et al. (36) have described a remarkable patient (case 21) who had surgery for bronchiectasis at ages 14 years and 25 years, after which only her right upper lobe remained. The lung had enlarged to 3–4 times its predicted volume, and the diffusing capacity for carbon monoxide was about 70% of that predicted for both lungs, suggesting that tissue proliferation, and perhaps alveolar multiplication, had occurred.

It has been suggested that the lung changes in shape as it grows. Using excised lung specimens, Hieronymi noted that the lung grew more in height than it did in width (28, 29). Other observers using chest roentgenograms have noted a more rapid rate of growth in lung height than lung width between the ages of 5 and 19 years (37).

Growth of Other Structures in Lungs

Airways Because airways do not increase in number, they must increase in dimension. The increase in dimension parallels the increase in stature, as shown by the measurement of anatomical dead space in children (38). Tracheal diameter increases directly with the increase in chest circumference (28). However, there are discrepant views about the relative rate of growth of central and peripheral airways. This is of more than trivial interest—it has been shown that the conductance of peripheral airways in children up to the age of 4 is considerably lower than in older children and in adults (39). It has been suggested that this is why bronchiolitis is a life-threatening disease in small children; inflammation and narrowing of airways with low conductance would produce marked air flow obstruction. Hislop et al. (40) considered that all airways grew proportionately and in parallel with lung volume changes. Cudmore et al. (41) thought that the proximal airways grew faster than the distal airways. On the contrary, Hogg et al. (39) found that there was a disporportionate increase in the diameter of distal airways compared to central airways up to the age of 5 years. It has also been suggested that the rate of growth depends on age and that length and diameter may differ. The most complete study, by Hieronymi (28), indicated that proximal and distal airways enlarged equally but that their diameters increased slightly more than their lengths up to the age of 5 months. After 1 year, distal airways increased 12–30% more than the proximal airways, and the increase in diameter was consistently less than the increase in length.

Qualitative differences may also exist between the lungs of children and the lungs of adults. The peripheral airways show increasing amounts of muscle in their walls in the postnatal period (42). This is unlikely to account for the change in conductance, because the increase in muscle is gradual over childhood, whereas the increase in conductance is rather sharp, occurring between the ages of 3 and 5 years. In addition, the Reid index of mucous gland size (43) and the proportion of mucous glands in the central airways (42) are greater in children than in adults.

Vascular System At birth, the pulmonary circuit suddenly changes from a high resistance one in utero to the low resistance one of extrauterine life. There are sudden morphological changes, and the vessels appear much less muscular soon after birth. This is brought about primarily by dilatation of pulmonary arteries (44). In addition to this change, there must be growth of the arterial and venous trees to supply and drain the newly developed lung parenchyma. It is important to recognize that there are two categories of blood vessel in the lung—"supernumerary" and "conventional" (45). Conventional arteries accompany the airways, whereas supernumerary ones do not. The latter are usually smaller, more numerous, and join the pulmonary arteries at right angles. Conventional branches of the pulmonary vein (46) form an axial pathway which is separate from the bronchopulmonary sheath. Supernumerary veins resemble supernumerary arteries in that they are more numerous, smaller, and join the main venous system at right angles. The main conventional branches of the pulmonary artery and vein parallel bronchial development in utero, and most of the conventional branches are present at birth. However, conventional branches continue to appear until about 18 months of age, perhaps paralleling the small increase in the number of airway generations within the acinus. Supernumerary branches of the arteries and veins are present in utero, but in relatively small numbers, and following birth there is a marked increase in their number, reflecting alveolar multiplication. These branches occur not only in the developing lung parenchyma, but also in the pulmonary arteries proximal to the acinus. These supernumerary arteries continue to develop until about 5 years of age when the adult ratio of supernumerary to conventional branches is found. The ratio of alveoli to pulmonary arteries provides useful information. At birth, 141 alveoli per artery were noted and, at 4 months of age, 98 alveoli per artery. After this time, the ratio remained fairly constant at 30–50 alveoli per artery. This suggests that alveolar multiplication preceded arterial development. Pulmonary artery volume changed directly with lung volume, and length and diameter of the vessels increased proportionately. As is the case with bronchioles, there were qualitative changes in the pulmonary arteries. No muscular arteries are found in the acinus at birth, and, during childhood, muscle gradually extended into the acinus, reaching respiratory bronchioles at 4 months of age, alveolar ducts at 3 years of age, and alveolated tissue at 10 years of age. Muscle continued to develop until 19 years of age.

Alterations in Postnatal Lung Growth

Resection of Lung Tissue A large number of papers (18) have been published on this topic, dating back more than 50 years and using a variety of measurements of lung growth, often subjective. As might be anticipated, there is some conflict of opinion, but overall there is a reasonable consensus, particularly from experimental studies in the rat (47, 48) and the rabbit (49, 50). Following resection of lung tissue, the remaining lung increases both in volume and weight to approximate the volume and weight of both lungs in the control animals (47–59). The first response is overexpansion of the remaining lung tissue, followed by cellular proliferation that starts within days of the operation, reaches a maximum at about 5–7 days following resection of lung tissue, and returns to normal some 10–12 days later (49, 53, 54). The contralateral lung after pneumonectomy may not expand isotropically. It has been claimed that the lower lobe expands more than the upper lobe (55). The response is greater in young animals than in old animals. The real controversy is whether or not resection of lung tissue results in alveolar multiplication in the opposite side. Older observations suggested that alveolar multiplication occurred in puppies and kittens, because alveolar dimensions remained the same in the contralateral lung following pneumonectomy (56, 57).

Other authors have counted the number of alveoli and suggested that alveolar multiplication occurred (48, 51, 58). In one study, alveolar multiplication occurred in young, but not adult, guinea pigs (58), whereas alveolar multiplication occurred in both young and adults rats, being slower and less marked in the adults (51). More recent studies using modern morphometric techniques have produced conflicting results. Two studies suggested that alveolar multiplication did not occur (50, 52), but the most recent study has presented indirect evidence from the average interalveolar wall distance that multiplication of surface alveoli occurred following pneumonectomy, but not multiplication of the more central alveoli (47).

The factors which control lung growth following resection of lung tissue are unknown. However, it is clear that mechanical factors and stretch probably play a much more important role in the lung than in the liver or the kidney, which have been well studied. The response in the contralateral lung following pneumonectomy can be altered by placing a sponge or wax in the contralateral side (49, 51, 54). In the former instance, the mitotic response was suppressed or delayed (54), and in the latter the increases in weight and in collagen synthesis were almost abolished (49).

Very little is known about the effect on the contralateral lung following pneumonectomy in humans. We have previously referred to the case reported by Bates et al. (36) that suggested that lung regeneration might occur following resection of lung tissue. Studies on living subjects indicate that the remaining lung increases about 30–40% in volume following pneumonectomy rather than doubling, as might be anticipated from the animal experiments (36). One detailed morphometric study on the contralateral lung following pneumonectomy suggested that only overinflation occurred and that alveolar multiplication was absent (60).

Diminution of Lung Volume   Following injections of wax into the pleural cavity, thoracoplasty, or phrenic nerve section, the ipsilateral lung has been found to be small in weight, but the same author did not think that this process interfered with the total number of alveoli (51, 61). Alteration of the configuration of the thoracic cavity, by production of experimental diaphragmatic hernias in lambs, resulted in severely hypoplastic lungs and alterations in alveolar development (62).

In humans, severely hypoplastic lungs occur in congenital diaphragmatic hernia (63, 64). Not only is alveolar development altered, but there are too few airways and vessels. In kyphoscoliosis, there is gross distortion of the shape of the lungs as the lungs fit the distorted thorax. After removal and inflation of the lungs at necropsy, the deformed shape persists (65, 66). In kyphoscoliosis of childhood onset, too few alveoli have been noted in two different studies (60, 66). In one instance, the diminution in alveolar number was so great as to be well outside the bounds of biological variation noted above.

Growth Hormone   The effects of administration of growth hormone or hypophysectomy are difficult to interpret (67–69). Somatic growth is interfered with, as is lung growth, and the question is whether or not there is some specific effect on the lung. In general terms, lung growth increased after administration of growth hormones or tumors which secrete growth hormone and diminished in size and weight after hypophysectomy. However, the alterations in lung size are less that the alteration of body size. One author has suggested that growth hormone produces alveolar multiplication as well as an increase in lung volume (67).

Hypoxia and Hypobaric Conditions   Because hypobaric conditions are also associated with hypoxia, it is not always clear how these two effects can be separated. Furthermore, there is conflict in the results of both experiments which use hypoxia and hypobaric conditions. The problem is likewise complicated by the fact that both hypoxia and hypobaric conditions affect somatic growth, so that it is difficult to separate a specific lung growth effect. One author has noted no effect of hypoxia on lung growth (70), but another group of investigators (71) has noted an increase in lung weight and in alveolar number in young animals exposed to hypoxic conditions.

Similar controversy surrounds hypobaric conditions. Some authors have concluded that there were no differences in structure between the lungs of guinea pigs and sheep brought up at high altitude and those raised at near sea level (72). However, other authors have suggested an increase in lung volume, lung weight, and alveolar number under hypobaric conditions (61, 73, 74). Once again, man has been studied very little. It is well known that, for a given stature, lungs are larger in subjects living at high altitudes than in those living at sea level (75). High altitude residents also have an increased D_{LCO} , which has been interpreted as meaning both an increased capillary blood volume and an increase in alveolar surface area (76, 77). One author has examined lungs at postmortem and suggested that high altitude residents have a larger surface area and more alveoli than a small group of comparable lowlanders (78). However, this information is contained in an abstract, and it is not clear whether or not the subjects were matched for stature.

Hyperoxia   Oxygen is a notable lung poison, and it is thus not surprising that lung growth is hampered in animals exposed to high levels of oxygen. Lung volumes, lung weight, alveolar surface area, and probably the number of alveoli are decreased under these experimental conditions (70, 73).

LUNG EXPANSION

The way in which the lung expands has recently received considerable attention, and the exact ways in which airways, capillaries, and alveoli change in dimension have all been examined. Perhaps the most interesting is recent work (79) which has suggested that the lung expands by recruitment of alveoli (opening up of previously closed alveoli) with resultant large increase in alveolar surface area. Alternatively, the lung may expand by the smoothing out and unwrinkling of alveolar walls (80), in which instance alveolar surface area would change little. It may be that the general view that alveoli expand like rubber balloons does have to be discarded. Certainly, this is the time to review the information that has led us to believe that this is the case.

Alveolar Expansion

The notion that alveoli behave as paper bags rather than as balloons was first clearly expressed by the great pulmonary anatomist C. C. Macklin (81). In his review of the structure and function of the musculature of the lung, he noted that, in some species at any rate, alveolar ducts had a central spiral of muscle. He felt that contraction of this muscle would open up the mouths of alveoli. He further amplified this idea 20 years later (82), when he compared the shape of an alveolus to a cup on expiration and a saucer on inspiration. He felt that there was little, if any, stretching of the alveolar wall and that the alveolar size remained constant. He felt that it was the lumen of the alveolar ducts and sacs, internal to the alveolar mouth, that enlarged on inspiration.

As will be seen below, there is considerable difference in opinion, and reasons for this difference should be examined. It is possible, perhaps likely, that the lung may expand differently at different lung volumes. For example, the gas-free lung must have apposed alveolar walls, and they must initially, at least, expand by opening up alveoli, as in opening up empty paper bags. Whether or not this is a major method of expansion is another matter. It should be noted at this point that if the lung expanded as a paper bag, then alveolar surface area would not change with inflation and alveolar volume and alveolar surface area would not be related. An increase in surface area with lung expansion does not necessarily imply alveolar wall stretching; it can also be accomplished by other means, such as alveolar recruitment. If alveoli expand by stretching only, then the surface area of the lung should change to the 2/3 power of lung volume. An additional notion should be introduced at this point. Macklin felt that the alveolar wall, because of its structure, should not be distensible. However, direct experimentation has shown that the wall is sufficiently elastic to account for the lung volume changes that occur in the intact lung (83).

Secondly, the lung probably behaves differently on inflation and on deflation. Radford (84) has pointed out that one of the possible causes of hysteresis in the lung is alveolar recruitment on the inflation limb of the pressure-volume curve. Certainly, this must occur in the first inflation of a degassed lung or of a lung that starts from a very low lung volume. Thus, observers would probably get different results if the inflation limb rather than the deflation limb were studied. At this point, it should be noted that the alveolar surface area should be greater at the same transpulmonary pressure on the deflation limb of the pressure-volume curve than on the inflation limb, given a significant hysteresis loop in the lung. This has been shown by morphometric techniques (79). In addition, linear or area measurements within the lung or on its surface should show differences on the inflation and deflation limbs ("geometric hysteresis" and "irreversibility"). This has also been demonstrated by some observers (80, 85), but not by all (86).

Interpretation might also differ depending on the resolution of the test system. Electron microscopy indicates a much more irregular alveolar epithelial surface than does light microscopy. Hence, the surface area measured by electron microscopy is much larger than that measured by light microscopy, in much the same way that the surface area of the small intestine is much greater when measured by light microscopy than by gross inspection. Electron microscopically, it would be even larger. Smoothing and flattening of airway epithelium seen by electron microscopy is probably an important way of increasing surface area when seen at that level, but the observation might have little relevance to the way in which alveoli expand.

It is also thought possible that alveoli may expand differently within the chest than they would expand when removed from the body. It is fortunate that a study has addressed itself to this problem. The evidence is that expansion is the same in situ and ex situ, other than for some minor exceptions in particular situations (87). The criticism can also be made that the standard ways of preparing the lung for histological examination are unphysiological. However, when freezing techniques have been used (87–90), they have produced results similar to those found by more conventional methods.

Another cause for difference of opinion is that much of the data depends on counting and measurements of dimensions of lung structures. These techniques are often not easy and are always tedious so that, frequently, only small groups of animals have been used. Finally, biological variation may produce anomalous results. It is possible that lungs from different species may expand differently, and certainly there are wide within-species variations in dimension, in part related to differences in size and age. The within-species variations often lead to relatively large standard errors, and apparent relationships between inflation and morphometric variables may be obscured.

Lung Inflation Primarily by Alveolar Enlargement and Stretching

The first important evidence for this phenomenon came as long ago as 1962 when Storey and Staub (88) rapidly froze cat lungs at approximately functional residual capacity (FRC) and at about 80% of total lung capacity (TLC). They were able to measure an increase in alveolar and alveolar duct diameter and noted that alveoli and alveolar ducts expanded to about the same degree. Kuno and Staub (89) indicated that surface area changed directly with alveolar volume from 18% of TLC to TLC. On the basis of a statistical fit, it appeared that alveolar surface area expanded to the 2/3 power of lung volume, and, therefore, alveoli were thought to enlarge by expansion through this volume range. In a subsequent, more detailed study, Klingele and Staub (90) measured the maximum depth (D) and the maximum mouth diameter (MD) of alveoli at various levels of inflation. They expressed their results as the ratio $D{:}MD$; thus, if alveoli

changed shape and became flatter and more like a bag, this ratio would change and increase. They found that at 50% of maximum lung volume (V) and above, D:MD remained constant at about 0.89; at 37% of V, it was 1.17; at 25% of V, it was 1.24; and at 20% V, it was 1.41. They thus concluded that "... alveolar shape is nearly constant over the useful range of lung volume during normal breathing. Shape does change progressively below the physiological range. The alveoli become narrow and finally fold up from side to side as an accordion or concertina folds, rather than by uniform decrease in all dimensions." Whimster (91), in his description of the microanatomy of the alveolar ducts, indicated how this might happen (Figure 13). He pointed out that a thick spiral of elastin and collagen (there is little muscle in the human) traverses in lumen of the alveolar duct, and alveoli open through the turns of the spiral. As the spiral opens out, so

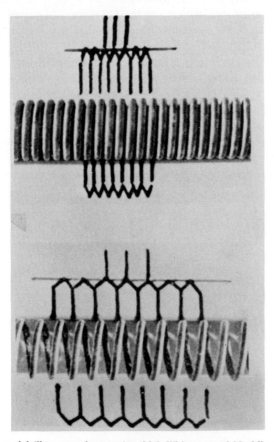

Figure 13. This model illustrates the way in which Whimster and Macklin envisage expansion of alveolar ducts and sacs. The coiled spring (top) represents the central spiral of elastic tissue of the alveolar duct. As the spring is stretched (bottom), the alveoli open up through the spirals of the spring. This method of expansion requires no increase of alveolar surface area. Reprinted with permission of Thorax 25:141 (1974).

the alveoli unfold. He, however, envisaged this process as occurring throughout inspiration to TLC, rather than only at low lung volumes. He, therefore, projected primarily an unfolding of alveoli, with little or no increase in alveolar surface area throughout expansion.

Dunnill (92) provided the first detailed morphometric study of lung expansion with the use of dog lung. He found that the alveolar air proportion expanded directly with lung volume and that the proportion that respiratory duct air formed of the lung actually decreased, i.e., the respiratory duct actually expanded less than the whole lung or alveoli, in direct contradistinction to Macklin's notion. He also plotted the log of alveolar surface area against the logs of both lung volume and alveolar volume. He found significant relationships for both and found regression lines with slopes of 0.81 and 0.77, respectively. Because these slopes were not significantly different from a slope of 2/3, he thought that surface area changed to the 2/3 power of lung volume in the range of inflation studied. He concluded, therefore, that alveoli enlarged by isotropic expansion.

Forrest (93) studied lung inflation in guinea pigs by using similar morphometric techniques. He found that total alveolar volume expanded directly with lung volume, but that the fraction that alveolar volume formed of lung volume changed with inflation. Below 30% TLC, the alveolar fraction was 0.52; between 30–60% TLC, it was 0.62; and greater than 60% TLC, it was 0.51. This increase and decrease in the alveolar volume fraction was mainly due to the fact that alveolar duct volume changed little to 40% TLC and then increased rapidly (Figure 14). The relationship between alveolar surface area and lung volume that

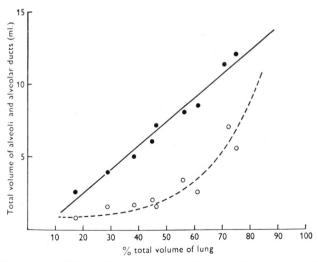

Figure 14. Comparison of the total volume of alveoli (•) and alveolar ducts (○) as the lung expands. Alveolar volume shows a linear relationship with lung volume. Alveolar duct volume, however, shows relatively little change from 18% of lung volume to 50% of lung volume and then a rapid increase. Reprinted with permission of J. Physiol. (Lond.) 210:533 (1970).

Forrest found is difficult to interpret because of a 2-fold difference in the size of the animals he used. The relationship appears linear, but recalculation of the data (87) has suggested that surface area changed to the 2/3 power of TLC. Forrest also found that there was no change in average geometric shape of the alveoli, which also suggests uniform alveolar enlargement. He noted that both alveoli and alveolar ducts increased about 40% in diameter from 17.5% TLC to 75.1% TLC and that this enlargement is consistent with the 3-fold increase in alveolar volume that he observed. He also made the observation that the alveolar surface membrane was smooth whether or not lungs were inflated. He used only nine guinea pigs, and the wide scatter in his data might obscure results reflecting the narrowing and folding of alveoli at low lung volumes suggested by Klingele and Staub (90). Nonetheless, Forrest provided clear evidence of alveolar enlargement when the lung expanded. Other authors (87, 94), primarily interested in the effects of the pleural pressure gradient, have provided supporting data. Glazier et al. (94) found alveolar volumes to be 3.7 times greater near the apex of the lung in upright dogs than at the base. Similarly, D'Angelo (87) showed an increase in alveolar size (as measured by the volume to surface ratio) with increasing lung volume. Indeed, the linear change in alveolar dimension is almost directly related to the cube root of lung volume. When he plotted alveolar surface area against alveolar volume, he found that the surface area changed to $V^{0.68}$. This once again is support for the notion of isotropic alveolar expansion, paralleling lung volume.

Lung Inflation by Alveolar Recruitment or Unfolding

The above views have been challenged by Gil and Weibel (79). They studied the lungs of rats on both the inflation and deflation limbs of the pressure-volume $(P\text{-}V)$ curve. They found that surface area changed directly with lung volume, and not to the 2/3 power, suggesting that factors other than alveolar expansion were involved. When they examined the lung with the use of light and transmission electron microscopy, they noted that on the inflation limb of the $P\text{-}V$ curve at a transpulmonary pressure of 7 Torr there were large areas of obvious atelectasis. In addition, they saw "thickened interalveolar septa" with several capillary layers (Figures 15 and 16). They pointed out that this had to represent collapse and pleating of alveolar walls and confirmed this by electron microscopy (Figure 17). They observed hysteresis of alveolar surface area and specifically stated that collapsed alveoli were seen on the deflation limb of the curve. They also felt that the major part of the increase and decrease in alveolar surface area with inflation and deflation was due to recruitment and derecruitment of alveoli. This was because the alveolar surface density (surface area per unit of volume), the surface area to volume ratio, and the mean alveolar diameter were unchanged in the inflation limb from 12−16 Torr and on the deflation limb from 16 to 17 Torr. These variables should change if alveoli changed in diameter. They saw no transition between collapsed and open alveoli and thus envisaged an all-or-none recruitment phenomenon. (The findings in the animals at a transpulmonary pressure of 7 Torr on the inflation limb were different. In these,

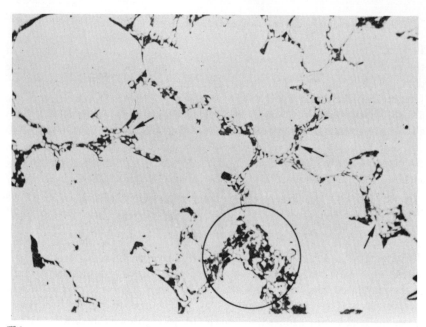

Figure 15. Although on casual inspection this lung appears inflated, closer examination at the *arrows* shows areas where there is a double capillary layer. These represent collapsed alveoli. Within the *circle,* it is apparent that there is a considerable amount of atelectactic lung tissue X 160. Reprinted with permission of Respir. Physiol. 15:190 (1972).

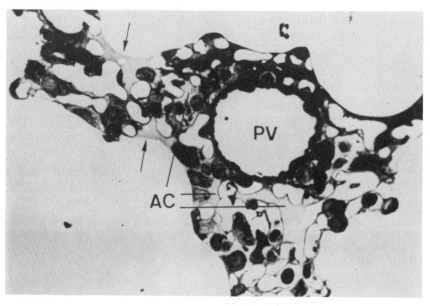

Figure 16. An area similar to that in the circle in Figure 15 but at a higher power (X 600). Collapsed alveoli (AC) are readily apparent. In the center is a small pulmonary vein (PV), around which the alveolar septa have folded. The *arrows* point to an area of hypophase. Reprinted with permission of Respir. Physiol. 15:190 (1972).

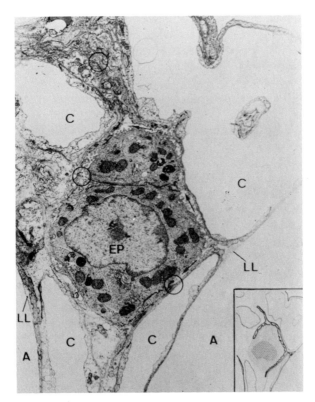

Figure 17. An electron micrograph shows a small area of collapse. The *circled areas* indicate the collapsed alveolar lumen, as do the *arrows*. (See insert.) C, capillaries; A, alveoli; LL, lining layer. (× 11,000.) Reprinted with permission of Respir. Physiol. 15:190 (1972).

alveolar diameters were smaller, surface to volume ratio was larger, and the alveolar surface density was greater, all suggesting that alveoli were smaller in this group of animals.) Specific confirmatory work from other laboratories is lacking, but Assimacopoulos et al. (95) have done similar work and are purported to support the observations of Gil and Weibel. However, examination of their data shows that alveolar surface density decreases with expansion, suggesting alveolar enlargement as well as recruitment, if the latter occurs. The relationship between alveolar surface area and alveolar volume described by them (95) is consistent with the linear relationship, but a significant relationship also exists with the 2/3 power of alveolar volume.

Daly et al. (80) have been able to examine the surface alveoli in rapidly breathing rats by using videomicroscopy. They observed that alveolar mouths expanded more than other parts of the alveoli. They were primarily interested in the cause of the hysteresis loop and measured linear dimensions of alveoli. They found that "geometric irreversibility" (the linear dimensions which changed on inflation did not reverse exactly in magnitude or sequence on deflation) was a characteristic of alveolar wall motion. They noted that there were folds in the alveolar walls, both by videomicroscopy and conventional light microscopy and histological sections. They felt that alveolar expansion involved smoothing of the walls as well as alveolar enlargement (which they showed). They also noted that the alveolar wall varied in the details of expansion and deflation from breath to breath.

Thus, it appears that the majority of observers, but not all, feel that alveoli enlarge on inspiration. The nature of the expansion at low lung volumes is not certain, but it appears that there may be narrowing and folding of alveoli. The balance of evidence is that at high volumes the change is primarily one of alveolar expansion. It may also be that there are alveolar wall folds, so that smoothing of the alveolar wall may occur with inflation. Finally, recruitment and derecruitment play an uncertain role, which may augment to a variable extent the increase in surface area brought about by alveolar expansion. An investigator of considerable stature attributes the greater part of surface area enlargement in the lung to recruitment (79).

Effects of Lung Inflation on Capillary Bed

A recent study (95) has described in detail the morphological and morphometric events that occur in lung capillaries as the lung expands, and it has made interesting observations about the general morphology of the pulmonary capillary bed. The authors examined the effects of the lung and its capillary bed by using distending transpulmonary pressures of between 0 and 20 cm H_2O. At low transpulmonary pressures, they found that the thin part of the alveolar walls collapsed and appeared as thin clefts squeezed between capillaries. The alveolar walls were plicated in such a way that lung tissue flaps projected into the capillary space, dividing it into intercommunicating chambers. They felt that the thick parts of the blood-air barrier (with interstitial cells and type II cells) were more rigid and the thick layers of the alveolar walls folded over on it in much the same way "as the cloth is folded over the spokes of an umbrella." They also described the "posts" or "pillars" in the capillaries connecting the two alveolar wall sheets envisaged by Sobin et al. (96). Of particular interest is the observation that the pillars contained the newly described "contractile" interstitial cells (97). These cells are attached to the basement membrane of two adjacent alveoli and are thought to be capable of folding the blood-air barrier. These authors have speculated that the contractile interstitial cells could regulate blood flow. Their morphometric observations included the finding that lungs expanded only a little when a transpulmonary pressure of 15 cm H_2O was exceeded. The capillary volume (Figure 18) remained constant between a transpulmonary pressure of 0 and 5 cm H_2O and showed a small, insignificant fall between 5 and 15 cm H_2O. There was a large and significant fall between 15 and 20 cm H_2O. Capillary surface area was constant throughout the transpulmonary pressure range. The surface to volume ratio of the capillaries showed a sudden increase between 15 and 20 cm H_2O, indicating a marked capillary narrowing at this stage, which they could also visualize microscopically. They believed that these

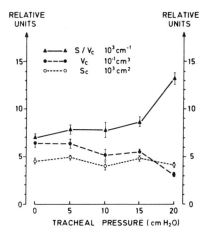

Figure 18. As a greater tracheal pressure is applied and the lung expands, no change occurs in the surface area of the capillaries (S_c). There is no significant change in capillary volume (V_c) to 15 cm H_2O transpulmonary pressure, when there is a sudden drop from this pressure to 20 cm of pressure. Similarly, the surface to volume ratio of the capillary bed remains the same until a transpulmonary pressure of 15 cm H_2O is reached. Beyond this, the surface to volume ratio increases (representing a marked narrowing of the pulmonary capillary bed). Reprinted with permission of Lab. Invest. 34:10 (1975).

changes were the cause of the increase in pulmonary vascular resistance at high transpulmonary pressure.

Expansion of Airways

This topic is discussed only briefly and mainly for the sake of completeness. It will become apparent that the data are old and incomplete, reflecting the difficulty of making the required measurements. It is generally agreed that bronchi increase in dimension much more in intact lungs than when they are dissected free from lungs (98–102). The most recent study is that of Hughes et al. (103) who studied airways 0.1–1.17 cm in diameter and 0.82–4.74 cm in length in dogs. They found that airway length changed in proportion to the cube root of lung volume. On inflation and deflation, the bronchial dimensions were the same at the same lung volume, irrespective of transpulmonary pressure, thus following the hysteresis loop of the lung. They felt that this reflected the interdependence of the lung tissue and bronchi. They also noted that bronchial dimensions in intact lungs were much greater than predicted for given pressures than for airways dissected free of lung tissue. The relationship between volume and diameter was less clear, but in the majority of instances diameter varied approximately with the cube root of lung volume. They also noted that large and small airways expanded proportionately. Klingele and Staub (104) had previously noted that the best fit between the diameter of the terminal bronchioles and lung volume in the cat was a cube root function with a correlation coefficient of 0.90. This suggests that small airways behave in the same way as the larger airways observed by Hughes et al. and are a good deal easier to measure. It was true, however, that significant correlations existed between terminal bronchiolar diameter and lung volume with the use of linear and square root functions and that the correlation coefficient with a cube foot function, although higher, was not significantly different. It has been suggested that airways of different size may enlarge to different degrees in man in vivo. Marshall and Holden (105) found that airways 1.7–7.0 mm in diameter increased 14–15% in diameter between FRC and TLC, whereas airways less than 1.7 mm in diameter increased 28%. Fraser (106) found that the diameter of airways 2.7–5.9 mm increased about the same (26–33%) from residual volume to TLC, the exception being the bronchus to the basal segments, which increased 44%. Extrapolation from findings in bronchi of excised lungs to intact humans is particularly hazardous, because bronchomotor tone plays an important part and regional differences in expansion and pressure must also have a role to play.

LUNG AND ITS NERVES

There is considerable interest currently in the nerve supply of the lung, and some preliminary information about lung nerves was discussed briefly in the last edition of this book. The reason for the recent work is in part due to the interest in afferent receptors in the lung and their possible role as irritant and J receptors. Clinical interest is also involved. It is now clear that airway receptors, probably of the irritant type (as the afferent limb), and the vagus (as the efferent limb) may play important roles in experimental bronchoconstriction (107, 108). This may be relevant to the pathogenesis of asthma in humans. The most interesting recent observation, however, is the discovery of a nonadrenergic inhibitory nervous system in the trachea of the guinea pig (109, 110) and the airways of the human lung (111).

Airways and Nonadrenergic Inhibitory Nervous System

The nonadrenergic nervous system is the dominant inhibitory nervous system in the gastrointestinal tract and is responsible for the relaxation of the esophago-gastric junction and the internal anal sphincter, as well as for the relaxation phase of peristalsis (112–114). The chemical mediator of the system has not been identified, but the role of ATP has been argued. The lung and the gastrointestinal tract have a common embryological origin, and it is, therefore, logical to anticipate that this nonadrenergic inhibitory nervous system may play a significant role in the lung. Indeed, there is evidence for this in the guinea pig. The most recent work has clearly shown the presence of a nonadrenergic inhibitory nervous system in the guinea pig trachea (110). Electrical field stimulation of the guinea pig trachea caused initial contraction, followed by relaxation during stimulation and then a further relaxation following cessation of stimulation. The adrenergic β-blocking drug propranolol prevented relaxation during the stimulation, but did not prevent the subsequent relaxation. Atropine abolished the initial contraction brought about by cholinergic fibers, and, after both drugs had been given, stimulation brought about relaxation. Stimulation of this system produced relaxation of smooth muscle contracted by experimentally-induced immediate hypersensitivity or by histamine. Tetrodotoxin, a drug which blocks nervous conduction, abolished the response, suggesting that it was nerve-mediated, but hexamethonium, a ganglion blocker, had no effect. This indicates that the nerves concerned were not preganglionic.

Even more interesting is the demonstration of the nonadrenergic inhibitory nervous system in the bronchi and bronchioles of human lungs removed at surgery (111). In contrast to the guinea pig, no evidence was found of the presence of adrenergic fibers in the airways with either pharmacological or histochemical techniques. Stimulation of the inhibitory system inhibited histamine- or cholinergic-induced contraction. Tetrodotoxin also abolished the response, and high stimulus frequencies were needed for the inhibitory response. It has been suggested that this may represent the paucity of ganglion cells in the airways and their deep position in these tissues.

Loss of the nonadrenergic inhibitory system has been shown in Hirshsprung's disease (115), a condition characterized by marked inhibition of peristaltic relaxation. A similar lack of nonadrenergic inhibitory system in the bowel has been shown in an experimental model of Hirshsprung's disease (116). Although there is no direct evidence that this system plays a role in airway disease, it is possible that a defect in it may be responsible for hyperactivity of the airways, a condition present in asthma and chronic bronchitis.

Nerves in Alveoli and Airway Epithelium

In the last edition of this book, mention was made of the recent observations of nerves in the alveolar walls, in both rats and mice, thought to represent J receptors. The information about mice was then limited only to an abstract and this has now been described more completely. Hung et al. (117) found nonmeylinated axons surrounded by Schwann cells in the alveoli and alveolar ducts of mice. They were regularly seen in the alveolar wall of mice but rarely occurred in rats. Two types of nerves were seen—one with many mitochondria which resembled the mitochondrion-rich afferent nerve endings in other organs. These nerve endings were seen close to the cell bodies or processes of type I pneumonocytes, and these nerves were then thought to be afferent, probably type J, receptors. The other type of nerve endings were packed with dense core vesicles, approximately 120 nm in diameter, and were in close association with type II pneumonocytes. These were thought to be cholinergic fibers, and the authors suggested that surfactant secretion by the type II cells might be under neuronal control.

Jeffery and Reid (118) made a quantitative study of the airway epithelium in rats and found that nerves were only found in the epithelium of extrapulmonary airways and not in intrapulmonary airways. Nerves were seen more frequently proximally than distally and were more frequent anteriorly than posteriorly. Based on ultrastructural criteria, about half the axons were thought to be afferent, one-third efferent and adrenergic, and the remaining fibers cholinergic. Nerves were found in association with all epithelial cell types and most strikingly with basal cells. The occurrence of nerve fibers with goblet cells and ciliated cells raises the question of neural control of these cells. Although these authors did not find nerves in intrapulmonary airways, other authors have found nerves in bronchioles in association with the Kultschitzky (K) type cells (119) and with the neuroepithelial bodies (120). (These cells and bodies were described in the previous edition of this book.) The arrangement of the nerve fibers and the cells was very reminiscent of the carotid bodies, muscle spindles, and taste buds, and thus it seems likely that the bodies have a receptor function. Both afferent and efferent nerve fibers have been seen in the bodies (121). Fenestrated capillaries are present at the base of the neuroepithelial bodies, and it is postulated that the granules in the cells are secreted into the capillaries, exiting via the bronchial veins and pulmonary veins. Secretion of the dense core vesicles in the cells of the neuroepithelial bodies has been observed in experimental animals following hypoxia (121). It has been suggested that they are intrapulmonary hypoxia-sensitive neuro(chemo)receptors modulated by the central nervous system and that they may influence the pulmonary vasoconstrictor response. There is some question whether the cells in the neuroepithelial bodies represent clusters of K cells (122) or whether they are different (120). The consensus seems to be that the cells are essentially the same in appearance and perhaps in function.

REFERENCES

1. Thurlbeck, W. M., and Wang, N. S. (1974). The structure of the lungs. *In* A. C. Guyton and J. G. Widdicombe, (eds.), MTP International Review of Science Physiology Series I, Vol. 2, Respiratory Physiology, pp. 1–30. Butterworths, London; University Park Press, Baltimore.
2. Etherton, J. E., Conning, D. M., and Corrin, B. (1973). Autoradiographical and morphological evidence for apocrine secretion of dipalmitoyl lecithin in the terminal bronchiole of the mouse lung. Am. J. Anat. 138:11.
3. Etherton, J. E., and Conning, D. M. (1971). Early incorporation of labelled palmitate into mouse lung. Experientia 27:554.
4. Smith, P., Heath, D., and Moosari, H. (1974). The Clara cell. Thorax 29:147.
5. Wang, N. S., Huang, S. N., Sheldon, H., and Thurlbeck, W. M. (1971). Ultrastructural changes of Clara and type II alveolar cells in adrenalin-induced pulmonary edema in mice. Am. J. Pathol. 62:237.
6. Petrik, P., and Collet, A. J. (1974). Quantitative electron microscopic autoradiography of *in vivo* incorporation of 3H-choline, 3H-leucine, 3H-acetate and 3H-galactose in non-ciliated bronchiolar (Clara) cells of mice. Am. J. Anat. 139:519.
7. Macklem, P. T., Proctor, D. F., and Hogg, J. C. (1970). The stability of peripheral airways. Respir. Physiol. 8:191.
8. Gil, J., and Weibel, E. R. (1971). Extracellular lining of bronchioles after perfusion-fixation of rat lungs for electron microscopy. Anat. Rec. 169:185.

9. Azzopardi, A., and Thurlbeck, W. M. (1969). The histochemistry of the non-ciliated bronchiolar epithelial cell. Am. Rev. Respir. Dis. 99:516.
10. Burri, P. H., Dbaly, J., and Weibel, E. R. (1974). The postnatal growth of the rat lung. I. Morphometry. Anat. Rec. 178:711.
11. Burri, P. H. (1974). The postnatal growth of the rat lung. III. Morphology. Anat. Rec. 180:77.
12. Amy, R., Bowes, D., Burri, P., Haines, J., and Thurlbeck, W. M. Postnatal growth of the mouse lung. J. Anat., in press.
13. Short, R. H. D. (1951). Alveolar epithelium in relation to growth of the lung. Philos. Trans. R. Soc. Lond. (Biol. Sci.) 235:35.
14. Collet, A. J., and Des Biens, G. (1974). Fine structure of myogenesis and elastogenesis in the developing rat lung. Anat. Rec. 179:343.
15. Kaufman, S. L., Burri, P. H., and Weibel, E. R. (1974). The postnatal growth of the rat lung. II. Autoradiography. Anat. Rec. 180:63.
16. Emery, J. L. (1970). The postnatal development of the human lung and its implication for lung pathology. Respiration (Suppl.), 27:41.
17. Emery, J. L,, and Fagan, D. G. (1970). New alveoli . . . where and how? Arch. Dis. Child. 45:145.
18. Thurlbeck, W. M. (1975). Postnatal growth and development of the lung. Am. Rev. Respir. Dis. 111:803.
19. Dingler, E. C. (1958). Wachstum der Lunge nach der Geburt. Acta Anat. (Basel) (Suppl.), 30:1.
20. Boyden, E. A., and Tompsett, D. H. (1961). The postnatal growth of the lung in the dog. Acta Anat. (Basel) 47:185.
21. Stigol, L. C., Vawter, G. F., and Mead, J. (1972). Studies on elastic recoil of the lung in a pediatric population. Am. Rev. Respir. Dis. 105:552.
22. Dunnill, M. S. (1962). Postnatal growth of the lung. Thorax 17:329.
23. Willson, H. G. (1928). Postnatal development of the lung. Am. J. Anat. 41:97.
24. Boyden, E. A. (1969). The pattern of the terminal air spaces in a premature infant of 30–32 weeks that lived nineteen and a quarter hours. Am. J. Anat. 126:31.
25. Reid, L. (1967). The embryology of the lung. In A. V. S. deReuck and R. Porter (eds.), Development of the Lung, pp. 109–124. Churchill, London.
26. Davies, G., and Reid, L. (1970). Growth of the alveoli and pulmonary arteries in childhood. Thorax 25:669.
27. Thurlbeck, W. M., and Angus, G. E. (1972). Number of alveoli in the human lung. J. Appl. Physiol. 32:483.
28. Hieronymi, G. (1961). Uber den durch das Alter bedingten formwandel menschlicher Lungen. Ergeb. Allerg. Pathol. Anatl. 41:1.
29. Hieronymi, G. (1960). Veranderungen der Lungenstruktur in verschiedenen Leibensalteren. Verh. Dtsch. Ges. Pathol. 44:129.
30. Boyden, E. A. (1967). Notes on the development of the lung in infancy and childhood. Am. J. Anat. 121:749.
31. Davies, G., and Reid, L. (1970). Growth of the alveoli and pulmonary arteries in childhood. Thorax 25:669.
32. Emery, J. L., and Mithal, A. (1960). The number of alveoli in the terminal respiratory unit of man during late intrauterine life and childhood. Arch. Dis. Child. 35:544.
33. Emery, J. L., and Wilcock, P. F. (1966). The postnatal development of the lung. Acta Anat. (Basel) 65:10.
34. Nakamura, T., Takizawa, T., and Morone, T. (1967). Anatomic changes in lung parenchyma due to aging process. Dis. Chest 52:518.

35. Angus, G. E., and Thurlbeck, W. M. (1972). Number of alveoli in the human lung. J. Appl. Physiol. 32:483.
36. Bates, D. V., Macklem, P. T., and Christie, R. (1971). V. Respiratory Function in Disease: An Introduction to the Integrated Study of the Lung. W. B. Saunders Co., Philadelphia.
37. Simon, G., Reid, L., Tanner, J. M., Goldstein, H., and Benjamin, B. (1972). Growth of radiologically determined heart diameter, lung width and lung length from 5–19 years with standards for clinical use. Arch. Dis. Child. 47:373.
38. Wood, L. D. H., Prichard, S., Weng, T. R., Kruger, K., Bryan, A. C., and Levison, H. (1971). Relationship between anatomic dead space and body size in health, asthma and cystic fibrosis. Am. Rev. Respir. Dis. 104:215.
39. Hogg, J. C., Williams, J., Richardson, J. B., Macklem, P. T., and Thurlbeck, W. M. (1970). Age as a factor in the distribution of lower airway conductance and in the pathologic anatomy of obstructive lung disease. N. Engl. J. Med. 282:1283.
40. Hislop, A., Muir, D. C. F., Jacobsen, M., Simon, G., and Reid, L. (1972). Postnatal growth and function of the pre-acinar pathways. Thorax 27:265.
41. Cudmore, R. E., Emery, J. L., and Mithal, A. (1962). Postnatal growth of bronchi and bronchioles. Arch. Dis. Child. 37:481.
42. Matsuba, K., and Thurlbeck, W. M. (1972). A morphometric study of bronchial and bronchiolar walls in children. Am. Rev. Respir. Dis. 105:908.
43. Field, W. E. H. (1968). Mucous gland hypertrophy in babies and children aged 15 years or less. Br. J. Dis. Chest 62:11.
44. Hislop, A., and Reid, L. (1973). Pulmonary arterial development during childhood: branching pattern and structure. Thorax 28:129.
45. Elliot, F. M., and Reid, L. (1965). Some new facts about the pulmonary artery and its branching pattern. Clin. Radiol. 16:193.
46. Hislop, A., and Reid, L. (1973). Fetal and childhood development of the intrapulmonary veins in man–branching pattern and structure. Thorax 28:313.
47. Nattie, E. E., Wiley, C. W., and Bartlett, D., Jr. (1974). Adaptive growth of the lung following pneumonectomy in rats. J. Appl. Physiol. 37:491.
48. Romanova, L. K. (1961). Regenerative hypertrophy of the lungs in rats after one-stage removal of the entire left lung and the diaphragmatic lobe of the right lung. Bull. Exp. Biol. Med. 50:1192.
49. Cowan, M. J., and Crystal, R. G. (1975). Lung growth after unilateral pneumonectomy: quantitation of collagen synthesis and content. Am. Rev. Respir. Dis. 111:267.
50. Sery, Z., Keprt, E., and Obrucnik, M. (1969). Morphometric analysis of late adaptation of the residual lung following pneumonectomy in young and adult rabbits. J. Thorac. Cardiovasc. Surg. 56:549.
51. Cohn, R. (1940). The postnatal growth of the lung. J. Thorac. Surg. 9:274.
52. Buhain, W. J., and Brody, J. S. (1973). Compensatory growth of the lung following pneumonectomy. J. Appl. Physiol. 35:898.
53. Romanova, L. K., Leikina, E. M., and Antipova, K. K. (1967). Nucleic acid synthesis and mitotic activity during development of compensatory hypertrophy of the lung in rat. Bull. Exp. Biol. Med. (USSR) 63:303.
54. Fisher, J. M., and Simnett, J. D. (1973). Morphogenetic and proliferative changes in the regenerating lung of the rat. Anat. Rec. 176:389.
55. Edwards, F. R. (1939). Studies in pneumonectomy and the development

of a two-stage operation for the removal of a whole lung. Br. J. Surg. 27:392.

56. Bremer, J. L. (1937). The fate of the remaining lung tissue following lobectomy or pneumonectomy. J. Thorac. Surg. 6:336.

57. Longacre, J. J., and Johansmann, R. (1940). An experimental study of the fate of the remaining lung following total pneumonectomy. J. Thorac. Surg. 10:131.

58. Gmavi, M., Pansa, E., and Anselmetti, G. (1970). L'accrescimento e la rigenerazione del pulmone (Ricerche sperimentali). Minerva Chir. 25: 1491.

59. Addis, T. (1928). Compensatory hypertrophy of the lung after unilateral pneumonectomy. J. Exp. Med. 47:51.

60. Dunnill, M. S. (1965). Quantitative observations on the anatomy of chronic non-specific lung disease. Med. Thorac. 22:261.

61. Cohn, R. (1939). Factors affecting the postnatal growth of the lung. Anat. Rec. 75:195.

62. deLorimer, A. A., Tierney, D. F., and Parker, H. R. (1967). Hypoplastic lungs in fetal lambs with surgically produced congenital diaphragmatic hernia. Surgery 62:12.

63. Areechon, W., and Reid, L. (1963). Hypoplasia of lung with congenital diaphragmatic hernia. Br. Med. J. 1:230.

64. Kitagawa, M., Hislop, A., Boyden, E. A., and Reid, L. (1971). Lung hypoplasia in congenital diaphragmatic hernia: a quantitative study of airway, artery and alveolar development. Br. J. Surg. 58:342.

65. Dunnill, M. S. (1970). The anatomy of restrictive lung disease. Human Pathol. 1:265.

66. Davies, G., and Reid, L. (1971). Effect of scoliosis on growth of alveoli and pulmonary arteries and on right ventricle. Arch. Dis. Child. 46:623.

67. Bartlett, D., Jr. (1971). Postnatal growth of the mammalian lung: influence of excess growth hormone. Respir. Physiol. 12:297.

68. Brody, J. S., and Buhain, W. J. (1972). Hormone-induced growth of the adult lung. Am. J. Physiol. 223:1444.

69. Brody, J. S., and Buhain, W. J. (1973). Hormonal influence on post-pneumonectomy lung growth in the rat. Respir. Physiol. 19:344.

70. Bartlett, D., Jr. (1970). Postnatal growth of the mammalian lung: influence of low and high oxygen tensions. Respir. Physiol. 9:58.

71. Cunningham, E. L., Brody, J. S., and Jain, B. (1974). Lung growth induced by hypoxia. J. Appl. Physiol. 37:362.

72. Tenney, S. M., and Remmers, J. E. (1966). Alveolar dimensions in the lungs of animals raised at high altitude. J. Appl. Physiol. 21:1328.

73. Burri, P. H., and Weibel, E. R. (1971). Morphometric estimation of the diffusion capacity. II. Effect of pO_2 on the growing lung. Respir. Physiol. 11:247.

74. Bartlett, D., Jr., and Remmers, J. E. (1971). Effect of high altitude exposure on the lungs of young rats. Respir. Physiol. 13:116.

75. Hurtado, A. (1932). Respiratory adaptation in the Indian natives of the Peruvian Andes: studies at high altitude. Am. J. Phys. Anthropol. 17:137.

76. Dempsey, J. A., Reddan, W. G., Birnbaum M. L., Forster, H. V., Thoden, D. S., Grover, R. F., and Rankin, J. (1971). Effects of acute though lifelong hypoxic exposure on exercise pulmonary gas exchange. Respir. Physiol. 13:62.

77. Guleria, J. S., Pande, J. N., Sethi, P. K., and Roy, S. B. (1971). Pulmonary diffusing capacity at high altitude. J. Appl. Physiol. 31:536.
78. Saldana, M., and Garcia-Oyola, E. (1970). Morphometry of the high altitude lung. Lab. Invest. 22:509.
79. Gil, J., and Weibel, E. R. (1972). Morphological study of pressure–volume hysteresis in rat lungs fixed by vascular perfusion. Respir. Physiol. 15:190.
80. Daly, B. D. T., Parks, G. E., Edmonds, C. H., Hibbs, C. W., and Norman, J. C. (1975). Dynamic alveolar mechanics as studied by videomicroscopy. Respir. Physiol. 24:217.
81. Macklin, C. C. (1929). Musculature of bronchi and lung. Physiol. Rev. 9:1.
82. Macklin, C. C. (1950). Alveoli of mammalian lung: anatomical study with clinical correlation. Proc. Inst. Med. Chic. 18:78.
83. Fukaya, H., Martin, C. J., Young, A. C., and Katsura, S. (1968). Mechanical properties of alveolar walls. J. Appl. Physiol. 25:689.
84. Radford, E. P. (1964). Some mechanical properties of mammalian lungs. In XXII International Congress of Science, Vol. I, pp. 275–280.
85. Hills, B. A. (1971). Geometric irreversibility and compliance hysteresis of lung. Respir. Physiol. 13:50.
86. Ardila, R., Horie, T., and Hildebrandt, J. (1974). Macroscopic isotropy of lung expansion. Respir. Physiol. 20:105.
87. D'Angelo, E. (1972). Local alveolar size and transpulmonary pressure in situ in isolated lungs. Respir. Physiol. 14:251.
88. Storey, W. F., and Staub, N. C. (1962). Ventilation of terminal air units. J. Appl. Physiol. 17:391.
89. Kuno, K., and Staub, N. C. (1968). Acute mechanical effects of lung volume changes on artificial microholes in alveolar walls. J. Appl. Physiol. 24:83.
90. Klingele, T. G., and Staub, N. C. (1970). Alveolar shape changes with volume in isolated, air-filled lobes of cat lung. J. Appl. Physiol. 28:411.
91. Whimster, W. F. (1970). The microanatomy of the alveolar duct system. Thorax 25:141.
92. Dunnill, M. S. (1967). Effect of lung inflation on alveolar surface area in the dog. Nature (Lond.) 214:1013.
93. Forrest, J. B. (1970). The effect of changes in lung volume on the size and shape of alveoli. J. Physiol. (Lond.) 210:533.
94. Glazier, J. B., Hughes, J. M. B., Meloney, J. E., and West, J. B. (1967). Vertical gradient of alveolar size in lungs of dogs frozen intact. J. Appl. Physiol. 23:694.
95. Assimacopoulos, A., Guggenheim R., and Kapanci, Y. (1975). Changes in alveolar capillary configuration at different levels of lung inflation in the rat. Lab. Invest. 34:10.
96. Sobin, S. S., Tremer, H. M., and Fung, Y. C. (1970). Morphometric basis of the sheet flow concept of the pulmonary alveolar microcirculation in the cat. Circ. Res. 26:397.
97. Kapanci, Y., Assimacopoulos, A., Irle, C., Zwahlen, A., and Sabbiani, G. (1974). Contractile interstitial cells in pulmonary septa: a possible regulator of ventilation/perfusion ratio? Ultrastructural, immunofluorescence and in vitro studies. J. Cell Biol. 60:375.
98. Martin, H. B., and Proctor, D. F. (1958). Pressure-volume measurements on dog bronchi. J. Appl. Physiol. 13:337.
99. Marshall, R. (1962). Effect of lung inflation on bronchial dimensions in the dog. J. Appl. Physiol. 17:596.

100. Hyatt, R. E., and Flath, R. E. (1966). Influence of lung parenchyma on the pressure-diameter behavior of dog bronchi. J. Appl. Physiol. 21:1448.

101. Olsen, C. R., Stevens, A. E., and McIlroy, M. B. (1967). Rigidity of tracheae and bronchi during muscular constriction. J. Appl. Physiol. 23:27.

102. Hyatt, R. E., Sittipong, R., Olafsson, S., and Potter, W. A. (1970). Some factors determining pulmonary pressure-flow behaviour at high rates of airflow. *In* A. Bouhays (ed.), Airway Dynamics, pp. 43–60. Thomas, Springfield, Illinois.

103. Hughes, J. M. B., Hoppin, F. G., Jr., and Mead, J. (1972). Effect of lung inflation on bronchial length and diameter in excised lungs. J. Appl. Physiol. 32:25.

104. Klingele, T. G., and Staub, N. C. (1971). Terminal bronchiole diameter changes with volume in isolated, airfilled lobes of cat lung. J. Appl. Physiol. 30:224.

105. Marshall, R., and Holden, W. J. (1963). Changes in calibre of the smaller airways in man. Thorax 18:54.

106. Fraser, R. G. (1961). Measurements of the calibre of human bronchi in 3 phases of respiration by cinebronchography. J. Can. Assoc. Radiol. 12:102.

107. Mills, J. E., and Widdicombe, J. G. (1970). Role of the vagus nerves in anaphylaxis and histamine induced broncho-constriction in guinea pigs. Br. J. Pharmacol. 39:724.

108. Gold, W. M., Kessler, G. F., and Yu, D. Y. C. (1972). Role of vagus nerves in experimental asthma in allergic dogs. J. Appl. Physiol. 33:719.

109. Coleman, R. A. (1973). Evidence for a non-adrenergic inhibitory nervous pathway in guinea pig trachea. Br. J. Pharmacol. 48:360.

110. Richardson, J. B., and Bouchard, T. (1975). Demonstration of a non-adrenergic inhibitory nervous system in the trachea of the guinea pig. J. Allergy Clin. Immunol. 56:473.

111. Richardson, J. A non-adrenergic inhibitory nervous system in human airways. J. Appl. Physiol., in press.

112. Burnstock, G., and Costa, M. (1973). Inhibitory innervation of the gut. Gastroenterology 64:141.

113. Crema, A., Figo, G. M., and Lecchini, S. (1970). A pharmacological analysis of the peristaltic reflex in the isolated colon of the guinea pig or cat. Br. J. Pharmacol. 39:334.

114. Furness, J. B., and Costa, M. (1973). The nervous release and the action of substances which affect interstitial muscle through neither adreno-receptors nor cholinoreceptors. Phil. Trans. R. Soc. Lond. (Biol. Sci.) 265:123.

115. Frigo, G. M., del Tacca, M., Lechlini, S., and Crema, A. (1973). Some observations on the intrinsic nervous system in Hirschsprung's disease. Gut 14:35.

116. Richardson, J. (1974). Pharmacologic studies on murine megacolon. Can. Fed. Biol. Soc. 17:88.

117. Hung, K. S., Hertweck, M. S., Hardy, J. D., and Loosli, C. G. (1973). Electron microscopic observations of nerve endings in the alveolar walls of mouse lungs. Am. Rev. Respir. Dis. 108:328.

118. Jeffery, P., and Reid, L. (1973). Intra-epithelial nerves in normal rat airways: a quantitative electron microscopic study. J. Anat. 114:35.

119. Hung, K. S., Hertweck, M. S., Hardy, J. D., and Loosli, C. G. (1973).

Ultrastructure of nerves and associated cells in bronchiolar epithelium of the mouse. J. Ultrastruct. Res. 43:426.

120. Lauweryns, J. M., and Goddeeris, P. (1975). Neuroepithelial bodies in the human child and adult lung. Am. Rev. Respir. Dis. 111:469.

121. Lauweryns, J. M., and Cokelaere, M. (1973). Hypoxia-sensitive neuroepithelial bodies. Intrapulmonary secretory neuroceptors, modulated by the CNS. Z. Zellforsch. Mikrosk. Anat. 145:521.

122. Cutz, E., Chan, W., Wong, V., and Conen, P. E. (1974). Endocrine cells in rat fetal lungs: ultrastructural and histochemical study. Lab. Invest. 30:458.

International Review of Physiology
Respiratory Physiology II, Volume 14
Edited by John G. Widdicombe
Copyright 1977   University Park Press   Baltimore

2
Gas Mixing
and Distribution
in the Lung

L. A. ENGEL AND P. T. MACKLEM

McGill University, Montreal, Canada

MIXING OF GASES DURING INSPIRATION   38
    Taylor-type Dispersion   38
    Axial Convection, Diffusion, and Anatomical Dead Space   44
    Cardiogenic Mixing   50

INTERREGIONAL VENTILATION DISTRIBUTION   52
    Quasi-static   53
    Dynamic   57
        Effect of Inspiratory Flow   57
        Effect of Expiratory Flow   57
        Mechanisms   59

INTRAREGIONAL VENTILATION DISTRIBUTION   62
    Experimental Evidence of Ventilation Nonuniformity   62
    Stratified Versus Parallel Inhomogeneity   63
    Model Analyses   64
    Single Breath Inert Gas Washouts   65
    Sequential Filling and Emptying   66
    Dynamic Factors   66
    Single Breath Studies with Two Tracer Gases   67
    Functional and Structural Basis   69

INTER- AND INTRAREGIONAL
    CONTRIBUTIONS TO INERT GAS WASHOUTS   70
    Single Breath Washouts   70
        Bolus Studies   71
        Tidal Breath Studies   72

Cardiogenic Oscillations   73
Multiple Breath Washouts   73

The distribution and mixing of inspired gases in the lung are vital processes which frequently become impaired early in the development of many diseases of the lung. The nonuniformity of ventilation distribution and gas mixing in the normal lung have been the subject of research for the last 50 years. The introduction of gaseous radioisotopes by Knipping et al. (1), West and Dollery (2), and Ball et al. (3) allowed a topographical localization of ventilation distribution in the lung and was a major advance on studies using expired gas analyses in which the lung was treated as a black box. In this context, the subject has been partitioned into gas distribution among topographical lung zones or regions (see under "Interregional Ventilation Distribution") and within such regions (see under "Intraregional Ventilation Distribution"). Under "Inter- and Intraregional Contributions to Inert Gas Washouts," the interregional and intraregional contribution to inert gas washouts measured at the mouth are discussed.

Because of space limitation, all aspects of gas mixing and distribution could not be adequately covered and we have been necessarily selective. In this selection, we were guided by previous reviews, current research trends, and personal interests. The reader is referred to the excellent review of pulmonary statics by Milic-Emili (4) and to accounts of stratified inhomogeneity and models of gas mixing by Piiper and Scheid (5) and Cumming (6), respectively. Collateral ventilation, lung interdependence, and the frequency dependence of pulmonary dynamic compliance have been comprehensively reviewed by Macklem (7) and are only briefly mentioned here.

Recently, there has been considerable interest in the application of basic fluid dynamic concepts to gas flow in the conducting airways. Consequently, the subject of Taylor-type dispersion as it applies to the lung is reviewed in some detail, even though its importance to pulmonary gas transport has not yet been defined. The diffusion of alveolar gas against a convection current during inspiration is reviewed in detail and a detailed account of cardiogenic mixing is given because no previous reviews are available and because much of the work was done in our laboratories. Throughout the chapter, an attempt has been made to be provocative, with the intention of stimulating ideas and further research.

MIXING OF GASES DURING INSPIRATION

Taylor-type Dispersion

When a fluid flows in a tube, the fluid molecules in the center travel faster than those near the wall, resulting in a radial gradient of velocities. Consequently, a nondiffusible fluid tracer introduced into the stream at time t_0 undergoes axial dispersion such that, at time t, the tracer molecules in the center are ahead of a point moving with the mean flow, whereas those near the wall are behind the point.

The study of flow-induced axial dispersion stems from two papers by Taylor (8, 9), who was the first to identify the opposing action of the velocity gradient and radial mixing on longitudinal spread. The velocity gradient produces a radial concentration gradient at the interface between two fluids with consequent radial mixing. In laminar flow, mixing is by random molecular motion. In turbulent flow, molecular diffusion is negligible relative to the mixing property of turbulence. Mixing due to diffusion or turbulent eddies inhibits axial dispersion by randomizing the position of molecules across the tube. This causes each molecule to spend more nearly the same amount of time under the influence of the different velocities present in a nonuniform velocity profile. Under certain conditions, the interaction between axial convection and radial mixing may be represented as the sum of convection at the mean flow rate and an apparent axial diffusion with an effective diffusion coefficient, D_{eff}, greater than that for molecular diffusion (Figure 1).

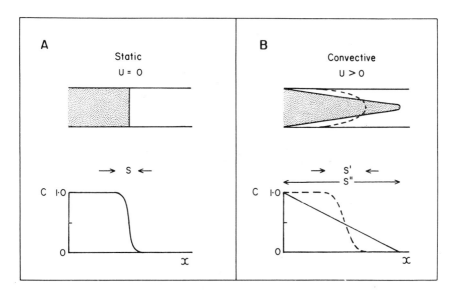

Figure 1. Radial concentration profiles (*upper panels*) and axial concentration gradients (*lower panels*) between two gases in a tube. *A*, static conditions; spread is by molecular diffusion only and concentrations are uniform across the diameter of tube. After time t spread, $S \alpha \sqrt{t\, D_{mol}}$, where D_{mol} is molecular diffusion coefficient of the gases. *B*, convection with average velocity u and molecular diffusion coefficient D_{mol}, where $D_{mol} > 0$ (*dashed line*) or $D_{mol} \approx 0$ (*solid line*). Note elongated "spike" of gas in the absence of diffusion, where spread (S'') after time t is given by $S'' = 2\,t\,u$. When $D_{mol} > 0$, radial diffusion diminishes axial spread (S') such that $S' = \sqrt{t\, D_{eff}}$, where D_{eff} is an effective diffusion coefficient. Note that $D_{eff} > D_{mol}$ and $S'' > S' > S$.

The mathematical expression for this diffusion coefficient, as modified by Aris (10), is

$$D_{\text{eff}} = D_{\text{mol}} + \frac{a^2 u^2}{K D_{\text{mol}}}$$

(1)

where D_{eff} is the effective axial diffusion coefficient under conditions of laminar flow with average velocity u in a tube radius a, and where D_{mol} is the molecular diffusivity. The value of constant K depends on the velocity profile and has a minimum of 48 when the profile is parabolic. The degree of axial spread is sensitive to the shape of the velocity profile, the blunter the profile, the smaller the dispersion. The inverse relationship between D_{eff} and D_{mol} implies that the smaller the molecular diffusivity of the fluid the greater the axial spread. Maximum spread occurs when dense fluids flow at high velocities through wide bore channels.

Although Taylor's analysis (8) applies to straight, smooth pipes at some distance from the site of introduction of the tracer fluid, the general principles apply to any fluid flowing in a conduit. The concept was first applied to gas flow in the airways of the lung early this century (11). Henderson et al. (11) speculated that a small volume of inspired gas traveled with a cone-front, thus penetrating deeply into the lung.

Wilson and Lin (12) applied Taylor's formulation in a quantitative way to a symmetrical model of the human lung (13) and concluded that Taylor dispersion is the dominant form of gas transport between generations 8 and 12. This conclusion must be treated with some reservation, however. The velocity profiles in the airways are almost certainly not parabolic due to the frequent branching (14), as well as the presence of cardiogenic flow pulses (15, 16). Also, Wilson and Lin (12) ignored the effect of turbulence in the larger airways. This would substantially diminish axial dispersion compared to that during laminar flow. In spite of these limitations, their analysis was the first rigorous description of axial dispersion in the lung. Most other models of gas transport have assumed that molecular diffusion was the only mixing mechanism.

Recently, Scherer et al. (17) measured the spread of a bolus of benzene vapor flowing through a five generation, branched, glass model of the human airways. The calculated effective diffusivity, D_{eff}, increased approximately linearly with flow over the range of Reynolds number 30–2,000, up to values three orders of magnitude higher than the molecular diffusivity of the gases used. The authors expressed the ratio of effective diffusivity, D_{eff}, to the molecular diffusivity, D_{mol}, during inspiration by the equation

$$D_{\text{eff}}/D_{\text{mol}} = 1 + 1.08 \, N_{P_e}$$

(2)

where N_{P_e} is the Peclet number (diameter × velocity/molecular diffusivity) (see under "Convection, Diffusion, and Anatomical Dead Space"). They expressed the relationship during expiration as

$$D_{\text{eff}}/D_{\text{mol}} = 1 + 0.37 \, N_{P_e}$$

(3)

The smaller axial dispersion coefficient during expiration was attributed to greater radial mixing at bifurcations and led to the conclusion that gas transport during inspiration is not identical to that during expiration. Although the analysis and conclusions were based on many simplifying assumptions, the equations offered the first empirical quantitation of Taylor-type dispersion in the study of gas transport in the lung.

There are few direct physiological data with which to test the mathematical and physical models discussed above. The rapid transit time of a bolus of gas from larynx to the pleural surface (18) is consistent with the presence of axial dispersion in the living lung. Engel et al. (16) used retrograde catheters through which to sample gas simultaneously in the trachea and a peripheral airway in dog lungs. During inspiration of 100% oxygen, the spread of the oxygen/nitrogen front was measurably increased during the transit between the trachea and an airway 4 mm in diameter (16). The authors calculated that the leading edge of the front moved ahead of its mean position by about 5 cm between the two sampling sites. Because the time of transit was of the order of 0.2 s, molecular diffusion would have accounted for only a small fraction of this spread. Taylor-type dispersion seems a likely mechanism to explain this observation. Using the same technique, Engel et al. (19) measured the spread of boli of oxygen between the trachea and a peripheral airway during inflation at different constant flow rates. Assuming that the axial spread, reflected in the concentration time profile at each sampling site, could be due to an effective diffusion process, an effective diffusivity at different flow rates was calculated. The results of one study in which the peripheral sampler was in a 4.4-mm airway 19 cm from the tracheal site are shown in Figure 2. The similarity to the findings of Scherer et al. (17) is striking, especially in view of the different experimental situations. The relationship between D_{eff} and inspiratory flow rate was roughly linear in this case (Figure 2), although in some lungs no clear relationship with flow was observed. In all airways, however, D_{eff} was at least 100 times greater than D_{mol}.

When a mixture containing two gases with differing diffusivities is made to flow through an air-filled tube, the two tracer gases separate at the interface between the mixture and the air, the denser gas being detectable slightly ahead of the lighter one (20). This behavior is predictable from the inverse relationship between D_{eff} and D_{mol} (equation 1). The slower radial diffusion of the denser gas leads to its greater axial dispersion. That such a separation may take place in the lung was suggested by Hogg et al. (21). They insufflated excised dog lobes with beads and inflated them with a gas mixture of 50% helium and sulfur hexafluoride (SF_6). Successive gas samples taken during expiration showed a progressive decrease in the He:SF_6 ratio, suggesting a deeper penetration of the denser gas into the lung. Recently, similar observations have been made in human subjects with induced bronchoconstriction after inspiration of 1 liter of a gas mixture containing 5% of each tracer (22). In the same subjects under control conditions, the He:SF_6 ratio increased progressively during expiration, in line with previous studies (23–25) (see under "Single Breath Studies with Two Tracer Gases"). The interpretation of these results is difficult. To evaluate from

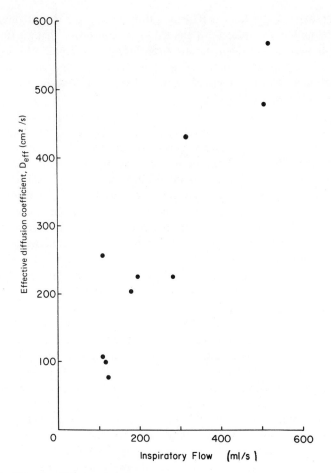

Figure 2. Effective diffusion coefficient (D_{eff}) measured at different flow rates between trachea and a 4.4-mm airway of excised dog lung. Note that D_{eff}, which is much greater than molecular diffusivity, increases with flow.

expired gas analysis the effect of Taylor dispersion during inspiration, one needs to assume a negligible dispersion during expiration. To the degree that Taylor dispersion may be less on expiration (17), the expired gas analysis will allow the detection of dispersion, but it will be underestimated.

These considerations may be relevant to conclusions drawn from aerosol studies. Aerosol particles 0.5 μm in diameter are said to trace out the convective movement of gases in the lung (26, 27). Indeed, in the absence of Taylor dispersion, penetration of inspired gas into the lung by convective movement should be represented by the behavior of the aerosol. In the presence of radial diffusion, however, the axial convective transport of the inspired gas is very much less than that of aerosol particles. According to equation 1, as $D_{mol} \rightarrow 0$,

$D_{eff} \rightarrow \infty$. Thus, aerosol particles, which diffuse several orders of magnitude more slowly than gases, must spread out axially considerably more than gases. Hence, the distribution of the inspired gas molecules with respect to the anatomy of the airways must differ from that of aerosol particles.

Although there is little doubt that Taylor-type dispersion takes place in the airways, little is known about how it influences overall gas transport and gas exchange. The Taylor effect increases the forward transport of inspired gas mainly during the first part of each breath. Once the conducting airways are filled with the inspirate, no more dispersion can take place there. Furthermore, in the largest airways, where D_{eff} is greatest, the volume per unit of distance and the transit time of the interface are least. Thus, both linear spread and its volume equivalent are minimized. In the study of Engel et al. (16), the advancing front moved ahead of its mean position by only 15 ml between the trachea and an airway of 4 mm diameter. Of this volume, only a small fraction constituted pure inspirate. Thus, the amount of inspirate transported by this means was minimal. A similar conclusion was reached from a computer simulation analysis in which D_{eff} was allowed to vary from 63 cm^2 s^{-1} in generation 7 to 0.22 cm^2 s^{-1} in generation 13 (28). The dead space remained almost unchanged when the effect of Taylor dispersion was included.

On the other hand, because of the inverse relationship between D_{eff} and D_{mol} (equation 1), it is tempting to explain the improved or unimpaired gas exchange present under conditions in which dense gases are breathed (29–33) by an enhanced axial dispersion. The value of D_{mol} is inversely related to the square root of density. A reduced D_{mol} should impair gas exchange if the latter were limited by diffusion gradients in the gaseous phase. Yet the $(A - a)D_{O_2}$ decreases substantially both in dogs (30, 33) and in man (31) when gas density is highest. Similarly, the uptake of carbon monoxide is enhanced when breathing SF_6 as compared to helium (32), although the single breath D_{CO} is unchanged (33). The $P_{A_{CO_2}}$ and V_D/V_T increase (30, 31) or do not change (33), however, suggesting that gas density acts differently on the pulmonary exchange of oxygen and carbon dioxide. It is not easy to see how Taylor dispersion could account for this difference.

A specific kind of Taylor-type dispersion is that which might occur within the alveolated zone. Radial diffusion from the alveolar ducts into the alveoli must retard the axial equilibration of concentration gradients (5, 24, 34–37), as can be experimentally demonstrated in a simple mechanical model with and without partitions (35). In the presence of axial convection along the duct lumen, a Taylor-type dispersion could take place if radial diffusion equilibration with the gas in the alveoli were not virtually instantaneous. Under these circumstances, if a gas mixture containing two tracer gases with different diffusivities were inhaled, the heavier, more slowly diffusing gas would be concentrated in the central core of the stream in comparison to the more rapidly diffusing gas. This would result in a deeper penetration into the lung by the heavier gas. Lacquet et al. (28) have simulated simultaneous axial convection and axial radial diffusion in a model of an alveolar duct with realistic boundary conditions and concluded that this mode of dispersion plays only a minor role. Nevertheless, it is possible that under certain conditions, e.g., airway obstruction with collateral ventilation, Taylor-type dispersion would be important. Indeed, it may account for the apparently deeper penetration of SF_6 relative to helium when a mixture of the two gases is used to inflate beaded dog lobes (21) (see above). If the effect is also appreciable when breathing respiratory gases, the collaterally ventilated space would be better ventilated than could be predicted from considerations not involving Taylor-type dispersion. It is possible that the efficient gas exchange measured within a collaterally ventilated segment of a dog lung (38) is partly due to this phenomenon.

Axial Convection, Diffusion, and Anatomical Dead Space

The study of convective and diffusive gas transport between the mouth and alveoli is simplified by assuming instantaneous equilibration of radial concentration differences in the conducting airways. The relative contribution of the two types of transport is given by the Peclet number (N_{P_e}). This is a ratio of the convective (velocity $\times$ diameter) to diffusive (D_{mol}) characteristics in an airway. At low flows the average gas velocity in an airway depends on its cross section, the flow at the mouth, and the relative compliance of that portion of lung ventilated by the airway. In a symmetrical model of the lung (13), N_{P_e} in all airways may be calculated for a given flow at the mouth (Table 1). Due to the enormous increase in total cross-sectional area, as well as the decrease in diameter in successive generations of branching, the Peclet number decreases by a factor of 100,000 from trachea to generation 22 (Table 1). The generation in which the Peclet number is equal to one (the terminal bronchiole at a flow of 400 ml/s) constitutes a "critical zone" in which mechanical motion and molecular diffusion contribute to the same extent to the transport of gas molecules (39).

Consequently, the volume to which the front separating freshly inspired gas from residual gas penetrates into the lung is much less than the volume of the breath. During inspiration of 100% oxygen at a constant, slow flow rate, the oxygen/nitrogen front moves into the lung until it reaches the critical zone. At that point, the front becomes stationary in spite of continuing oxygen flow into the lung (16, 36, 40–42) (Figure 3). On expiration, the interface moves rapidly mouthward. Measurements made within small airways have shown that the nitrogen concentration becomes fixed with relatively little change during the latter part of inspiration (16, 42) (Figure 4). This constant nitrogen concentration represents one point on the stationary front and is a direct confirmation of the prediction made from several theoretical analyses.

Most of these analyses consist of solutions of a second order differential equation describing simultaneous convection and diffusion in a symmetrical model of the lung (36, 41, 43). One such equation is

$$\frac{\delta c}{\delta t} + \frac{\dot{V}\delta c}{A\delta x} - \frac{D}{A} \cdot \frac{\delta A}{\delta x} \cdot \frac{\delta c}{\delta x} = D \cdot \frac{\delta^2 c}{\delta x^2} \qquad (4)$$

Table 1. Values of Peclet number (N_{Pe}) in different generations of symmetrical lung model (13) at a flow of 400 ml/s at mouth

Generation	Velocity (cm/s)	Diameter (cm)	N_{Pe}	Generation	Velocity (cm/s)	Diameter (cm)	N_{Pe}
0	160	1.8	1,152	12	13.8	0.095	5.24
2	190	0.83	631	14	5.80	0.074	1.72
4	160	0.45	288	16	2.22	0.060	0.533
6	100	0.28	112	18	0.755	0.050	0.151
8	57.1	0.19	43.4	20	0.250	0.045	0.045
10	30.8	0.13	16.0	22	0.0678	0.041	0.011

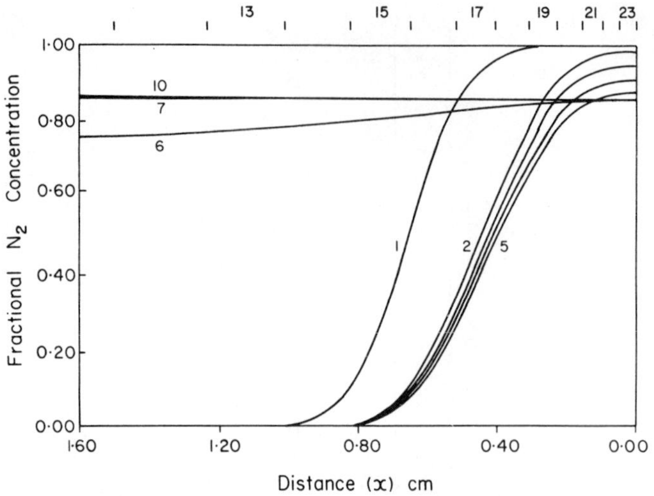

Figure 3. Fractional nitrogen concentration (F_{N_2}) in the last 12 generations (12–23) of a symmetrical lung model during a single breath of oxygen at a constant flow rate. Numbers 1–10 refer to F_{N_2} at 0.4s intervals during a cycle of 4-s duration. The oxygen/nitrogen front becomes relatively stationary during inspiration (nos. 2 to 5). Note that in generations 16–23 differences in F_{N_2} are present during inspiration but disappear rapidly after onset of expiration. Reprinted with permission of J. Appl. Physiol. 35:401 (1973).

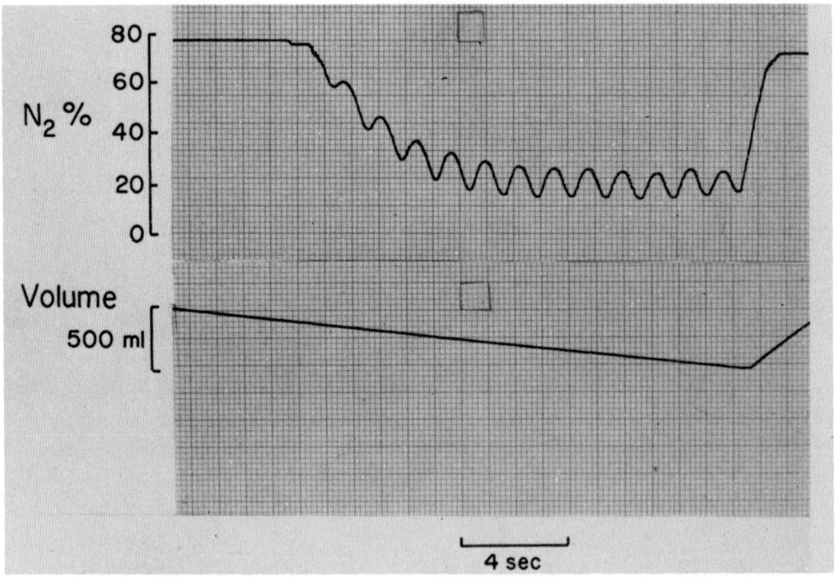

Figure 4. Changes in nitrogen concentration (*upper trace*) in a 4.1-mm airway of a living dog during inspiration of oxygen at a constant flow rate. *Lower trace*, lung volume change. Mean nitrogen concentration remains constant during the second part of the inspiration. Note cardiogenic oscillations. Reprinted with permission of Respir. Physiol. 26:77 (1976).

where c is the concentration of a gas at time t, V is the volume flow at the mouth, A the summed cross-sectional area at a distance x from the trachea, and D is the diffusion coefficient, which is assumed not to vary as a function of x. The right hand side of equation 4, together with the first term on the left, constitute the Fick equation governing unidimensional diffusion under static conditions. The second term on the left side introduces the convective component of gas transport. The third term takes account of the changing cross-sectional area and is dimensionally similar to the convective term. Because $\delta A/\delta x$ is positive, i.e., cross-sectional area increases with distance from the trachea, this term has a negative value, effectively resulting in a decreased convective component. This is the mathematical basis for the front becoming stationary at a point in the airways where the value of $\delta A/\delta x$ is large enough for the second and third terms to be equal and opposite.

The stationary oxygen/nitrogen front represents a balance between the convective transport of nitrogen toward the alveoli and the diffusive nitrogen transport toward the mouth (16, 42). Putting $\delta c/\delta t$ equal to zero and integrating, equation 4 reduces to

$$\dot{V} F_{N_2} = D A \frac{\delta F_{N_2}}{\delta x} \tag{5}$$

where F_{N_2} is the nitrogen concentration and $\delta F_{N_2}/\delta x$ is the axial concentration gradient at any point on the stationary front (42). Alternatively, for oxygen, integration results in the equation

$$\dot{V} = \dot{V} \cdot F_{O_2} - D A \frac{\delta F_{O_2}}{\delta x} \tag{6}$$

where F_{O_2} is the oxygen concentration and $\delta F_{O_2}/\delta x$ is the axial concentration gradient (42). This equation allows one to partition the oxygen transport to the alveoli into convective ($V \cdot F_{O_2}$) and diffusive ($DA\delta F_{O_2}/\delta x$) components. At any point on the stationary interface, the magnitude of F_{O_2} determines the proportion of total oxygen transport due to convection.

The configuration of the oxygen/nitrogen front may be derived by solving equation 4 (Figure 3). A simpler approach is first to calculate the linear velocity as a function of distance from the 23rd generation, and then, starting with an assumed F_{N_2} in the terminal generation, to calculate F_{N_2} at more proximal points by an iterative technique using equation 5 (42, 44).

The stationary interface demarcates the transition from the conducting airways filled with inspired gas to the alveolar compartment where rapid equilibration results in nearly uniform gas concentrations. It thus represents the internal limit of "the volume of the conducting airways down to the location at which a large change in gas composition occurs," which describes the Fowler dead space (45). On expiration, the front corresponds to phase II of the single breath nitrogen washout and is the basis for measuring anatomical dead space with this technique. Because of continuing diffusion during the expiration, the dead space measured at the mouth is less than the volume down to the position of the interface at end inspiration. Nevertheless, under standardized conditions of flow, lung volume, and gases breathed, the measured Fowler dead space (V_D) must reflect the position of the stationary front.

From equation 5 it is possible to predict qualitatively the influence of changes in flow, lung volume, and diffusivity on the position of the front, and hence the magnitude of the V_D. An increase in flow enhances the convective nitrogen transport, displacing the front distally, where the larger cross-sectional area favors diffusion and restores a new equilibrium. Decreases in flow have the opposite effect. Similarly, when lung volume is increased, A at a given point in the airways increases, favoring diffusive nitrogen transport mouthward. A shift of the front to a point of smaller total cross-sectional area restores the balance. These predictions are consistent with simulations of gas transport in the lung with the use of the general convection/diffusion equation (36, 41, 43) and have been confirmed by direct sampling of gases from intrapulmonary airways (16, 42). Predictably, the Fowler dead space (V_D) increases as inspiratory flow increases. This is especially apparent when that portion of the V_D located peripheral to a small airway is measured (Figure 5). In normal subjects breathing at high frequencies, the measured V_D increases markedly (46).

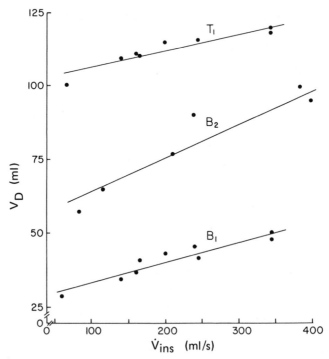

Figure 5. Fowler dead space (V_D), measured in the trachea (T_1) and two small airways (B$_1$, B$_2$) of excised dog lungs. When expiratory flows are identical, V_D increases with inspiratory flow ($\dot{V}_{ins}$). The increase is proportionately greater in small airways than in trachea. Reprinted with permission of J. Appl. Physiol. 35:18 (1973).

During an end-inspiratory pause, the diffusive nitrogen transport mouthward is no longer opposed by convective flow, resulting in a mouthward movement of the front (16, 40). Consequently, the V_D measured at the mouth decreases progressively with breathholding (11, 45, 47, 48) (see Figure 6). Because A in a given airway is approximately proportional to the 2/3 power of volume, equation 5 indicates that the position of the front is less dependent upon lung volume than upon flow and diffusivity. Nevertheless, for large volume changes at a given flow, the interface is actually situated more peripherally at low lung volumes than at high volumes (16), i.e., as lung volume increases during inspiration the interface tends to move mouthward. When the changes are small (e.g., during tidal breathing) the influence of volume on the position of the front can probably be neglected.

From equation 5 it is apparent that the diffusivity of the gases also influences the position of the stationary front. The latter is situated more peripherally when dense gases are breathed or when ambient pressure is increased (decreased D_{mol}). Predictably, the V_D for SF_6 is greater than that for helium (28). However, whereas the larger V_D suggests impairment of gas exchange, the alveolar-arterial oxygen difference is in fact less than SF_6 is breathed. Clearly, other factors must play a role (see under "Taylor-type Dispersion").

In the above account of convection and diffusion, the inspiratory flow was assumed to be constant. During normal quiet breathing, a cyclic flow pattern results in the advancement and recession of the front during the course of an inspiration (36, 41). Nevertheless, all the relationships between flow, the position of the front, and size of V_D discussed above are essentially unchanged.

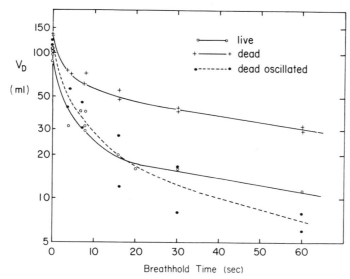

Figure 6. Fowler dead space (V_D) after breathholding, measured in trachea of dog lung. In vivo V_D decreases more rapidly than postmortem. Manual oscillation of the heart after death simulates the rapid decrease in V_D seen in vivo. Reprinted with permission of J. Appl. Physiol. 35:9 (1973).

Another assumption in the above description is that gas mixing takes place by molecular diffusion alone. Recently, the effect of convective dispersion has been incorporated into gas transport model analyses (12, 28, 49). In these cases, D_{mol} is replaced by an effective diffusion coefficient, D_{eff}, which varies as a function of distance from the trachea. This refinement involves the addition of another term into equation 4, reflecting the influence of $\delta D_{eff}/\delta x$ (43). Computer simulations suggest that this does not influence in a major way the position of the stationary front or the size of the dead space (28). Cardiogenic mixing also influences the front between inspired and alveolar gas and is discussed in detail under "Cardiogenic Mixing." Finally, most analyses deal with a fictitious symmetrical model of the lung (13, 50). Because the accurate geometry of the lung is not known, the conclusions may be subject to error. For example, the asymmetry of the bronchial tree and the range of path lengths contribute to the configuration of phase II (51). Furthermore, sequential emptying of lung units with differing ventilation to volume ratios also decreases the slope of phase II (46). However, the influence of these factors is probably small. In any case, the experimental measurements in the airways (16, 42, 52) suggest that the predictions of the model analyses are qualitatively correct.

Cardiogenic Mixing

Observations of the effect of heart action on lung and airways date back to the middle of the last century (53, 54), and many investigators correlated the pressure and flow variations at the mouth with the cardiac events during each cycle (55). West and Hugh-Jones (15) observed pulsatile gas flows caused by the heart in lobar and segmental bronchi of supine human subjects. The authors noted that at a given instant in the cardiac cycle the phase of the pulsations differed in different parts of the lung and that the magnitude of these pulses was out of proportion to the pulsatile flow at the lips. West and Hugh-Jones foresaw that gas mixing between the anatomical dead space and alveolar gas must be accelerated by these pulsations and speculated that this influence may be greater than that of gaseous diffusion in the reduction of anatomical dead space during breathholding.

The mechanism responsible for the reduction of V_D during breathholding has been a matter for dispute. Horsfield and Cumming (51) inferred that alveolar nitrogen must advance to the main bronchi during 30 s of breathholding and concluded that the linear distance (8 cm) is too great to explain in terms of simple gaseous diffusion. Bartels et al. (47) found that the rate of decrease of V_D with breathhold time was the same for helium as for the respiratory gases. They concluded that the decrease could not be due to diffusion alone, because the rapidly diffusing helium should have resulted in a smaller V_D. Roos et al. (46) disagreed with this conclusion, claiming that because of the geometry of the bronchial tree significant differences, in terms of length, between obliteration of concentration differences for the two gases were in fact small when expressed in terms of volume. In other words, changes in V_D volume were insensitive indicators of longitudinal mixing within the airways.

Recently Engel et al. (52) showed in experimental animals that during breathholding after an inspiration of oxygen, the nitrogen concentration in small airways rises nearly 5 times more rapidly in vivo than in identical maneuvers postmortem. The authors attributed this difference to the action of the heart and were able to reproduce in dead lungs both the rhythmic oscillation in F_{N_2} and the enhancement of gas mixing by manually oscillating the heart with an attached thread. The Fowler dead space, measured in the trachea, decreased during breathholding more rapidly in vivo than postmortem (Figure 6). When the heart was manually oscillated in the dead animals, V_D decreased at a rate similar to that seen in vivo. Cardiac action accounted for only one fourth of the reduction in V_D with breathholding, in spite of a 2-fold enhancement of gas mixing in the pulmonary airways. This supports the contention that changes in V_D are insensitive indicators of longitudinal mixing in the airways. Nevertheless, measurements of V_D with gases of different diffusivities do differ (20, 28). Although the V_D for helium is smaller than that for SF_6, during breathholding in man the difference decreases, whereas in excised dog lungs the difference increases (56). Because the mechanical basis for cardiogenic gas mixing is probably a convective dispersion similar to that described by Taylor (see under "Taylor-type Dispersion"), the more rapid mixing of the denser gas in vivo suggests that cardiac mixing is more important than molecular diffusion in equilibrating alveolar and dead space gas during breathholding.

The influence of cardiac action on gas mixing is also apparent during inspiration. The position of the stationary interface separating the inspired and alveolar gas extends into much larger airways than predicted from model analyses using molecular diffusion coefficients. For a given flow, the interface is invariably more peripherally situated postmortem than in vivo (16, 42). The calculated effective diffusion coefficient in vivo is approximately 5 times greater than that postmortem (42).

The mechanism by which cardiac action influences gas mixing is not well understood, but probably the effect is due to the heart motion itself. Obstruction of blood flow in a lobar branch of the pulmonary artery has no influence on intralobar gas mixing during breathholding (52) or during inspiration. On the other hand, a small volume of saline solution introduced into the pericardial sac effectively dampens a major proportion of the cardiogenic mixing with little change in the lobar pulmonary arterial pulse pressure (57).

The manner in which the lung transmits a pressure impulse has received little attention in the past. The asymmetric motion of the heart wall during each cycle probably creates a pressure wave which is transmitted through the lung. Whether the lung units exposed to the pressure impulse deflate or not may depend on their time constants. When these are sufficiently short relative to the duration of a heart beat, transient partial deflation of the units enhances gas mixing in the presence of concentration differences, probably by a mechanism akin to Taylor dispersion (52).

The intrapulmonary mechanical events discussed above are reflected in the pattern of cardiogenic oscillations on expired gas tracings. The oscillations seen at the mouth are probably due to asynchronous contributions from apical and basal lung regions when these contain different gas concentrations (58–60). This explanation obviously cannot account for the oscillations observed on alveolar plateaus recorded within intrapulmonary airways. Several investigators have made such observations (61–64). Although the size of the units whose asynchronous emptying gives rise to the oscillations is unknown, the units must be smaller than those subtended by airways 3 mm in diameter (64).

Cardiogenic oscillations are present on tracings of expired gases from most normal subjects, but not on those from patients with emphysema (58, 65, 66). Patients with bronchial asthma also have diminished or absent oscillations which increase in amplitude following partial relief of the bronchial obstruction by bronchodilator drugs (66, 67). Intrapulmonary sampling studies in patients with chronic obstructive lung disease indicate that the oscillations are not present in the trachea unless they are also seen within the lobes (63). Because sublobar as well as lobar time constants are likely to be prolonged in obstructive lung disease, it is possible that the mechanical response of the lung parenchyma to the cardiogenic pressure impulse is diminished, resulting in smaller flow transients, and consequently diminished or absent cardiogenic oscillations both in the trachea and smaller airways (35).

The influence of cardiac mixing on pulmonary gas exchange is not known. In normal lungs, the component of alveolar ventilation due to cardiac mixing is probably quite small (52). Under conditions of severe hypoventilation with oxygen-enriched mixtures, however, the cardiogenic effect may be important. In all cases, the persistence of alveolar gas in major airways throughout inspiration tends to make the composition of gas in different alveoli more homogeneous. This is similar to the buffering effect of a common dead space on limiting the possible range of gas compositions in alveoli (68). The cardiogenic enhancement of gas mixing necessarily minimizes any limitation to gas diffusion which may exist in the lung. Model analyses or calculations which ignore the cardiogenic component must overestimate the degree of inhomogeneity existing in the lung. The observation that the effective diffusion coefficient, which incorporates cardiogenic mixing, is on the average 5 times greater than the molecular diffusion coefficient, suggests that the error may be substantial.

INTERREGIONAL VENTILATION DISTRIBUTION

The measurement of intrapulmonary radioactive gas concentrations by scintillation counters placed externally over the chest (2, 3) has greatly clarified the topographical distribution of gas in the lung (4). The lung field detected by each counter consists of a slice or cylinder of tissue whose size depends on the degree of collimation. These fields bear little relationship to anatomical subdivisions of the lung. Recently, many investigators have adopted the term "regional" to describe measurements made among such counter fields. This convention will be followed in this chapter. In this context, the title "interregional gas distribution" refers to the distribution of volume and inspired gas among lung zones which are macroscopic in size and topographically distributed, usually in the direction of gravity. Conventionally, the volume of a region is expressed as a fraction of the regional volume at total lung capacity.

Quasi-static

This subject has recently been elegantly reviewed by Milic-Emili (4). The regional distribution of volume may be usefully described by a relatively simple model: briefly, the lung in situ is viewed as being exposed to a vertical gradient in pleural pressure which is gravity-dependent and essentially the same at different lung volumes. The stress-strain relationships of the lung are assumed to be uniformly distributed; hence, all regions in the same horizontal plane are expanded to the same degree, whereas vertically distributed regions exhibit a gradient of expansion corresponding to the vertical range of transpulmonary pressure (69). Due to the curvilinear pressure-volume relationship of the lung, the dependent, less expanded regions have a higher compliance than the non-dependent, more expanded zones. During slow changes in lung volume, the distribution of gas above "closing volume" may be accounted for by the distribution of regional pulmonary compliance (69). In this volume range, filling and emptying of all regions takes place essentially in a uniform manner.

In fact, when apex-to-base concentration differences are large, dependent regions are seen to empty preferentially at higher lung volumes (70). Although this volume-dependent, sequential emptying represents only a small deviation from the model described above, it is instructive to examine the possible mechanisms which may account for these deviations (70).

1. Differences in lobar pressure-volume (P-V) curves. If the upper lobes were relatively more expanded at a given translobar pressure than the lower lobes, their contribution to the expirate would progressively increase, as observed experimentally (see Figure 11). This could explain the sequential emptying observed in upright and supine postures. However, in the prone posture in man, the upper lobes are located below the lower lobes due to the course of the oblique fissures. Hence, the gravity-dependent sequential emptying observed also in this posture cannot be readily explained by different lobar P-V curves.

2. Nonmonoexponential P-V curve of the lung. A P-V relationship described by a single exponential is the only one (besides a linear one) which allows regions at different degrees of expansion to fill and empty nonsequentially so that the contribution of each region to the gas appearing at the mouth is constant (69, 71). Above functional residual capacity (FRC), the P-V curve of the lung conforms closely to a single exponential (72, 73). However, other functions have been proposed (74), and small departures from a single exponential could be responsible for the observed sequential behavior.

3. Different changes in applied pleural pressure. If during expiration the pleural pressure over apical regions increased initially more slowly and later more rapidly than that over basal lung zones, the vertically distributed regions would empty sequentially. This possibility is discussed in greater detail later.

The assumption of a constant pleural pressure gradient at all lung volumes implies equal changes in pleural pressure in all parts of the thorax. Thus, inhomogeneity in the stress-strain relationships of the chest wall should play little role in gas distribution. Indeed, regional volume distribution in man is not influenced by a wide range of changes in thoracoabdominal shapes (75). Similar deforming forces applied to animals substantially alter the gradient in pleural pressure (76) as well as the gradient in regional alveolar size as measured by frozen sections (77). This difference between animals and man was interpreted to be due to a relatively stiffer rib cage in humans, resulting in a greater resistance to deformation (75). The same explanation may account for the observations that, contrary to the findings in experimental animals (78), in upright man neither the weight of the abdominal contents (79) nor passive inflation of the respiratory system (80) influences the distribution of gas within the lungs.

Predictably, more extreme deformations produced either by externally applied force or by muscle action can be associated with changes in regional volume and, by inference, in pleural pressure (81, 82).

Selective use of different respiratory muscles may alter the distribution of pleural pressure between lung apex and base, independent of the influence of gravity. In the dog, electrophrenic stimulation produces markedly more negative pleural surface pressure over the lower lobes than over the upper lobes both in the supine (83) and erect postures (84). After phrenicotomy the swings in pleural pressure during spontaneous breathing are greater over the upper lobes (83). Consistent with these observations, the esophageal pressure gradient in upright human subjects may be enhanced during Muller maneuvers performed mainly with the rib cage musculature, whereas similar efforts produced by diaphragmatic contraction have the opposite effect (85).

In man, voluntary selective contraction of either inspiratory intercostal and accessory muscles or the diaphragm measurably changes the apico-caudal distribution of gas in the lung. A bolus inspired at FRC in upright subjects is more evenly distributed when the rib cage muscles are used selectively than during inspiration achieved by contraction of the diaphragm (86). Helium bolus washouts both in the erect (86) and horizontal postures (87) differ when the thoracic and abdominal portion of the chest wall are deflated in differing sequences. It is possible, therefore, that during "spontaneous," slow expirations the gravity-dependent emptying sequence may also be due to configurational changes. Certainly the demonstration that very small differences in pleural pressure swings could influence gas distribution (88) makes this possibility an attractive one.

In the horizontal posture, the vertical distribution of regional volume, as well as of inspired gas, depends on the state of contraction of the diaphragm. At all lung volumes in the lateral decubitus posture, voluntary diaphragmatic contraction greatly reduces the vertical gradient in regional volume (89), abolishing it completely in some subjects (Figure 7). Analysis of helium bolus washouts in both the supine and lateral decubitus postures also indicates a more homogeneous pattern of volume change among vertically distributed zones when the transdiaphragmatic pressure (P_{di}) is high (82). Even relatively modest increases in P_{di} (20 cm H_2O) make the sequence of lung emptying more homogeneous. In anesthetized, paralyzed, and mechanically ventilated subjects in the lateral posture, the inspired gas is preferentially distributed to the nondependent lung (90), whereas, in spontaneously breathing man, inspired gas goes predominantly to the dependent lung. This is consistent with the observations that during spontaneous breathing in both supine and lateral postures the dependent portion of the diaphragm moves more, whereas during positive pressure inflation it is the nondependent portion which is displaced most (91). Recently, Engel and Roussos (92) demonstrated that awake subjects in the lateral decubitus posture could voluntarily distribute a bolus of tracer gas at FRC preferentially to the

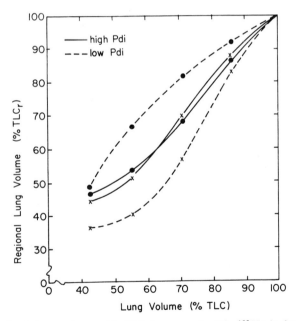

Figure 7. Regional lung volumes (% TLC$_r$) measured with ^{133}Xe in lateral decubitus posture and plotted against overall volume (% TLC). -•-, mean of two regions 5 and 10 cm from lung top; -x-, mean of two regions 25 and 30 cm from lung top. Voluntary contraction of the diaphragm (high P_{di}) eliminates the vertical gradient in regional expansion observed when the diaphragm is relaxed (low P_{di}).

nondependent lung when they inspired predominantly with the rib cage. This was done by selective contraction of the intercostal and accessory muscles. In contrast, when the subjects inspired by contracting the diaphragm the tracer gas went preferentially to the dependent lung.

The above observations support the hypothesis that in the horizontal posture the hydrostatic pressure gradient in the abdomen influences the vertical gradient of expansion in the lung (93). A more rigid, contracting diaphragm tends to insulate the thorax from the influence of the hydrostatic gradient in the abdomen, reducing the gradient of regional volumes and, by inference, the pleural pressure gradient. However, the effect of abdominal weight may not be the only factor changed by contracting the diaphragm. It is possible that diaphragmatic contraction also flares the lower rib cage (94) and elevates the mediastinum in the lateral posture. The former would tend to stiffen the rib cage making it less deformable, and thus minimize the gravity-induced deflation of the dependent, weight-bearing half. Elevation of the mediastinum would necessarily inflate the dependent lung at the expense of the upper one. Both of these effects would decrease the vertical gradient in regional expansion. To the degree that diaphragmatic contraction abolishes this gradient (Figure 7), lung weight should contribute only minimally to its presence.

Because during spontaneous breathing the diaphragm contracts on inspiration and relaxes during expiration, in the horizontal posture the swings of pleural pressure over the dependent regions must be greater than those over the nondependent zones (82). Thus, preferential distribution of inspired gas to dependent zones takes place not only due to the greater pulmonary compliance but also due to greater applied pressures.

Although direct measurements in animals have failed to show any differences in pleural pressure in the same horizontal plane at end expiration (95), a gradient of regional volume is present between lung apex and base both in supine man (75, 88, 96) and in the dog (97). In fact, Grassino et al. (75) observed that apex-to-base differences in regional volume in the supine posture were approximately 70% of those found in the same subjects in the erect position. Differences in mechanical properties between upper and lower lobes could theoretically account for these findings. No information is available on P-V curves of human lobes, but differences exist between upper and lower lobes in dogs (98) and rabbits (77), although not in monkeys (99). Indeed, in the dogs studied (97), the apex-to-base gradient of expansion (1.4% total lung capacity (TLC)/cm) fell within the range calculated from published differences between canine lobar P-V curves. However, if the results in supine human subjects were entirely due to differences in lobar P-V curves, these differences ought also to influence regional volumes in the erect position. In that case, the vertical gradient in pleural pressure compatible with the distribution of lung volumes would need to be smaller than that directly measured in animals (78) or in the human esophagus (100). Clarification of this apparent paradox awaits further investigations.

Dynamic

In contrast to the distribution of regional volume under quasi-static conditions, no simple model has been proposed which describes regional volume changes under dynamic conditions. In fact, studies of dynamic ventilation distribution have been carried out only recently and our knowledge of this subject is still relatively scant.

Effect of Inspiratory Flow   During quiet breathing, topographical gas distribution approximates the simple model proposed by Milic-Emili (69). Below flow rates of 0.2 liter/s, flow has a negligible influence on distributing the tidal volume (101). At high inspiratory flow rates (2.4–5.7 liter/s), the distribution of a bolus of tracer gas inhaled at FRC differs from the quasi-static distribution, with an increase in the apical and a decrease in basal concentrations (88, 102, 103). In fact, in some subjects the rate of change of regional distribution with inspiratory flow is greatest between 0.2 and 0.5 liter/s, indicating a marked sensitivity of regional ventilation distribution to flow rates present during quiet breathing (88, 103). The influence of flow is even more noticeable when the boli of tracer gas are introduced into the trachea (101): distribution at low flows (0.1 liter/s) is relatively more to the base, whereas at higher flows (1.0 liter/s) the bolus goes more preferentially to apical zones. When the tracer gas is inhaled through a 500-ml added dead space, basal distribution exceeds apical at all flow rates (101). Similarly, the regional distribution of tidal volumes of air inspired from FRC is less flow-dependent than that of boli inhaled at the onset of the breath (104). Nevertheless, the observation that ventilation during exercise is much more evenly distributed than during quiet breathing (105) suggests that the redistribution may be important.

In the supine posture, in spite of a more uniform gradient of expansion, the apico-caudal distribution of a bolus of ^{133}Xe inspired from FRC is even more flow-dependent than in the upright position (88). Figure 8 shows that at high flow rates in the supine posture more of the bolus is inspired into apical regions than into lung bases (88), whereas in the erect posture the distribution becomes more even (88, 102, 103).

Flow also influences the distribution of gas inspired from residual volume (RV). In erect subjects, boli of ^{133}Xe inhaled from RV at low flow rates (0.2–0.3 liter/s) distribute preferentially to apical lung regions (102, 106). At flows of 3 liters/s, a more even regional distribution is obtained (102). Above about 3.0 liters/s, changes in inspiratory flow rate appear to have no further effect on regional distribution of the gas (102).

Effect of Expiratory Flow   The pattern of regional volume change during expiration at low flow rates is approximated by the model proposed by Milic-Emili (4, 69, 71). However, as discussed under "Quasi-static," the regional fractional contributions to the expirate are not constant. Apical lung regions contribute a progressively greater proportion of their initial volume in the course of expiration. If an apicobasal gradient in gas concentration is established in upright subjects, this volume-dependent sequential emptying results in a gently

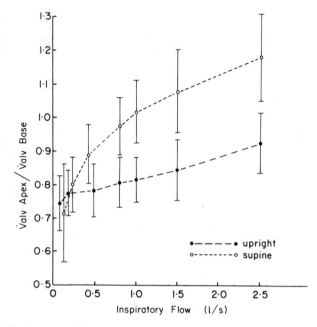

Figure 8. Distribution of inspired bolus of ^{133}Xe at different flow rates (abscissa). The *ordinate* is the ventilation of the upper two regions (5 and 10 cm from lung apex) relative to that of lower two regions (25 and 30 cm from lung apex). *Bars* represent ± 1 S.E. in seven subjects. Bolus distribution while supine is more dependent upon flow than in erect subjects. Reprinted with permission of J. Appl. Physiol. 41:489 (1976).

sloping alveolar plateau (70). An increase in expiratory flow decreases the slope of the nitrogen plateau after a breath of oxygen (107, 108), whereas the total amount of nitrogen in the expirate increases (108). Similar observations can be made from washouts of boli of tracer gas inhaled at RV (109). Furthermore, after maximally rapid expirations, regional volumes above 30% vital capacity (VC) are essentially uniform from apex to base (110). This contrasts with the static vertical gradient of expansion and indicates a marked departure from elastic equilibrium conditions. Thus, not only does each region contribute a constant fraction of the expirate, which in itself would be sufficient to produce a horizontal plateau, but the fractions are equal! However, since at RV the regional volumes are independent of the preceding rate of emptying (110), considerable redistribution of volume must occur as the static end point (elastic equilibrium at RV) is approached. Indeed, in the presence of apex-to-base differences in tracer gas concentrations, this redistribution is reflected in the pattern of expired gas concentrations at low lung volumes. The steep terminal portion (phase IV) of a nitrogen washout is first flattened, then partly reversed (phase V) in some subjects at progressively higher expiratory flows (111). Presumably, phase V represents diminishing contributions from apical lung regions, in spite of "rising" airway closure, due to the preceding preferential emptying of these regions at higher lung volumes.

During a single breath nitrogen washout, transient increases in expiratory flow are associated with transient increases in expired F_{N_2} (112). This pattern is consistent with enhanced emptying of apical lung regions and is also demonstrable with other tracer gases (113). Recently, Roussos et al. (114) showed that involuntary transient increases in flow, produced by manipulation of an expiratory resistance, did not influence the pattern of expired F_{N_2}. In contrast, "active" flow transients, produced by voluntary efforts, resulted in transient increases in the expired F_{N_2}, as shown previously (112, 113). Roussos et al. (114) related the changes in expired F_{N_2} to changes in transdiaphragmatic pressure (P_{di}) which increased during the active flow transients but not when the flow changes were produced passively. When expiratory flow was kept constant, transient increases in P_{di}, produced by voluntary increases in abdominal pressure, gave rise to transient changes in expired F_{N_2} similar to those after active flow transients. The authors proposed that the altered pattern of lung emptying was not due to flow changes per se, but consequent upon configurational changes in the chest wall produced by the associated contraction of the diaphragm.

Mechanisms The mechanisms responsible for the distribution of ventilation under dynamic conditions are not well understood. The model which has been most extensively examined is based on differences in mechanical time constants between pulmonary units.

If one considers the topographically distributed lung regions to be ventilated in parallel, then by analogy with the theory of parallel electrical circuits, the product of air flow resistance (R) and lung compliance (C) determines the rate of entry of gas into each lung unit (115). Regions whose product (RC), or time constant, is low should fill and empty faster than regions with a high RC.

It is probable that RC inequalities do exist within the normal lung. Because lower pulmonary resistance varies inversely with lung volume (116, 117), one would expect the resistance to the more expanded upper regions to be less than that to the less expanded lower zones. Because of the shape of the P-V curve, the more expanded upper regions also have a lower compliance. Consequently their time constant is shorter than that of the dependent zones. Accordingly, RC discrepancies among vertical regions may differ by more than a factor of 2 due to the pleural pressure gradient alone (31).

Pedley et al. (118) extended the theoretical analysis of Otis et al. (115) by incorporating the alinearity of P-V curves and of resistances, as well as the volume-dependence of resistance, into a two-compartment model representing upper and lower lung regions. The authors solved for the distribution of a bolus of gas inspired at different flow rates and lung volumes. The results of this analysis correspond reasonably well to experimental findings (101–104) supporting the hypothesis that under dynamic conditions topographical ventilation distribution may be determined by regional time constants.

An implicit assumption in the above analyses was that the swings in pleural pressure were the same everywhere. Recently, several experimental findings have led to a re-examination of this assumption and a re-evaluation of the time constant model as a mechanism for the dynamic distribution of ventilation. When appropriate compliance values are assigned to two compartments representing upper and lower lung regions, the distribution of boli at different flow rates is simulated most closely by a model which assumes that regional resistances to the upper and lower lung zones are equal (103). This is surprising as the airway dimensions in the more expanded upper regions are greater than in the dependent lung zones in the upright posture (119). Secondly, the analysis of Pedley et al. (118) predicts that changes in the density and viscosity of gases should alter gas distribution under dynamic conditions. Yet, the distribution of ^{133}Xe boli inhaled at different flow rates while breathing 80% SF_6 does not differ systematically from that while breathing air (103). Similarly, a tidal volume of ^{133}Xe-labeled gas is distributed in the same manner when breathing air as it is while breathing 80% helium at a comparable flow rate (104). Finally, the greater flow-dependence of gas distribution in supine subjects (88), when regional resistance and compliance should be more uniform than in the upright posture (Figure 8) is difficult to explain on the basis of time constant differences alone.

The above observations suggest that swings in pleural surface pressure (ΔP) may not be identical everywhere in the chest. Two distinct mechanisms may be responsible for differences in ΔP. When different lung zones fill asynchronously due to differences in time constants, the pleural pressure over the lagging lung regions may become more negative than that over regions which are leading. This inequality of ΔP reflects the resistance of the chest wall to deformation and acts so as to minimize the difference between dynamic and quasi-static gas distributions. This mechanical interdependence between lung regions and the overlying chest wall was proposed by Bake et al. (103) to explain why boli inhaled at high flow rates did not go preferentially to lung apices as predicted by the time constant model (118).

For reasons already discussed, there is an alternative mechanism for ΔP inequality. The evidence (reviewed above) that selective contraction of chest wall musculature alters the pattern of lung filling and emptying (82, 86, 87, 89) strongly suggests that ΔP values in different lung regions may differ not merely as a consequence of time constant discrepancies, but because chest wall expansion differs.

Differences in ΔP need not necessarily make gas distribution dependent on flow. If the tidal pressure swing (ΔP_T) is greater over lung region A than over region B, the relative inflation of the former will be greater than predicted from the ratio of regional pulmonary compliances. But if at all points during the inflation $\Delta P/\Delta P_T$ is the same over both regions, then, ignoring differences in time constants, the distribution of gas will be independent of flow. Thus, not only must there be a difference in ΔP between lung regions for the distribution to be flow-dependent, but the ratio of the ΔP values must be changing during inflation. Assigning different values of ΔP to two regions in a two-compartment model, Sybrecht et al. (88) were able to simulate the distribution of boli of ^{133}Xe at different flow rates in both upright and supine postures. Although a model based on time constant differences alone could not be made to fit the data, incorporation into the model of only small differences in ΔP substantially changed the bolus distribution (Figure 9). At the highest flow rate of 2.5 liter/s, a difference of only 0.6 cm H_2O in pleural pressure produced a 25% change in bolus distribution. To match the experimental results at lower inspiratory flows, smaller differences in ΔP were sufficient.

Differences in pleural pressure swings greater than this have been demonstrated both in animals (83, 84, 120) and in man (121). Changes in the esophageal gradient of pressure are also readily demonstrable (85, 103). The analysis of Sybrecht et al. (88) makes it apparent that these differences may exert a major influence on the distribution of inspired gas and could account for its flow-dependence.

During a rapid inspiration from FRC, the motion of the rib cage and abdomen differs from that during quiet breathing (122, 123). At progressively faster inspirations, the rib cage expansion is progressively greater relative to that of the abdomen (123). That this may be the cause rather than a consequence of the preferential distribution of inspired gas to the lung apices is suggested by the observation that voluntary selective motion of the rib cage and diaphragm/

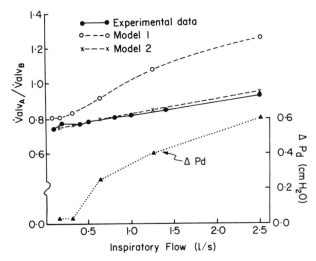

Figure 9. Distribution of inspired bolus of ^{133}Xe at different flow rates. *Left ordinate* and *abscissa* as in Figure 8. *Right ordinate* is the difference in applied pleural pressure between upper and lower lung regions (ΔP_d) required to simulate the experimental results in erect posture (Model 2). Model 1, equal pressures applied to two compartments with differing time constants. Note small magnitude of ΔP_d required to simulate experimental results. Reprinted with permission of J. Appl. Physiol., in press.

abdomen influenced the distribution of inspired gas at flow rates of up to 2 liter/s (124). During rapid inspiratory maneuvers abdominal pressure falls (125). This may be explained by contraction of the inspiratory intercostal and accessory muscles lifting the rib cage and pulling up the diaphragm/abdomen. In contrast, during a quiet inspiration, abdominal pressure increases, reflecting diaphragmatic contraction (126). The above observations are compatible with an increased involvement of intercostal and accessory musculature at higher inspiratory flow rates, resulting in a redistribution of inspired gas toward lung apices. This hypothesis could account for the flow-dependence of ventilation distribution independent of any differences in time constants. What the mechanisms are that would initiate and regulate the different patterns of contraction of respiratory muscles under varying dynamic conditions is at present unknown.

INTRAREGIONAL VENTILATION DISTRIBUTION

In this section, the ventilation distribution among lung zones situated within the lung field detected by a single scintillation counter is discussed. The term "intraregional" has, therefore, no anatomical connotations and merely refers to a small portion of lung tissue.

The concept that gas concentrations within small regions of the lung may not be uniform was first clearly proposed by Krogh and Lindhard (127) to explain the observation that after a single breath of an inert gas the expired concentration changed progressively at different points in the expiration (127, 128). Because of the technical difficulties involved in sampling gas within small lung zones, experimental observations on intraregional ventilation inhomogeneity have been necessarily indirect.

Experimental Evidence of Ventilation Nonuniformity

During multiple breath nitrogen washouts, when gas is sampled in small airways, the curves obtained by plotting expired nitrogen concentration against breath number are not single exponentials, indicating nonuniformity of mixing between inspired and residual gas (129). Using a multicompartmental analysis of such curves, Suda et al. (129) found a wide dispersal of compartmental volumes (V_0) and volume to ventilation ratios $(V_0 : \Delta V)$ within lobes, segments, and subsegments of lungs in normal subjects. Furthermore, neither the mean value nor the range of $V_0 : \Delta V$ differed between these anatomical units. In fact, the dispersion of $V_0 : \Delta V$ was not demonstrably different between upper and lower lobes even in the erect posture. From these observations, Suda et al. (129) concluded that gravitational forces cannot be the major factor responsible for ventilation inhomogeneity in the lung. These conclusions were supported by the findings of Engel et al. (64) who studied dogs whose chests had been widely opened, thus eliminating the gradient in pleural pressure. After a breath of 100% oxygen, the magnitude of the slope of the nitrogen plateau, recorded within airways 3 mm in diameter, constituted a major proportion of that recorded in the trachea of intact dogs. Furthermore, measurement of the magnitude of the cardiogenic oscillations revealed $V_0 : \Delta V$ differences of *at least* 2 to 1 in several small airways. The findings in the above studies indicate that 1) within lung units subtended by 3-mm airways there exists a range of gas concentration, and 2) the concentration differences must be due to intrinsic mechanical properties of the lung itself.

Stratified Versus Parallel Inhomogeneity

The mechanisms responsible for ventilation inhomogeneity within small lung regions are poorly understood. Krogh and Lindhard (127) proposed that gas diffusion along each pulmonary pathway is incomplete during the time of a respiratory cycle, causing the most distal alveoli to receive less of the inspired gas than those more proximally situated. The concentration differences would thus be serially arranged, and subsequent investigators have referred to this as "stratified or series inhomogeneity."

An alternative distribution of concentration differences is that among alveoli ventilated by separate pathways. If different amounts of inspired gas enter different units and/or if the initial volumes of the units differ, then the volume to ventilation ratio ($V_0 : \Delta V$) and end-inspiratory concentrations will not be the same. This type of nonuniformity may be referred to as "parallel inhomogeneity" and has already been discussed with reference to interregional ventilation distribution. Curiously, there has been a tendency to regard the latter as the only type of parallel inhomogeneity, and the possibility that within small lung regions respiratory units in parallel may differ in their gas concentrations has not received adequate attention. This has led to some unjustified conclusions regarding the presence of stratified inhomogeneity and will be discussed below.

When elastic properties of units ventilated in parallel differ, then, even if the pathway resistances are identical, the filling and emptying of the units may be asynchronous due to differences in time constants (115). Similarly, if resistances of the pathways differ, the short time constant units fill and empty before those with long time constants. This time-dependent sequential filling and emptying could theoretically account for the pattern of ventilation observed in lung subsegments (61, 62, 64).

It is possible that the nonuniformity in alveolar gas concentrations is not readily described by a series or a parallel model. The two categories may not in fact constitute distinct entities, but one may merge with the other. For example, collateral ventilation of a unit whose airway has become obstructed may result in concentration differences which, in terms of gas transport, are serially arranged. Yet, mechanically, the units are in parallel. In the presence of partial obstruction, the situation may be different. Because of the interdependence between neighboring lung units (130), the pressure within a unit which is lagging is less than that in a unit which leads. Consequently, flow into the former is enhanced. If this enhancement occurs via the normal pathway, the gas concentration in the unit will increase. However, if the additional volume change is achieved by collateral flow, gas concentrations might be decreased. Insofar as the gas entering collaterally will be situated in the more distal alveoli, this may be thought of as stratification provoked by parallel inhomogeneity!

The intraregional inhomogeneity of alveolar gas concentrations has been investigated in two principal ways. One approach has been the use of mathematical models; the other has been the study of washouts of one or more inert tracer gases and the effect of breathholding on these.

Model Analyses

Mathematical models have been used to estimate whether or not gas concentrations within respiratory units equilibrate during the time of a respiratory cycle. In the previous edition of this book, Cumming (6) reviewed this work and commented on the potential value as well as the limitations of this approach. Since then several workers have solved the differential equation for simultaneous unidimensional diffusion and convection in a symmetrical lung model (36, 41, 43). These analyses are likely to constitute improvements on previous modeling attempts, as the computational techniques are probably more accurate, the geometry of the models more akin to that of the lung, and, because convection and diffusion are treated simultaneously, the boundary conditions are more realistic. The results of one such analysis are illustrated in Figure 3. Each curve represents the position of the front between an inspired breath of oxygen and alveolar gas at 0.4-s intervals in a respiratory cycle of 4-s duration. It is apparent that within the respiratory zone (generations 16–23) a gradient of concentrations persists during inspiration (see under "Convection, Diffusion, and Anatomical Dead Space"). However, on expiration, the gradient is rapidly eliminated. Indeed, Paiva's model predicts that the rapid disappearance of concentration gradients results in a horizontal alveolar plateau measured at the mouth (36). Because this prediction is not borne out by experimental observation, it is not possible to decide conclusively whether the quantitation of stratified inhomogeneity by the model is inadequate, or whether, indeed, stratification does not contribute to the slope of the alveolar plateau. Certainly the assumption that mixing takes place by molecular diffusion alone, thus ignoring Taylor diffusion and cardiogenic mixing, overestimates the persistence of concentration gradients. Consideration of both these mechanisms should enhance uniformity of gas concentrations and diminish stratification in the model. It is noteworthy that to account for a normally sloping alveolar plateau by stratified inhomogeneity, the pre-expiratory gradient of gas concentration must be extraordinarily large. This is due to the slope being quantitated as a function of expired volume, whereas intrapulmonary gas volume increases dramatically as a function of linear distance from the trachea. Thus, with the use of the model of Weibel (13) and assuming no mixing between serially arranged gas populations during expiration, a sloping nitrogen plateau of 3%/liter would require a concentration difference of 9.4% between the alveolar ducts (generation 20) and the alveolar sacs (generation 23), i.e., a nitrogen gradient of nearly 5%/mm. If gas mixing were included in the calculation, the stratification would need to be even greater. It seems unlikely that such large concentration differences could exist within the respiratory units.

Irrespective of whether stratification contributes to the slope of the alveolar plateau or not, the prediction that during inspiration a gradient of concentrations is maintained due to the opposing action of convection and diffusion (16, 36, 41) implies that, for the respiratory cycle as a whole, a mean value for stratified inhomogeneity can be calculated. It is ironic that the concept of stratification first proposed to explain the changing concentrations in expired gas (127) may be valid, yet it may not have any bearing on the slope of the alveolar plateau.

Single Breath Inert Gas Washouts

Much of the information about intraregional ventilation inhomogeneity has been obtained from the study of inert gas washouts. However, the full degree of inhomogeneity cannot be demonstrated by this means. To achieve this, the expirate would need to contain gas coming exclusively from the well-ventilated regions at one point in time, and only from poorly ventilated ones at another. Conversely, a horizontal alveolar plateau does not preclude the presence of significant nonuniformity of gas concentration within the lung.

The slope of the alveolar plateau is measurably decreased after an end-in-spiratory breathhold (21, 24, 46, 60, 64, 107, 113, 131–133). The reduction in slope is greatest during the first portion of the breathhold, the effect gradually diminishing as breathholding continues. A residual slope is often apparent, however, even after 60 s. Rauwerda (131) was the first to quantitate these changes. Sampling at two points during expiration, he found that a 17-s breathhold reduced the measured inhomogeneity to 16% of the initial value. He calculated the length of the tubular space in which molecular diffusion would reduce gas concentrations at a comparable rate and concluded that the concentration differences which were equalized during the first 20–30 s of breathholding were situated within individual lobules or between adjacent lobules.

Recently, Hogg et al. (21) studied single breath nitrogen washouts before and after insufflation of beads (2.9 mm diameter) into excised dog lobes. Collateral ventilation of lung segments subtended by obstructed airways produced a difference in nitrogen concentration, as evidenced by a steep slope of the alveolar plateau. Breathholding at end inspiration had to be maintained for as long as 5 min before the slope returned to control values. Because flattening of the slope occurs much more rapidly in normal lungs, these results suggest that most of the concentration differences responsible for the slope of the alveolar plateau recorded at the mouth are situated in lung units smaller than those subtended by 3-mm airways (see under "Tidal Breath Studies").

From the above observations, it is apparent that nonuniformity of gas concentrations within small lung zones contributes substantially to the changing gas concentrations recorded at the mouth during expiration. However, the results give no indication of the spatial or functional disposition of these zones. In particular, the findings do not distinguish between stratification and intraregional parallel inhomogeneity. Both types would be diminished by gas mixing during breathholding. Several authors have assumed that concentration differences which disappear on breathholding must necessarily be of the stratified type (60, 133). There seems to be little justification for such an assumption. Gas mixing both by molecular diffusion and cardiogenic mechanisms could take place via collateral channels, as well as along bronchial pathways between units in parallel, as first suggested by Rauwerda (131).

Sequential Filling and Emptying

Nitrogen washouts recorded within intrapulmonary airways clearly indicate that better ventilated lung units empty preferentially early in expiration (63, 64). Thus, emptying is sequential and not uniform. Whether during inspiration the units inflate homogeneously or sequentially has not been previously demonstrated. Studies in human subjects in which different portions of the inspirate have been labeled with a tracer gas are generally interpreted in terms of interregional inhomogeneity (102, 106, 134). Recently, Fukuchi et al. (135) studied washouts of helium boli, injected at different times during a VC inflation, in prone, open-chested dogs. Thus, both distribution and washout of boli were uninfluenced by a gradient in pleural pressure. The washouts sloped upward when the bolus was injected at 20% or 40% VC, were horizontal for boli injected at 60% VC, and sloped downward when the bolus was introduced at 80% VC. Furthermore, a qualitatively similar pattern was observed in washouts recorded from lobar bronchi. These results strongly suggest that, over the vital capacity range, filling as well as emptying throughout the lung is sequential. The "first in-last out" pattern first proposed by Fowler (136) seems to hold true in a lung devoid of the interregional inhomogeneity related to a gradient in pleural pressure. Although Rauwerda and Fowler explained this pattern by the unequal distribution of dead space gas, the mechanism remains unclear. Sequential filling and emptying of units in parallel as well as of units in series could produce identical experimental results.

Dynamic Factors

The influence of flow rate on intraregional filling or emptying is poorly understood. Theoretically, differences in time constants between intraregional units ventilated in parallel could give rise to maldistribution of inspired gas. Indeed, because interregional differences account for only a 7% reduction in dynamic compliance when breathing at 100 breaths/min (103) in normal subjects, most frequency-dependent behavior should have an intraregional basis. The fact that the reduction in dynamic compliance is density-dependent (137) suggests, however, that the relevant lung units are subtended by larger airways in which flow is not laminar. This is consistent with the observation that in dogs the slope of the alveolar nitrogen plateau recorded within small airways is not influenced by 4-fold changes in either inspiratory or expiratory flow rates (138).

These observations may be explained in one of two ways: either the time constants of units distal to the small airways are uniform, or they differ but are very short (139). We favor the latter possibility. If a stimulus with a sufficiently high frequency content were applied to the lung, these differences in time constants could become apparent. The pressure impulse due to the action of the heart may constitute such a stimulus. The units with the shorter time constants would then empty preferentially during systole. Cardiogenic oscillations are frequently superimposed on the alveolar plateau recorded within intrapulmonary airways (61–64). Presumably, the oscillations reflect asychronous emptying from units with different time constants and containing different alveolar gas concentrations. Most intrapulmonary cardiogenic oscillations reflect transient preferential emptying of the better ventilated units (64). This suggests that these have shorter time constants. Such units could be arranged in series or in parallel. In some cases, however, cardiogenic oscillations indicate preferential emptying of poorly ventilated units (64). In these cases, only a parallel arrangement of units with different alveolar concentrations could account for the findings.

Single Breath Studies with Two Tracer Gases

When a subject inhales a gas mixture containing equally small concentrations of two inert tracer gases differing in diffusivity, the washouts of the two gases differ. The first part of the expirate contains relatively more of the heavier gas, whereas the later portion is enriched by the lighter gas (23–25). Furthermore, the slope of the alveolar plateau of the heavier, less rapidly diffusing gas, is steeper than that of the tracer with the higher diffusivity. Breathholding flattens both slopes and tends to make them more alike. These results have been regarded as evidence favoring the presence of stratification within respiratory units (5, 23–25). Such an interpretation is based on at least two important assumptions: first, that the two tracer gases do not separate during inspiration through the conducting airways and, second, that the differences in concentration between the two gases are distributed in series.

Longitudinal, Taylor-type dispersion has been discussed under "Taylor-type Dispersion," where it was pointed out that enrichment of the central part of the stream with the heavier gas may indeed separate the two tracers. Under these conditions, the heavier, less rapidly diffusing gas would penetrate more deeply into the lung and should appear preferentially in the last part of the expirate. Except for some specific experimental conditions (21), the reverse is usually true, so that different degrees of axial dispersion of the two gases cannot be responsible for the experimental findings. Alternatively, the two tracers may separate in such a way that vertically distributed regions receive different proportions of each. This could be due to the effect of gravity on the heavier gas, distributing it preferentially to dependent zones. Up to now, no attempt has been made to justify the assumption that the concentration of one gas relative to the other is identical in vertically distributed regions. Nevertheless, this assumption is probably valid. After a 1-liter breath of a gas mixture containing 5% of helium and SF_6 in air, a phase IV is present on washouts of both tracers (Figure 10). Yet the plot of the ratio of the expired concentrations (He:SF_6) against expired volume shows no inflection point at the onset of phase IV. Because the latter reflects sequential emptying between lung base and apex, any interregional differences in He:SF_6 ratio should be apparent. The fact that they are not suggests that the interregional distribution of He:SF_6 concentration ratios is uniform.

The second assumption is that separation of the tracers within the terminal portion of the bronchial tree takes place in series within the respiratory unit. This need not necessarily be so. An alternative model is one of units ventilated in parallel, yet small enough and close enough to each other so that substantial gas mixing can take place between them during each cycle. If the units differ in their ventilation to volume ratios, concentration differences will be established between the two tracer gases from the instant the inspirate enters both units. Equilibration of these concentration differences will be more rapid for the lighter gas. Consequently, the ratio of the two tracer gas concentrations will

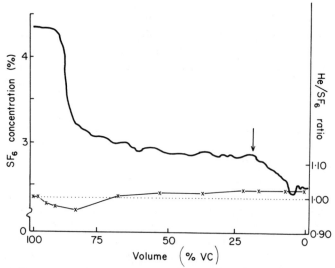

Figure 10. Expired SF_6 concentration and He:SF_6 ratio (*ordinates*), measured at the mouth, after a vital capacity inspiration of gas mixture containing 5% helium and 5% SF_6 in air. *Abscissa,* lung volume (% VC). *Arrow* indicates onset of sequential emptying from vertically distributed lung regions (phase IV). The He:SF_6 ratio remains relatively constant in this volume range, reflecting equal interregional distribution of helium relative to SF_6 (22).

differ in the 2 units throughout the respiratory cycle. If emptying is sequential, a pattern similar to that obtained experimentally is predictable. Breathholding, by allowing further equilibration of concentration differences between the units, will flatten the washouts of both gases. To the best of our knowledge, there is no evidence to date which would be incompatible with this model. Therefore, the interpretation of the dual tracer experiments, which favors the presence of stratification, is not unique. Intraregional inhomogeneity among units in parallel could equally well account for the results.

Functional and Structural Basis

Theoretically, differences in pressure-volume relationships between units in parallel could account for both the nonuniformity of gas concentrations as well as the pattern of sequential emptying demonstrable in small lung segments (64). An example is shown in Figure 11. If A and B are the P-V curves corresponding to 2 such units, then an inspiration from C to D will result in proportionately less of the inspirate entering unit A. Furthermore, due to the higher initial volume at C, the ventilation to volume ratio of A will be less, resulting in a smaller end-inspiratory concentration of the inspired tracer gas. On expiration, unit A contributes progressively more to the expirate, resulting in a progressive decrease in the expired concentration of the tracer gas.

There is some evidence for a structural basis for the above model. Using a standardized cycling pattern, Sugihara et al. (140) measured the stress-strain characteistics of individual alveolar walls. The length at infinite stress (L_{max}) was predicted from the length-tension curves, and the maximum extensibility ratio (λ_{max}) was calculated. $\lambda_{max} = L_{max}/L_0$ where L_0 is the length at which force first increases with extension. In 170 specimens from 36 lungs, λ_{max} ranged from 1.33–2.6. There was an inverse correlation of λ_{max} with age, and λ_{max} was lower at any age in patients with diffuse obstructive lung disease. However, within each lung there

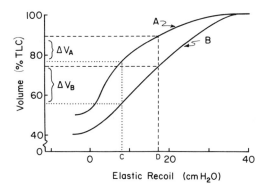

Figure 11. Theoretical volume-pressure curves of 2 units within a small lung region. Inspiration from C to D results in a smaller relative volume change in unit A (ΔV_A) than in unit B (ΔV_B). During expiration A and B empty sequentially. A similar analysis is pertinent to upper and lower dog lobes. See text for details.

was nonuniformity of λ_{max} (1.48–2.2) which was only slightly less than the range of means between different lungs. This nonuniformity was not topographically distributed. Sugihara et al. (140) pointed out that to the extent that variations in L_0 are responsible for the range of λ_{max} in each lung, there may exist a range of V_0 within small lung regions. Furthermore, the change in stress for a given change in length was greater for lung tissue with low λ_{max}. If these results are pertinent to the intact lungs, low λ_{max} units, having a higher V_0, are less compliant and less well ventilated by equal applied stresses than higher λ_{max} units.

Intraregional differences in dead space per unit of volume (V_D/V_0) may occur due to the asymmetry of the lung. In both human and canine lungs, the bronchial path to terminal bronchioles varies, such that the longer path has the wider diameter (51, 141). Consequently, the dead space volume should be preferentially distributed to respiratory units situated in the periphery of the lung. Calculations made on the human lung indicate that the inspired volume required to bring fresh inspirate into lobules subtended by different airways ranges from 102–271 ml (51). Thus, inspiration of 500 ml of oxygen would result in differences in alveolar nitrogen concentration of about 5% due to dead space distribution alone. The only experimental data pertinent to these predictions are measurements of the expired nitrogen concentrations in different airways of live dogs after single breaths of oxygen (64). These measurements reflected the ventilation to volume ratio of the segment subtended by the airway sampled and did not differ systematically between airways in the lung periphery and those near the hilum. However, the scatter of measurements was large, and the method may not have been sensitive enough to detect small differences.

INTER- AND INTRAREGIONAL
CONTRIBUTIONS TO INERT GAS WASHOUTS

Until recently, analyses of gas mixing in the lung were made predominantly from measurements of expired gases at the mouth. During the past 15 years, the distribution of ventilation among topographically distributed regions has been considerably clarified. It is of interest, therefore, to examine the intraregional and interregional contributions to the changes in expired gas concentration measured at the mouth.

Single Breath Washouts

During a slow expiration, vertically distributed lung regions do not empty in a perfectly uniform manner, the dependent regions tending to empty first (see under "Quasi-static"). This gravity-dependent sequential emptying, together with the interregional differences in alveolar gas concentration, contributes to the slope of the alveolar plateau (phase III) recorded at the mouth. The contribution is greatest when the apico-basal concentration differences are large.

The phase IV of the single breath washout reflects a progressive relative increase in emptying of the nondependent regions (70, 106). The degree of sequential emptying is far greater than in the volume range corresponding to phase III and has been attributed to progressive closure of airways "rising" from lung base to apex as RV is approached (69, 106). In the upright posture, the terminal concentration at RV corresponds closely to that measured within the apical lung zones (70). Consequently, the height of phase IV (i.e., the difference between the terminal concentration at RV and that at the onset of phase IV) correlates closely with the intrapulmonary apico-basal concentration gradient (31, 142, 143).

Bolus Studies When a bolus of gas containing ^{133}Xe is inhaled slowly at RV, the ^{133}Xe concentration in the apical lung regions, measured at TLC, is 5–10 times greater than that in the lung base (70, 102, 106, 110). If the concentration differences within any single region were much less than this, then the slope of the expired ^{133}Xe plateau would reflect the interregional distribution of the tracer. There is convincing evidence that this is indeed the case. If at end inspiration the subject reverses the direction of the gravity field on the lung by changing his posture, the alveolar plateau slopes in the opposite direction and appears as a mirror image of the control washout (59, 70). It is most unlikely that gravity influences the emptying pattern within small lung regions. Hence, these findings indicate that the washout of an RV bolus reflects almost exclusively gravity-dependent sequential emptying from vertically distributed lung regions. Of all maneuvers in which expired gas is sampled, single breath washouts of a bolus of tracer gas, inhaled slowly at RV, probably reflect most accurately interregional concentration differences and/or the pattern of interregional sequential emptying. Indeed, the RV bolus washouts have proved useful in the study of interregional patterns of lung emptying under various experimental conditions (59, 82, 86, 87, 109).

When the end-inspiratory differences in regional concentration are diminished, the bolus washout is no longer determined predominantly by interregional inhomogeneity. Wood et al. (142) studied subjects who inhaled boli of ^{133}Xe from FRC at different flow rates and observed that phase III was horizontal for all apico-basal concentration ratios studied (up to a factor of 2). They suggested that interregional emptying may not be sequential enough to produce a measurable slope of phase III when the concentrations differed by a factor of two or less. Even at low lung volumes, where emptying is much more sequential, no phase IV was observed when apical and basal concentrations differed by less than a factor of 1.25, i.e., airway closure during expiration went undetected. For concentration ratios between 2.0 and 1.25, the lung volume at which phase IV began (closing volume) was progressively underestimated.

Inert gas washouts of boli inhaled at different lung volumes were first studied by Fowler (134). Dollfuss et al. (106) measured intrapulmonary concentrations after inspiration of ^{133}Xe boli and showed a progressive decrease, leading to a reversal, of the apico-basal concentration difference when a ^{133}Xe bolus was inhaled at progressively higher lung volumes between RV and 26% VC. Above that volume, bolus distribution remained approximately constant. It is not known to what degree expired gas analyses reflect these differences in distribution. In dogs, the washout of a helium bolus inhaled at different lung volumes has an alveolar plateau whose slope is similar in the intact and open-chested animal, as well as within a single lobe (135) (see under "Sequential Filling and Emptying"). In fact, only when the bolus is introduced at trapped gas volume does the washout differ substantially between the intact and the open-chest situations.

These results are consistent with the view that when boli are inhaled at mid- and high-lung volumes, phase III of the washout reflects predominantly the intraregional inhomogeneity of concentrations and emptying rates.

Tidal Breath Studies   In normal subjects, after a tidal inspiration of a tracer gas, the phase III of the washout has a gentle slope. The respective contributions to this slope of interregional and intraregional concentration differences vary depending on the amount of the inspirate (ΔV) and the initial volume (V_0), as well as the flow rates used (104). A vital capacity breath of oxygen results in an apical nitrogen concentration twice that at the base, reflecting the vertical gradient of regional volumes (V_{or}) at residual volume. Although the flattening of the upward slope of the nitrogen plateau on breathholding (144) suggests a large intraregional component, the residual slope after a prolonged breathhold reflects the interregional contribution (see under "Single Breath Inert Gas Washouts"). The presence of the latter is further supported by the demonstration that the slope of phase III can be changed by voluntary thoracoabdominal deformation during the washout (114). The apico-basal concentration differences may be enhanced by taking the breath of oxygen from a higher initial volume (145, 146). This is due to a larger vertical gradient of V_{or} at or above the volume at which dependent airways close (69). In some cases, closing volume cannot be measured by the resident gas technique unless interregional concentration differences are enhanced in this way (145).

With the use of the simplified model proposed by Milic-Emili et al. (4), it is possible to calculate from the regional ventilation to volume ratio the difference in nitrogen concentration between any two regions after a breath of oxygen (31). Thus, after an inspiration from FRC of a volume of oxygen equivalent to 10% TLC, the difference between the upper two regions and the lowest two regions is 11.5% nitrogen, whereas the ratio of concentrations is 1.20. When bigger inspirates of oxygen are taken, the nitrogen concentrations diminish but the differences increase, so that after a 40% TLC breath the two lung zones differ by 18.3% nitrogen and the ratio is 1.6. These calculations suggest that the interregional contribution to the nonuniformity of expired gas concentrations may diminish the smaller the volume of tracer gas inspired. For supine dogs, Engel et al. (64) quantitated the contributions to the slope of the nitrogen plateau recorded in the trachea after 500-ml breaths of oxygen up to an end-inspiratory lung volume of 70% VC. Fourteen percent was attributed to differences in lobar elastic properties, 34% was due to the effects of gravity, and 52% was due to inhomogeneity within small subsegments distal to 3-mm airways.

Because high flow rates tend to distribute the inspirate more evenly among vertically distributed lung regions and to empty them more homogeneously (see under "Dynamic"), the minimal interregional contribution to changes in expired gas concentration may be expected when small breaths are taken at high flow rates. Indeed, exactly these types of maneuvers have been used in studies which claimed to show a negligible contribution of regional ventilation inhomogeneity to the expired plateau (24, 133).

Cardiogenic Oscillations During an inert gas washout in normal subjects, the alveolar plateau recorded at the mouth manifests oscillations in expired gas concentration due to the heart action (65, 107) (see under "Cardiogenic Mixing"). These are due to asynchronous emptying of apical and basal lung regions, and for a given expiratory flow rate the amplitude of the oscillations bears a close relationship to the difference in alveolar concentrations between lung apex and base (58–60). The amplitude does not decrease when a 2-min breathhold is interposed at end inspiration, even though the alveolar plateau becomes considerably flatter (60). This indicates that the time interval is too short to measurably diminish the regional concentration differences responsible for the oscillations. The observation strongly supports an interregional basis for the oscillations, because molecular diffusion alone could be expected to markedly diminish intraregional concentration differences during this time. Indeed, simultaneous recording of cardiogenic nitrogen oscillations in the trachea and small airways of living dogs clearly illustrates the effect of breathholding on concentration differences between lung zones situated close together and those far apart (Figure 12).

Multiple Breath Washouts

When the nitrogen in the lung is washed out during tidal breathing of 100% oxygen, the logarithm of the expired nitrogen concentration plotted against breath number reflects the nonuniformity of the mixing process (147). Perfect mixing produces a straight line (single exponential) indicating uniformity of ventilation to volume ratios ($\Delta V/V_0$). Alinear nitrogen clearance curves can be analyzed by a curve-stripping procedure into a sum of two or more exponential functions (147). In recent years, many sophisticated analyses have been proposed, all of which give quantitative descriptions of the process without regard to the mechanism of unequal distribution. They represent the lung as if it consisted of a number of parallel compartments with exponential ventilation rates. This model approach is legitimate and has been fruitful, especially in the comparison between normal subjects and those with obstructive lung disease (46, 148, 149). However, the nonlinearity of the clearance curves is due to all the factors which contribute to nonuniform ventilation distribution, and the

74   Engel and Macklem

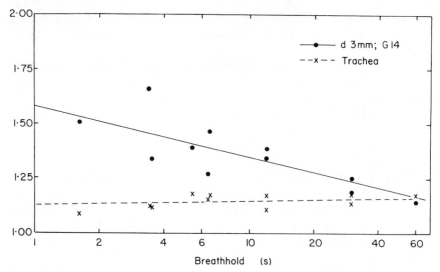

Figure 12. Dispersal of ventilation to volume ratios (*ordinate*) calculated from the amplitude of cardiogenic oscillations on a nitrogen plateau recorded in trachea (x−−−x) and 3-mm. 14 generation airway (●——●) after breathholding. The constant values in trachea reflect concentration differences between regions too far apart for gas mixing to have a measurable effect. The results in the small airway reflect the decrease in concentration differences within small lung regions due to gas mixing. Reprinted with permission of J. Appl. Physiol. 37:194 (1974).

compartments giving rise to the exponential components cannot be considered as having any anatomical or physiological reality.

It is now possible to evaluate the relative contribution of interregional and intraregional inhomogeneity to the multiple breath nitrogen clearance curve. The above analysis suggests that during tidal breathing interregional inhomogeneity should be relatively small. Experimental evidence supports this hypothesis. In some normal adults and many children, the washout is linear (150) in spite of nonuniform topographical ventilation distribution. In normal nonsmoking subjects, nitrogen washouts are not dependent on breathing frequency up to 60 breaths/min (151), yet regional ventilation distribution is influenced by comparable changes in flows (103). Finally, a 20-s breathhold at the end of each inspiration converts an alinear clearance curve to a single exponential (46), whereas concentration differences between apical and basal lung regions persist for longer than this (60, 70). All the above observations suggest that in upright subjects the multiple breath nitrogen washout is a measure of predominantly intraregional inhomogeneity. It, therefore, has some theoretical advantage over the single breath tests in evaluating the degree of ventilation maldistribution in diffuse lung disease.

REFERENCES

1. Knipping, H. W., Bolt, W., Venrath, H., Valentin, H., Ludes, H., and Endler, P. (1955). Eine neue Methode zur Prufung der Herz-und Lungenfunktion. Die regionale Funkionsanalyse in der Lungen-und Herzklinik mit Hilfe des radioaktiven Edelgases Xenon 133. Dtsch. Med. Wochenschr. 80:1146.
2. West, J. B., and Dollery, C. T. (1960). Distribution of blood flow and ventilation-perfusion ratio in the lung measured with radioactive CO_2. J. Appl. Physiol. 15:405.
3. Ball, W. C., Jr., Stewart, P. B., Newsham, L. G., and Bates, D. V. (1962). Regional pulmonary function studied with Xenon 133. J. Clin. Invest. 41:519.
4. Milic-Emili, J. (1974). Pulmonary statics. In J. G. Widdicombe (ed.), MTP International Review of Science, Physiology Series I, Vol. 2, Respiratory Physiology I. pp. 105–137. Butterworths, London; University Park Press, Baltimore.
5. Piiper, J., and Scheid, P. (1971). Respiration: alveolar gas exchange. Ann. Rev. Physiol. 33:131.
6. Cumming, G. (1974). Alveolar ventilation: recent model analysis. In A. C. Guyton, and J. G. Widdicombe (eds.), MTP International Review of Science, Physiology Series I, Vol. 2, Respiratory Physiology I. pp. 139–166. Butterworths, London; University Park Press, Baltimore.
7. Macklem, P. T. (1971). Airways obstruction and collateral ventilation. Physiol. Rev. 51:468.
8. Taylor, G. (1953). Dispersion of soluble matter in solvent flowing slowly through a tube. Proc. R. Soc. Lond. (Biol.) A 219:186.
9. Taylor, G. (1954). The dispersion of matter in turbulent flow through a pipe. Proc. R. Soc. Lond. (Biol.) A 223:446.
10. Aris, R. (1956). On the dispersion of a solute in a fluid flowing through a tube. Proc. R. Soc. Lond. (Biol.) A 235:67.
11. Henderson, Y., Chillingworth, F. P., and Whitney, J. L. (1915). The respiratory dead space. Am. J. Physiol. 38:1.
12. Wilson, T. A., and Lin, K. M. (1970). Convection and diffusion in the airways and the design of the bronchial tree. In A. Bouhuys (ed.), Airway Dynamics, pp. 5–19. Charles C Thomas, Springfield, Illinois.
13. Weibel, E. R. (1963). Morphometry of the Human Lung. Academic Press, New York.
14. Schroter, R. C., and Sudlow, M. F. (1969). Flow patterns in models of the human bronchial airways. Respir. Physiol. 7:341.
15. West, J. B., and Hugh-Jones, P. (1961). Pulsatile gas flow in bronchi caused by the heart beat. J. Appl. Physiol. 16:697.
16. Engel, L. A., Wood, L. D. H., Utz, G., and Macklem, P. T. (1973). Gas mixing during inspiration. J. Appl. Physiol. 35:18.
17. Scherer, P. W., Schendalman, L. H., Greene, N. M., and Bouhuys, A. (1975). Measurement of axial diffusivities in a model of the bronchial airways. J. Appl. Physiol. 38:719.
18. Wagner, W. W., Jr., Latham, L. P., Brinkman, P. D., and Filley, G. F. (1969). Pulmonary gas transport time: larynx to alveolus. Science 163:1210.
19. Engel, L. A., Sybrecht, G., and Savage, S., unpublished observation.

20. Mazzone, R. W. (1975). Intrapulmonary gas transport. Ph.D. thesis, State University of New York at Buffalo.
21. Hogg, W., Brunton, J., Kryger, M., Brown, R., and Macklem, P. (1972). Gas diffusion across collateral channels. J. Appl. Physiol. 33:568.
22. Siegler, D. I. M., Fukuchi, Y., and Engel, L. A., unpublished observations.
23. Georg, J., Lassen, N. A., Mellemgaard, K., and Vinther, A. (1965). Diffusion in the gas phase of the lungs in normal and emphysematous subjects. Clin. Sci. 29:525.
24. Cumming, G., Horsfield, K., Jones, J. G., and Muir, D. C. F. (1967). The influence of gaseous diffusion on the alveolar plateau at different lung volumes. Respir. Physiol. 2:386.
25. Power, G. (1969). Gaseous diffusion between airways and alveoli in the human lung. J. Appl. Physiol. 27:701.
26. Altschuler, B., Palmes, E. D., Yarmus, L., and Nelson, N. (1959). Intrapulmonary mixing of gases studied with aerosols. J. Appl. Physiol. 14:321.
27. Muir, D. C. F. (1967). Distribution of aerosol particles in exhaled air. J. Appl. Physiol. 23:210.
28. Lacquet, L. M., Van der Linden, L. P., and Paiva, M. (1975). Transport of H_2 and SF_6 in the lungs. Respir. Physiol. 25:157.
29. Saltzman, H. A., Salzano, J. V., Blenkarn, G. O., and Kylstra, J. A. (1971). Effects of pressure on ventilation and gas exchange in man. J. Appl. Physiol. 30:493.
30. Martin, R. R., Zutter, M., and Anthonisen, N. R. (1972). Pulmonary gas exchange in dogs breathing SF_6 at 4 ATA. J. Appl. Physiol. 33:86.
31. Wood, L. D. H. (1974). The effect of gas physical properties and flow rate on pulmonary ventilation and gas exchange. Ph.D. thesis, McGill University.
32. Kvale, P. A., Davis, J., and Schroter, R. C. (1975). Effect of gas density and ventilatory pattern on steady state CO uptake by the lung. Respir. Physiol. 24:385.
33. Worth, H., Takahaski, H., and Piiper, J. (1975). Alveolar gas exchange in anaesthetized dogs after replacement of air nitrogen by helium, argon or sulphur hexafluoride. Presented at INSERM Meeting on Distribution of Pulmonary Gas Exchange, Paris, September 23–24.
34. Altschuler, B. (1969). Behaviour of airborne particles in the respiratory tract. In Circulatory and Respiratory Mass Transport, CIBA Foundation Symposium, pp. 215–235. G. Wolstenholme and J. Knight (eds.), Churchill, London.
35. Engel, L. A. (1973). Ventilation distribution and gas mixing in the lung studied by intrapulmonary gas sampling. Ph.D. thesis, McGill University.
36. Paiva, M. (1973). Gas transport in the human lung. J. Appl. Physiol. 35:401.
37. Chang, H. K., Cheng, R. T., and Farhi, L. E. (1973). A model study of gas diffusion in alveolar sacs. Respir. Physiol. 18:386.
38. Flenley, D. C., Welchel, L., and Macklem, P. T. (1972). Factors affecting gas exchange by collateral ventilation in the dog. Respir. Physiol. 15:52.
39. Gomez, D. M. (1965). A physico-mathematical study of lung function in normal subjects and in patients with obstructive pulmonary disease. Med. Thorac. 22:275.
40. Cumming, G., Horsfield, K., and Preston, S. B. (1971). Diffusion equilibrium in the lungs examined by nodal analysis. Respir. Physiol. 12:329.

41. Scherer, P. W., Shendalman, L. H., and Greene, N. M. (1972). Simultaneous diffusion and convection in single breath lung washout. Bull. Math. Biophys. 34:393.
42. Fukuchi, Y., Roussos, C. S., Macklem, P. T., and Engel, L. A. (1976). Convection, diffusion and cardiogenic mixing; an experimental approach. Respir. Physiol. 26:77.
43. Baker, L. G., Ultman, J. S., and Rhoades, R. A. (1974). Simultaneous gas flow and diffusion in a symmetrical airway system: a mathematical model. Respir. Physiol. 21:119.
44. Macklem, P. T., and Engel, L. A. (1973). Diffusive mixing of gas within the lung. Presented at American Physiological Society, Fall Meetings, August 20–24, Rochester, N. Y.
45. Fowler, W. S. (1948). Lung function studies. II. The respiratory dead space. Am. J. Physiol. 154:405.
46. Roos, A., Dahlstrom, H., and Murphy, J. P. (1954). Distribution of inspired air in the lungs. J. Appl. Physiol. 7:645.
47. Bartels, J., Severinghaus, J. W., Forster, R. E., Briscoe, W. A., and Bates, D. V. (1954). The respiratory dead space measured by single breath analysis of oxygen, carbon dioxide, nitrogen or helium. J. Clin. Invest. 33:41.
48. Shepard, R. G., Campbell, E. J. M., Martin, H., and Enns, T. (1957). Factors affecting the pulmonary dead space as determined by single breath analysis. J. Appl. Physiol. 11:241.
49. Paiva, M., Lacquet, L. M., and Van der Linden, L. P. Gas transport in a model derived from Hansen-Ampaya anatomical data of the human lung. J. Appl. Physiol., in press.
50. Hansen, J. E., and Ampaya, E. P. (1975). Human air space shapes, sizes, areas and volumes. J. Appl. Physiol. 38:990.
51. Horsfield, K., and Cumming, G. (1968). Functional consequences of airway morphology. J. Appl. Physiol. 24:384.
52. Engel, L. A., Menkes, H., Wood, L. D. H., Utz, G., Joubert, J., and Macklem, P. T. (1973). Gas mixing during breath holding studied by intrapulmonary gas sampling. J. Appl. Physiol. 35:9.
53. Voit, C. (1865). Ueber Druckschwankungen im Lungenraum in Folge der Herzbewegungen. Z. Biol. 1:390.
54. Haycraft, B., and Edie, R. (1891). The cardiopneumatic movements. J. Physiol. (Lond.) 12:426.
55. Luisada, A. (1942). The internal pneumocardiogram. Am. Heart J. 23:676.
56. Wagner, P. D., Gaines, R. A., Mazzone, R. W., and West, J. B. (1972). Mechanism of intrapulmonary gas mixing during breathholding in man. Physiologist 15:295.
57. Fukuchi, Y., Cosio, M., Kelly, S., and Engel, L. A. Influence of pericardial fluid on cardiogenic gas mixing in the lung. J. Appl. Physiol. In press.
58. Fowler, K. T., and Read (1961). Cardiac oscillations in expired gas tensions and regional pulmonary blood flow. J. Appl. Physiol. 16:863.
59. Clarke, S. W., Jones, J. G., and Glaister, D. H. (1969). Change in pulmonary ventilation in different postures. Clin. Sci. 37:357.
60. Farber, J. P. (1969). Study of factors influencing regional emptying of the lung with soluble inert gas. Ph.D. thesis, State University of New York at Buffalo.
61. Fowler, W. S. (1951). Alveolar ventilation of individual pulmonary lobes in various postures. Am. J. Med. 222:602.

62. Martin, C. J., and Young, A. C. (1956). Lobar ventilation in man. Am. Rev. Tuberculosis 73:330.
63. Young, A. C., and Martin, C. J. (1966). The sequence of lobar emptying in man. Respir. Physiol. 1:372.
64. Engel, L. A., Utz, G., Wood, L. D. H., and Macklem, P. T. (1974). Ventilation distribution in anatomical lung units. J. Appl. Physiol. 37:194.
65. Dahlstrom, H., Murphy, J. P., and Roos, A. (1954). Cardiogenic oscillations in composition of expired gas: the "pneumocardiogram." J. Appl. Physiol. 7:335.
66. Langer, G. A., Bornstein, D. L., and Fishman, A. P. (1960). Cardiogenic oscillations in expired nitrogen and regional alveolar hypoventilation. J. Appl. Physiol. 15:855.
67. Siegler, D., Fukuchi, Y., and Engel, L. A. (1976). Influence of bronchomotor tone on ventilation distribution and airway closure in asymptomatic asthma. Am. Rev. Respir. Dis. 114:123.
68. Ross, B. B., and Farhi, L. E. (1960). Dead space ventilation as a determinant in the ventilation perfusion concept. J. Appl. Physiol. 15:363.
69. Milic-Emili, J., Henderson, J. A. M., Dolovitch, M. B., Trop, D., and Kaneko, K. (1966). Regional distribution of inspired gas in the lung. J. Appl. Physiol. 21:749.
70. Anthonisen, N. R., Robertson, P. C., and Ross, W. R. D. (1970). Gravity dependent sequential emptying of lung regions. J. Appl. Physiol. 25:589.
71. Sutherland, P. W., Katsura, F., and Milic-Emili, J. (1968). Previous volume history of the lung and regional distribution of gas. J. Appl. Physiol. 25:566.
72. Salazar, E., and Knowles, J. H. (1964). An analysis of pressure-volume characteristics of the lungs. J. Appl. Physiol. 19:97.
73. Glaister, D. H., Schroter, R. C., Sudlow, M. F., and Milic-Emili, J. (1973). Bulk elastic properties of excised lungs and the effect of a transpulmonary pressure gradient. Respir. Physiol. 17:347.
74. Paiva, M., Yernault, J. C., Van Eerdeweghe, P., and Englert, M. (1975). A sigmoid model of the static volume pressure curve of human lung. Respir. Physiol. 23:317.
75. Grassino, A., Bake, B., Martin, R. R., and Anthonisen, N. R. (1975). Voluntary changes of thoracoabdominal shape and regional lung volumes in humans. J. Appl. Physiol. 39:997.
76. Agostoni, E., and D'Angelo, E. (1971). Topography of pleural surface pressure during simulation of gravity effect on abdomen. Respir. Physiol. 12:102.
77. D'Angelo, E. (1972). Local alveolar size and transpulmonary pressure *in situ* and in isolated lungs. Respir. Physiol. 14:251.
78. Agostoni, E. (1972). Mechanics of the pleural space. Physiol. Rev. 52:57.
79. Greene, R., Hughes, J. M. W., Sudlow, M. F., and Milic-Emili, J. (1974). Regional lung volumes during water immersion to the xyphoid in seated man. J. Appl. Physiol. 36:734.
80. Lemelin, J., Ross, W. R. D., Martin, R. R., and Anthonisen, N. R. (1973). Regional lung volumes with positive pressure inflation in erect humans. Respir. Physiol. 16:273.
81. Grassino, A., and Anthonisen, N. R. (1975). Chest wall distortion and lung regional volume distribution in erect humans. J. Appl. Physiol. 39:1004.
82. Roussos, C. S., Fukuchi, Y., Macklem, P. T., and Engel, L. A. (1976).

Influence of diaphragmatic contraction on ventilation distribution in horizontal man. J. Appl. Physiol. 40:417.

83. D'Angelo, E., Sant'Ambrogio, G., and Agostoni, E. (1974). Effect of diaphragm activity or paralysis on distribution of pleural pressure. J. Appl. Physiol. 37:311.

84. Minh, V., Kurihara, N., Friedman, P. J., and Moser, K. M. (1974). Reversal of the pleural pressure gradient during electrophrenic stimulation. J. Appl. Physiol. 37:496.

85. Dosman, J., Grassino, A., Macklem, P. T., and Engel, L. A. (1975). Factors influencing the esophageal pressure gradient in upright man. Physiologist 18:194.

86. Roussos, C. S., Genest, J., Cosio, M. G., and Engel, L. A. (1975). Rib cage vs. abdominal breathing and ventilation distribution. Clin. Res. 23:648A.

87. Kelly, S., Roussos, C. S., and Engel, L. A. (1975). Gravity independent sequential emptying from topographical lung regions. Clin. Res. 23:645A.

88. Sybrecht, G., Landau, L., Murphy, B. G., Engel, L. A., Martin, R. R., and Macklem, P. T. (1976). Influence of posture on flow dependence of distribution of inhaled ^{133}Xe boli. J. Appl. Physiol. 41:489.

89. Roussos, C. S., Martin, R. R., and Engel, L. A. Diaphragmatic contraction and the gradient of alveolar expansion in the lateral posture. J. Appl. Physiol. In press.

90. Rehder, K., Hatch, D. J., Sessler, A. D., and Fowler, W. S. (1972). The functions of each lung of anesthetized and paralyzed man during mechanical ventilation. Anesthesiology 37:16.

91. Froese, A. B., and Bryan, A. C. (1974). Effects of anesthesia and paralysis on diaphragmatic mechanics in man. Anesthesiology 41:242.

92. Engel, L. A., and Roussos, C. S. (1976). Voluntary control of inspired gas distribution in the lateral posture. Am. Rev. Respir. Dis. 113:226.

93. Agostoni, E., D'Angelo, E., and Bonanni, M. V. (1970). The effect of the abdomen on the vertical gradient of pleural surface pressure. Respir. Physiol. 8:332.

94. D'Angelo, E., and Sant'Ambrogio, G. (1974). Direct action of the contracting diaphragm on the rib cage in rabbits and dogs. J. Appl. Physiol. 36:715.

95. D'Angelo, E., Bonanni, M. V., Michelini, S., and Agostoni, E. (1970). Topography of the pleural pressure in rabbits and dogs. Respir. Physiol. 8:204.

96. Bake, B., Bjure, J., Grimby, G., Milic-Emili, J., and Nilsson, N. J. (1967). Regional distribution of inspired gas in supine man. Scand. J. Respir. Dis. 48:189.

97. Lupi-Herrera, E., Prefaut, C., Grassino, A. E., and Anthonisen, N. R. (1976). Effect of negative abdominal pressure on regional lung volumes in supine dogs. Respir. Physiol. 26:213.

98. Frank, N. R. (1963). A comparison of static volume-pressure relations of excised pulmonary lobes in dogs. J. Appl. Physiol. 18:274.

99. Paré, P., Boucher, R., and Hogg, J. C. (1975). Pressure volume characteristics in excised primate lungs and lobes. Clin. Res. 23:646A.

100. Milic-Emili, J., Mead, J., and Turner, J. M. (1964). Topography of esophageal pressure as a function of posture in man. J. Appl. Physiol. 19:212.

101. Grant, B. J. B., Jones, H. A., and Hughes, J. M. B. (1974). Sequence of regional filling during a tidal breath in man. J. Appl. Physiol. 37:158.

102. Robertson, P. C., Anthonisen, N. A., and Ross, D. (1969). Effect of inspiratory flow rate on regional distribution of inspired gas. J. Appl. Physiol. 26:438.
103. Bake, B., Wood, L., Murphy, B., Macklem, P. T., and Milic-Emili, J. (1974). Effect of inspiratory flow rate on regional distribution of inspired gas. J. Appl. Physiol. 37:8.
104. Connolly, T., Bake, B., Wood, L., and Milic-Emili, J. (1975). Regional distribution of a [133] Xe labelled gas volume inspired at constant flow rate. Scand. J. Respir. Dis. 56:150.
105. Bryan, A. C., Bentivoglio, L. G., Beerel, F., Macleish, H., Zidulka, A., and Bates, D. V. (1964). Factors affecting regional distribution of ventilation and perfusion in the lung. J. Appl. Physiol. 19:395.
106. Dollfuss, R. E., Milic-Emili, J., and Bates, D. V. (1967). Regional ventilation of the lung studied with boluses of Xenon 133. Respir. Physiol. 2:234.
107. Fowler, W. S. (1949). Lung function studies. III. Uneven pulmonary ventilation in normal subjects, and in patients with pulmonary disease. J. Appl. Physiol. 2:283.
108. Bashoff, M. A., Ingram, R. H., Jr., and Schilder, D. P. (1967). Effect of expiratory flow rate on the nitrogen concentration vs. volume relationship. J. Appl. Physiol. 23:895.
109. Jones, J. G., and Clarke, S. W. (1969). The effect of expiratory flow rate on regional lung emptying. Clin. Sci. 37:343.
110. Millette, B., Robertson, P. C., Ross, W. R. D., and Anthonisen, N. R. (1969). Effect of expiratory flow rate on emptying of lung regions. J. Appl. Physiol. 27:587.
111. Urbanetti, J., Martin, R., and Macklem, P. T. (1973). Effect of expiratory flow rates on closing volume. Presented at Canadian Thoracic Society Meeting, Calgary, Canada, June 25–27.
112. Young, A. C., Martin, C. J., and Pace, W. R., Jr. (1963). Effect of expiratory flow patterns on lung emptying. J. Appl. Physiol. 18:47.
113. Read, J. (1966). Alveolar populations contributing to expired gas tension plateaus. J. Appl. Physiol. 21:1511.
114. Roussos, C. S., Siegler, D. I. M., and Engel, L. A. (1976). Influence of diaphragmatic contraction and expiratory flow on the pattern of lung emptying. Respir. Physiol. 27:157.
115. Otis, A. B., McKerrow, C. B., Bartlett, R. A., Mead, J., McIlroy, M. B., Selverstone, N. J., and Radford, E. P., Jr. (1956). Mechanical factors in distribution of pulmonary ventilation. J. Appl. Physiol. 8:427.
116. Blide, R. W., Kerr, H. D., and Spicer, W. S., Jr. (1964). Measurement of upper and lower airway conductance in man. J. Appl. Physiol. 19:1059.
117. Vincent, N. J., Knudson, R., Leith, D. E., Macklem, P. T., and Mead, J. (1970). Factors influencing pulmonary resistance. J. Appl. Physiol. 29:236.
118. Pedley, T. J., Sudlow, M. F., and Milic-Emili, J. (1972). A non-linear theory of the distribution of pulmonary ventilation. Respir. Physiol. 15:1.
119. Wilson, A. G., Jones, H. A., and Hughes, J. M. B. (1974). Effect of posture on airway length and diameter. Respir. Physiol. 22:381.
120. Farhi, L., Otis, A. B., and Proctor, D. F. (1957). Measurement of intrapulmonary pressure at different points in the chest of the dog. J. Appl. Physiol. 10:15.

121. Daly, W. J., and Bondurant, S. (1963). Direct measurement of respiratory pleural pressure changes in normal man. J. Appl. Physiol. 18:513.
122. Grassino, A. (1974). Influence of chest wall configuration on the static and dynamic characteristics of the contracting diaphragm. *In* Loaded Breathing, pp. 64–71. L. D. Pengelly, A. S. Rebuck, and E. J. M. Campbell (eds.), Logman Ltd., Canada.
123. Sharp, J. T., Golberg, N. B., Druz, W. S., and Danon, J. (1975). Relative contributions of rib cage and abdomen to breathing in normal subjects. J. Appl. Physiol. 39:608.
124. Fixley, M., Roussos, C. S., and Engel, L. A., unpublished observations.
125. Milic-Emili, J., Orzalesi, M. M., Cook, C. D., and Turner, J. M. (1964). Respiratory thoraco-abdominal mechanics in man. J. Appl. Physiol. 19:217.
126. Goldman, M. D., and Mead, J. (1973). Mechanical interaction between the diaphragm and rib cage. J. Appl. Physiol. 35:197.
127. Krogh, A., and Lindhard, J. (1917). The volume of the dead space in breathing and the mixing of gases in the lungs of man. J. Physiol. (Lond.) 51:59.
128. Sonne, C. (1918). On the possibility of mixing the air in the lungs with foreign air especially as it is used in Krogh and Lindhard's nitrous oxide method. J. Physiol. (Lond.) 52:75.
129. Suda, Y., Martin, C. J., and Young, A. C. (1970). Regional dispersion of volume-to-ventilation ratios in the lung of man. J. Appl. Physiol. 29:480.
130. Mead, J., Takishima, T., and Leith, D. (1970). Stress distribution in lungs: a model of pulmonary elasticity. J. Appl. Physiol. 28:596.
131. Rauwerda, P. E. (1946). Unequal ventilation of different parts of the lung. Ph.D. thesis, University of Groningen, the Netherlands.
132. Kjellmer, I., Sandqvist, L., and Berglund, E. (1959). "Alveolar plateau" of the single breath nitrogen elimination curve in normal subjects. J. Appl. Physiol. 14:105.
133. Sikand, R., Cerretelli, P., and Farhi, L. E. (1966). Effects of V_A and V_A/Q distribution and of time on the alveolar plateau. J. Appl. Physiol. 21:1331.
134. Fowler, K. T. (1964). Relative compliances of well and poorly ventilated spaces in the normal human lung. J. Appl. Physiol. 19:937.
135. Fukuchi, Y., Cosio, M., and Murphy, B. (1976). Intraregional basis for helium bolus washouts. Fed. Proc. 35:837.
136. Fowler, W. S. (1952). Intrapulmonary distribution of inspired gas. Physiol. Rev. 32:1.
137. Forkert, L., Wood, L. D. H., and Cherniack, R. M. (1975). Effect of gas density on dynamic pulmonary compliance. J. Appl. Physiol. 39:906.
138. Fukuchi, Y., Cosio, M., and Engel, L. A., unpublished observations.
139. Macklem, P. T., and Mead, J. (1967). Resistance of central and peripheral airways measured by a retrograde catheter. J. Appl. Physiol. 22:395.
140. Sugihara, T., Martin, C. J., and Hildebrandt, J. (1971). Length-tension properties of the alveolar wall in man. J. Appl. Physiol. 30:874.
141. Ross, B. B. (1957). Influence of bronchial tree structure on ventilation in the dog's lung as inferred from measurements of a plastic cast. J. Appl. Physiol. 10:1.
142. Wood, L., Bake, B., and Macklem, P. T. (1974). The effect of regional concentration on the expired concentration vs. volume relationships.

Presented at Canadian Thoracic Society Meetings, Ottawa, Canada, June 10–11.

143. Engel, L. A., Landau, L., Taussig, L., Martin, R. R., and Sybrecht, G. (1976). Influence of bronchomotor tone on regional ventilation distribution at residual volume. J. Appl. Physiol. 40:411.

144. Buist, A. S., and Ross, B. B. (1974). The effect of breathholding on the single breath nitrogen washout. Am. Rev. Respir. Dis. 109:693.

145. Mansell, A., Bryan, A. C., and Levison, H. (1972). Airway closure in children. J. Appl. Physiol. 33:711.

146. Kaneko, K., Mohler, J., and Balchum, O. (1975). Effect of preinspiratory lung volume on closing volume determination by nitrogen method. J. Appl. Physiol. 38:10.

147. Robertson, J. S., Siri, W. E., and Jones, H. B. (1950). Lung ventilation patterns determined by analysis of nitrogen elimination rates; use of the mass spectrometer as a continuous gas analyzer. J. Clin. Invest. 29:577.

148. Fowler, W. S., Cornish, E. R., and Kety, S. S. (1952). Lung function studies. VIII. Analysis of alveolar ventilation by pulmonary N_2 clearance curves. J. Clin. Invest. 31:40.

149. Briscoe, W. A., and Cournand, A. (1959). Uneven ventilation of normal and diseased lung studied by an open circuit method. J. Appl. Physiol. 14:284.

150. Chang, S. T., Wang, B. C., Chi, Y. L., and Hsieh, Y. S. (1971). Ventilatory components of lungs in relation to sex and age. Am. Rev. Respir. Dis. 104:175.

151. Bouhuys, A., Lichtneckert, S., Lundgren, C., and Lundin, G. (1961). Voluntary changes in breathing pattern and N_2 clearance from lungs. J. Appl. Physiol. 14:284.

International Review of Physiology
Respiratory Physiology II, Volume 14
Edited by John G. Widdicombe
Copyright 1977   University Park Press   Baltimore

3
Pulmonary
Gas Exchange

J. B. WEST

University of California San Diego, La Jolla, California

NUMERICAL PROCEDURES FOR
BLOOD-GAS DISSOCIATION CURVES   84
   O_2 Dissociation Curve   84
   CO_2 Dissociation Curve   85
   pH-P_{CO_2} Relationship   85

VENTILATION-PERFUSION RATIO EQUATION   86
   Description   86
   Solution by Means of R Lines   86
   Solution by Means of Fick Principle for Three Gases   87

GAS EXCHANGE IN LUNG MODELS OF
VENTILATION-PERFUSION INEQUALITY   88

MEASUREMENT OF CONTINUOUS
DISTRIBUTIONS OF VENTILATION-PERFUSION RATIOS   90
   Method   90
   Distributions During Air Breathing   92
   Distributions During Oxygen Breathing   95

INSTABILITY OF LUNG UNITS WITH
LOW VENTILATION-PERFUSION RATIOS   95

GAS EXCHANGE IN PRESENCE OF
HIGHLY SOLUBLE INERT GASES   98

GAS EXCHANGE WITH SERIES INEQUALITY   100

TIME COURSE OF P_{CO_2} IN PULMONARY CAPILLARIES   102

FORMAL ANALYSIS OF
GAS EXCHANGE IN NONHOMOGENEOUS LUNGS   102

The essential function of the lung is to allow gas exchange to occur between alveolar gas and pulmonary capillary blood. Under ideal conditions, approximately 1 liter of alveolar ventilation is matched with 1 liter of pulmonary blood flow, giving a ventilation-perfusion ratio of 1. The resulting partial pressures are those which result when a liter of air and a liter of mixed venous blood are mixed in a tonometer until equilibration takes place.

However, in the actual human lung, it is inevitable that some mismatching of alveolar ventilation and blood flow takes place. In part this is because of topographical differences of ventilation and blood flow caused by gravity. In part it may be ascribed to the mechanical impossibility of providing each of the 300 million alveoli with the appropriate share of the total ventilation and blood flow. As a consequence, the efficiency of gas exchange is impaired.

Quantitative analysis of gas exchange under these conditions of mismatched ventilation and blood flow is greatly complicated by the nonlinearity and interdependence of the O_2 and CO_2 dissociation curves. We can distinguish three phases of investigation in this area. The first was the realization by Krogh and Lindhard (1) and Haldane (2) that, indeed, it is the ratio of ventilation to blood flow which is the key variable. The second was the work of Fenn, Rahn, and Otis (see, for example, Rahn and Fenn (3)) and Riley and Cournand (4), who began a quantitative study of the problem. They applied graphical analysis to circumvent the algebraic difficulties of manipulating the O_2 and CO_2 dissociation curves. The third phase began with the introduction by Kelman (5, 6) of digital computer procedures for the O_2 and CO_2 dissociation curves and the pH-P_{CO_2} relationship. These procedures paved the way for the application of numerical methods to the analysis of pulmonary gas exchange (7–9) with the result that the last 5 years have seen extremely rapid progress.

It is not possible to cover all aspects of pulmonary gas exchange in this short review. Instead, recent work exploiting numerical analysis is described, including a method for determining continuous distributions of ventilation-perfusion ratios. In addition, a short section on the formal analysis of pulmonary gas exchange is included.

NUMERICAL PROCEDURES FOR BLOOD-GAS DISSOCIATION CURVES

O_2 Dissociation Curve

In Kelman's procedure (5), the input variables are P_{O_2}, pH, P_{CO_2}, and temperature. Recently an additional factor has been introduced (10) to take account of shifts of the dissociation curve caused by other factors such as 2,3-diphosphoglycerate. O_2 saturation is determined in two steps. First the "virtual" P_{O_2} is computed. This is the P_{O_2} which would obtain at a pH of 7.40, P_{CO_2} of 40 Torr, and temperature of 37°C. It is derived from the measured values of pH, P_{CO_2}, and temperature by applying appropriate correction factors. The choice of these factors from the various studies reported in the literature is discussed at length by Kelman (5) and Severinghaus (11).

The second step is the conversion of P_{O_2} to O_2 saturation. This is accomplished by an equation similar in form to that proposed by Adair (12),

$$S = (A_x + B_x{}^2 + C_x{}^3 + x^4)/(D + E_x + F_x{}^2 + G_x{}^3 + x^4) \qquad (1)$$

where S is the saturation and x is the virtual P_{O_2}. The coefficients A to G were chosen to fit the standard dissociation curve given by Severinghaus (11). Below a P_{O_2} to 10 Torr, the above equation is unsatisfactory, and it is then replaced by a quadratic function (13).

Other procedures for the O_2 dissociation curve have been described. That used by Gomez (14) should be mentioned, because it is more suitable for small computers for which Kelman's procedure may give erroneous results because the terms become so large.

CO_2 Dissociation Curve

Kelman's procedure for CO_2 content requires the P_{CO_2}, plasma pH, O_2 saturation, hematocrit, and temperature. The first step is to compute the total CO_2 content of the plasma from its pH and P_{CO_2} with the use of the Henderson-Hasselbalch equation. This requires the pK and solubility of CO_2 in plasma which are calculated from expressions given by Austin et al. (15). The second step is to calculate the CO_2 content of whole blood by means of the ratio $[CO_2]$ cells: $[CO_2]$ plasma, which was determined experimentally by van Slyke and Sendroy (16).

This subroutine gives results which agree closely with those given by Singer and Hastings (17). Alternative procedures have been described (7, 18) and are apparently equally satisfactory.

pH-P_{CO_2} Relationship

In practice, it is necessary to use this relationship in conjunction with the dissociation curves. Kelman's procedure (5) is based on the linear relationship between pH and $\log P_{CO_2}$. If the base excess is zero, the pH is calculated from a standard line which passes through the point (pH = 7.590, P_{CO_2} = 20 Torr) for fully oxygenated blood. An additional variable Y is included to take account of the shift of the buffer line by changes in O_2 saturation and hemoglobin concentration. If the base excess is not zero, four additional input values are required, these being two pairs of pH and P_{CO_2} values which locate the line on the pH-$\log P_{CO_2}$ diagram.

Because the value of Y depends on the O_2 saturation, but the calculation of the latter requires the pH, an iterative process is used. First, the hemoglobin is assumed to be fully saturated, and the pH and saturation are calculated. Y is then recalculated, and pH and saturation are determined again. Kelman showed that only one iteration is necessary to obtain acceptable accuracy (5).

VENTILATION-PERFUSION RATIO EQUATION

Description

The ventilation-perfusion ratio equation is the keystone of any analysis of gas exchange under steady state conditions. One derivation is as follows:

The amount of CO_2 leaving a lung unit in the expired gas is given by

$$\dot{V}_{CO_2} = \dot{V}_A \cdot P_{A_{CO_2}} \cdot K \tag{2}$$

where K is a constant which is appropriate for the units.

The amount of CO_2 which leaves the blood is given by

$$\dot{V}_{CO_2} = \dot{Q}(C_{\bar{v}CO_2} - C_{c'CO_2}) \tag{3}$$

where c' denotes end-capillary.

Because in a steady state these are equal, we have

$$\dot{V}_A/\dot{Q} = \frac{C_{\bar{v}CO_2} - C_{c'}{CO_2}}{P_{A_{CO_2}} \cdot K} \tag{4}$$

If $\dot{V}_A$ is in BTPS and the blood gas contents are in ml of STPD/100 ml, K is equal to 8.63^{-1}. This equation was originally derived independently by Rahn (19) and Riley and Cournand (4).

Although this equation looks simple, it is greatly complicated by the fact that O_2 saturation is an implicit variable, because it affects the relationship between P_{CO_2} and CO_2 content in blood. As a consequence, progress in understanding the quantitative aspects of pulmonary gas exchange was slow and labored until the introduction of numerical methods for dealing with the dissociation curves as described above.

Solution by Means of R Lines

This is the basis of the graphical methods used with the O_2-CO_2 diagram (3), and it was also the first numerical approach (13). The principle is that in any lung unit in a steady state, the R (respiratory exchange ratio) for gas and blood must be the same. In the graphical method, lines for a given R value are drawn for gas and blood, and the point of intersection gives the P_{O_2}, P_{CO_2}, and O_2 and CO_2 contents from which the ventilation-perfusion ratio can be calculated (3, 20). The numerical method is similar. A point is moved along a gas R line (given by the alveolar gas equation (3)) in a systematic way and blood R is calculated. When these are equal, the ventilation-perfusion ratio is derived.

An assumption of this method is that no nitrogen enters or leaves the blood in any lung unit. This is not strictly true, and important errors may occur when the ventilation-perfusion ratio is very low, particularly when the inspired O_2 concentration is increased. For this reason, an alternative method of solution is preferred.

Solution by Means of Fick Principle for Three Gases

Olszowka and Farhi (7) described a method based on the principle of conservation of mass (Fick principle) as applied simultaneously to O_2, CO_2, and N_2. The method sets up five equations. Three are of the form

$$\dot{V}_{A_I} \cdot F_{I_x} - \dot{V}_A \cdot F_{A_x} = \dot{Q}(C_{c_x} - C_{\bar{v}_x}) \tag{5}$$

where x refers to O_2, CO_2, and N_2, respectively. The other two equations state that the fractional concentrations of the three gases in both inspired and alveolar gas are equal to 1.0. This system of equations can be rapidly solved by a numerical procedure (10).

A disadvantage of this method is that it requires the value of the P_{N_2} in mixed venous blood, which is rarely known. However, in practice it is usually possible to estimate the value from the inspired P_{O_2} and P_{CO_2} with acceptable accuracy. Alternatively, it is not difficult to iterate the P_{N_2} until the mixed venous and arterial values are nearly identical.

This more complicated method of solving the ventilation-perfusion ratio equation is only necessary when the $\dot{V}_A/\dot{Q}$ is very low and the inspired O_2 concentration is raised. Under these circumstances, substantial errors can result from the use of the traditional method, as shown in Table 1.

Table 1. Alveolar P_{O_2} (in Torr) calculated from the traditional ventilation-perfusion ratio equation and allowing for nitrogen exchange.[a]

| $\dot{V}_A/\dot{Q}$ | $F_{I_{O_2}} = 0.21$ | | $F_{I_{O_2}} = 0.80$ | |
	Calculated from traditional $\dot{V}_A/\dot{Q}$ equation	Allowing for N_2 exchange	Calculated from traditional $\dot{V}_A/\dot{Q}$ equation	Allowing for N_2 exchange
1	104.0	104.0	526.3	526.9
0.1	45.3	45.4	416.2	430.9
0.01	40.5	40.6	53.7	118.6
0.001	40.1	40.2	41.1	61.3

[a]In all cases, the P_{O_2} and P_{CO_2} in mixed venous blood were 40 and 45 Torr, respectively, but the N_2 partial pressure was adjusted for no net transfer of this gas in a homogeneous lung. Note the much higher P_{O_2} at a V_A/Q of 0.01, $F_{I_{O_2}} = 0.8$ when nitrogen exchange is included.

GAS EXCHANGE IN LUNG MODELS
OF VENTILATION-PERFUSION INEQUALITY

A good deal has been learned about the gas exchange behavior of non-homogeneous lungs by studying numerical multicompartment models. First, a distribution of ventilation-perfusion ratios is set up. The logarithmic Gaussian distribution is particularly convenient and has been used extensively (9, 20–23). This is the simplest acceptable distribution in which the dispersion can be characterized by a single parameter, the log S.D. Note that a (linear) Gaussian distribution cannot be used because any substantial variance results in negative values which have no physiological meaning. Another useful feature of the log normal distribution is that a given log S.D. of either ventilation or blood flow has an identical effect on overall gas exchange (9, 24).

Once the multicompartment distribution of ventilation-perfusion ratios has been set up, the gas exchange in each compartment is determined from the ventilation-perfusion ratio equation, and overall gas exchange can be calculated by combining the expired ventilation and effluent blood flows from all the units. Numerical methods for doing this have been described in detail (10). In the simplest models, the gas composition of mixed venous blood is assumed, thus fixing the position of the ventilation-perfusion ratio line (3, 9). In a more general approach, the O_2 uptake and CO_2 output of the model are given, and the gas composition of mixed venous blood is found by an iterative process.

Some of the findings from this type of analysis can be summarized here. Mismatching of ventilation and blood flow in these models has always been found to cause a fall of P_{O_2} and a rise of P_{CO_2} in arterial and mixed venous blood. This statement assumes that other variables are held constant, such as total ventilation, total blood flow, O_2 uptake, and CO_2 output. However, if the composition of mixed venous blood is fixed while ventilation-perfusion inequality is imposed (such as occurs during the first few seconds of human exposure to high accelerations), a fall in O_2 uptake and CO_2 output is also observed.

An increase in either total ventilation or blood flow in a lung with ventilation-perfusion inequality increases the P_{O_2} and reduces the P_{CO_2} (Figure 1). The fall in P_{CO_2} accompanying an increase in ventilation is generally marked, whereas the rise in P_{O_2} may be minor, especially when the mismatching of ventilation and blood flow is severe. The difference in behavior can be attributed to the different shapes of the O_2 and CO_2 dissociation curves. This can be proved by carrying out the analysis when the O_2 dissociation curve has been artificially linearized. Under these circumstances, O_2 and CO_2 show similar behavior (9).

There has been some confusion about the effect of a rise in total blood flow on the arterial P_{O_2} in nonhomogeneous lungs. It is sometimes argued that as a result of the fall in overall ventilation-perfusion ratio (that is, total ventilation divided by total blood flow) the arterial P_{O_2} will fall. This argument overlooks

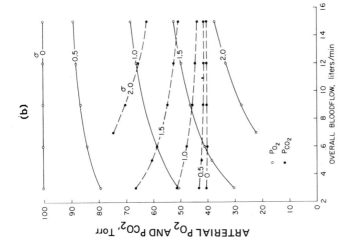

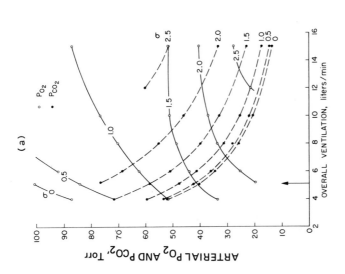

Figure 1. Effects of increasing overall ventilation (*a*) and blood flow (*b*) on the arterial P_{O_2} (○———○) and P_{CO_2} (●– – –●) in log normal distributions of ventilation-perfusion ratios. σ, the log standard deviation of the distribution. Reprinted with permission of Respir. Physiol. 7:88 (1969).

the increase in P_{O_2} in mixed venous blood and is fallacious. A rise in arterial P_{O_2} must occur, other things being equal.

The transfer of inert gases by nonhomogeneous lungs has also been studied (23). ("Inert" refers to gases with linear blood dissociation curves.) An interesting finding is the relationship between the gas solubility and the amount of reduction of transfer (Figure 2). Note that gases of medium solubility have their transfer (in this case, elimination) reduced much more than gases of very low or very high solubility. Figure 2 is drawn for a log Gaussian distribution of ventilation-perfusion ratios, and it is of interest that the minimum elimination occurs when the blood-gas partition coefficient is equal to the overall ventilation-perfusion ratio of the lung. It is possible to show formally that all distributions irrespective of their shape result in a reduced transfer of inert gases (25) (see under "Formal Analysis of Gas Exchange in Non-homogeneous Lungs") and that the shape of the curve is generally similar to that of Figure 2, that is, there is one minimum (24). However, the solubility at which the minimum occurs depends on the pattern of ventilation-perfusion inequality.

MEASUREMENT OF CONTINUOUS DISTRIBUTIONS OF VENTILATION-PERFUSION RATIOS

Method

Suppose an inert gas dissolved in saline is infused into the mixed venous blood at a constant rate. Then the "retention" of the gas, that is, the concentration in

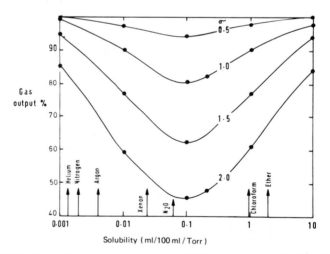

Figure 2. Elimination of inert gases of various solubilities by a lung model with a log normal distribution of ventilation-perfusion ratios. In each case, the elimination by a homogeneous lung is 100%. σ is the log standard deviation of the distribution. Note that gases of medium solubility have their elimination reduced most. Reprinted with permission of Respir. Physiol. 8:66 (1969–70).

end capillary blood divided by the concentration in the mixed venous blood in any lung unit, is a simple function of the solubility and the ventilation-perfusion ratio (26, 27). Thus,

$$R = \frac{C_{c'}}{C_{\bar{v}}} = \frac{\lambda}{\lambda + \dot{V}_A/\dot{Q}} \tag{6}$$

where λ is the blood-gas partition coefficient.

By infusing a mixture of six inert gases having a wide range of solubilities (sulfur hexafluoride, ethane, cyclopropane, halothane, diethyl ether, and acetone), a retention-solubility curve for the whole lung can be drawn (Figure 3). The retentions of the poorly soluble gases are very low, because they are almost completely eliminated from the blood, even by a lung with low ventilation-perfusion ratios, whereas the high solubility gases have much larger retentions. In practice the concentrations of the inert gases are measured by gas chromatography (28).

This retention-solubility curve contains information about the distribution of ventilation-perfusion ratios which gave rise to it. For example, completely unventilated (but perfused) alveoli particularly increase the retention of the least soluble gas, sulfur hexafluoride, while a group of units with very low (but not zero) ventilation-perfusion ratios will especially raise the curve in the region of ethane. Indeed, the solubility of the gas whose retention is most affected can be formally related to the ventilation-perfusion ratios of a simple two-compartment model (29). In the same way, the excretion-solubility curve (where excretion is defined as the partial pressure in mixed expired gas divided by that in mixed venous blood) gives information about the distribution of ventilation.

It is possible to transform the measured retention-solubility curve into a distribution of ventilation-perfusion ratios which is consistent with it (30) (Figure 3). This is done by numerical analysis with the use of a digital computer, and various techniques are available (31). The numerical procedure can be tested by generating retention-solubility curves from artificial distributions and then attempting to recover these. In practice, simple unimodal and bimodal distributions with and without shunt and dead space can be successfully recovered with a considerable degree of confidence (30, 31).

However, it is important to emphasize that other distributions may be compatible with the measured retentions, especially in the presence of inevitable experimental error (32, 33). In general, the numerical procedures recover the simplest smooth distribution which is consistent with the data. An extensive analysis of the confidence limits of the recovery techniques has recently been completed, and it is clear that, while the method is very successful with relatively narrow distributions such as are recovered in normal lungs, increasing uncertainty develops as the dispersion of ventilation-perfusion ratios is greatly broadened (34). An especially difficult problem is created by a lung with a substantial shunt, considerable blood flow to units with very low ventilation-perfusion ratios, and a broad dispersion outside this (33). In this case, there may be

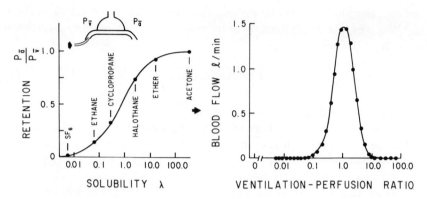

Figure 3. Diagram to show how the retention-solubility curve can be used to derive a distribution of ventilation-perfusion ratios compatible with it. For description, see text.

a range of distributions which are compatible with the measured retentions. However, in the normal and nearly normal lung, the method clearly gives additional information about the pattern of ventilation-perfusion ratios.

Distributions During Air Breathing

Figure 4 shows an example of the retention-solubility and excretion-solubility curves and the derived distribution of ventilation-perfusion ratios from a 22-year-old, normal volunteer studied in the semirecumbent position. Note that the observed inert gas retentions lay very close to the retention-solubility curve for a homogeneous lung (no ventilation-perfusion inequality). This is reflected in the narrow distribution of ventilation-perfusion ratios. Both the distributions of blood flow and ventilation are tight, and there was no blood flow or ventilation outside the range of 0.3–2.5. In addition, although not shown in this diagram, there was also no blood flow to the extremes of the range (0.005 and 100). Note also that there was no blood flow to unventilated alveoli (shunt).

In a series of young, normal subjects, the results were very consistent (35). The 95% limits for blood flow and ventilation were between ventilation-perfusion ratios of 0.3 and 2.1. For the blood flow distributions, the log mean and standard deviation were 0.78 and 0.43, whereas for ventilation the values were 1.03 and 0.35, respectively. These results are consistent with the small alveolar-arterial difference for P_{O_2} in young, normal subjects (36).

Figure 5 shows the results obtained in an older (44 years) apparently normal volunteer. It can be seen that the measured inert gas retentions lay somewhat above those for a homogeneous lung having the same total ventilation and blood flow. This was especially true of the retentions of ethane and cyclopropane. As a consequence, the derived distribution of ventilation-perfusion ratios shows important differences compared with that found in the young normal subject

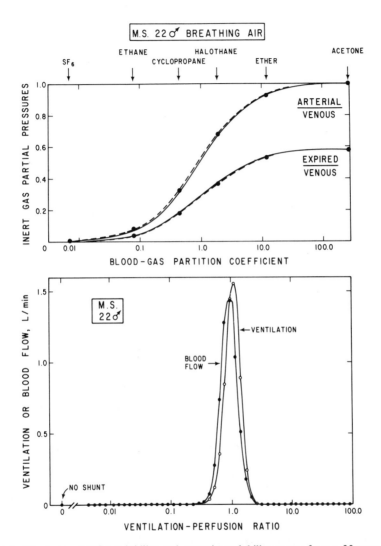

Figure 4. Measured retention-solubility and excretion-solubility curves from a 22-year-old, normal volunteer (*top panel, broken lines*). The *solid lines* are the curves which would be given by a homogeneous lung with the same total ventilation and blood flow. It can be seen that the observed data deviated little from these. The derived distribution of ventilation-perfusion ratios is shown in the *bottom panel*. Note that both the distributions of ventilation and blood flow were narrow and that there was no shunt. Reprinted with permission of J. Clin. Invest. 54:54 (1974).

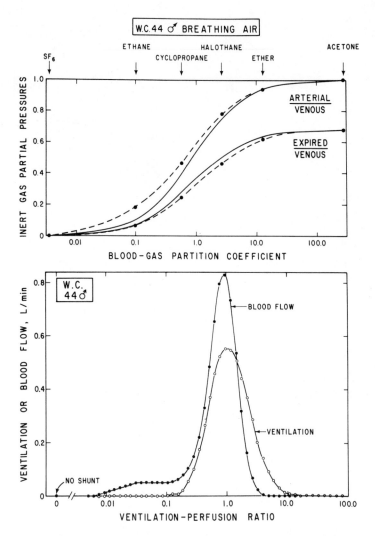

Figure 5. Data similar to those shown in Figure 4, but in this case from a 44-year-old, apparently normal subject. Note that the measured retentions lie well above the curve for the homogeneous lung. These differences are reflected in the broader distributions of ventilation and blood flow shown in the *bottom panel*. Note especially the shoulder on the left side of the blood flow distribution. Reprinted with permission of J. Clin. Invest. 54:54 (1974).

(Figure 4). There was more dispersion in the older man, so that the main body of the distribution covered approximately 2 decades of ventilation-perfusion ratios from 0.1 to 10. In addition, there was a definite shoulder to the left-hand side of the distribution of blood flow with appreciable amounts of flow to lung units in the range 0.1–0.01. However, again no shunt was detected.

In general, there was a consistent broadening of the distributions with age in the 12 normal subjects who were studied. Although there were insufficient data to derive a regression equation, the standard deviation of the blood flow distributions approximately doubled from 0.43 to 0.85 over the age range from 20 to 60 years. This increasing dispersion of ventilation-perfusion ratios is consistent with the almost linear fall in arterial P_{O_2} which occurs with increasing age (36, 37).

Distributions During Oxygen Breathing

A remarkable change occurs in some of the retention-solubility curves and distributions of ventilation-perfusion ratios following a 30-min period of 100% O_2 breathing. Figure 6 shows an example from the same normal subject of Figure 5. It can be seen that the shape of the retention-solubility curve changed because the retention of the least soluble gas, sulfur hexafluoride, was increased by O_2 breathing, whereas the retention of the slightly more soluble gas, ethane, fell a little. These changes must mean an increase in the amount of shunted blood but a decrease in the blood flow to poorly ventilated alveoli.

The derived distributions of blood flow reflect this. Note that, following the period of O_2 breathing, the left-hand shoulder of the distribution was abolished, but in its place a shunt of approximately 11% of the cardiac output appeared. This finding was observed in eight of the nine normal subjects who were studied while breathing air and O_2, although the shunts which developed were generally in the range of 1–3% and the magnitude of the shunt shown in Figure 6 was exceptional. In one subject, measurements were made during air breathing after a period of O_2 breathing, and the shunt was shown to disappear.

This phenomenon has also been observed in dogs in which ventilation-perfusion inequality was induced (38). This was done by infusing oleic acid into the right ventricle, thus causing hemorrhagic pulmonary edema (39), or by experimental glass bead embolism of the pulmonary circulation. In these animals, striking degrees of shunting often followed a period of O_2 breathing. Similar findings have been reported in patients with acute respiratory failure (40).

INSTABILITY OF LUNG UNITS WITH LOW VENTILATION-PERFUSION RATIOS

In the previous section, it was seen that lung units with low $\dot{V}_A/\dot{Q}$ may be transformed into unventilated areas following a period of 100% O_2 breathing. Such a possibility was predicted by Briscoe and his colleagues (41). It is now recognized that these very low $\dot{V}_A/\dot{Q}$ units may be inherently unstable because of a disparity between the volumes of gas entering and leaving them. This is particularly likely to occur during the inspiration of enriched O_2 mixtures.

Traditionally, alveolar ventilation is defined in terms of expired gas. However, in low $\dot{V}_A/\dot{Q}$ units it is important to distinguish between inspired and expired alveolar ventilations, because these may be very different. Figure 7

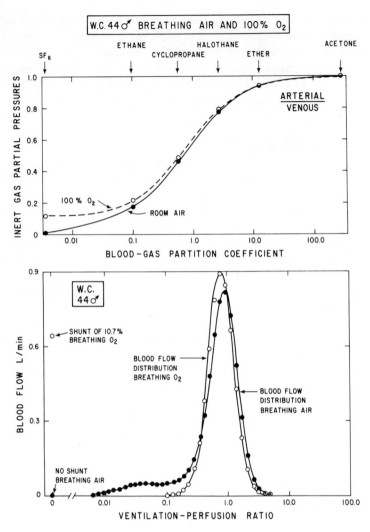

Figure 6. Retention-solubility curves measured in the subject of Figure 5 before and after a period of 100% oxygen breathing. Note the marked increase in the retention of sulfur hexafluoride following oxygen. The distributions of blood flow (*bottom*) show that the shoulder of blood flow to low ventilation-perfusion ratios disappeared and in its place a shunt of 10.7% developed. Reprinted with permission of J. Clin. Invest. 54:54 (1974).

shows calculated values for units with low $\dot{V}_A/\dot{Q}$ when the inspired O_2 concentration is 80%. These calculations were made by using the Fick principle for O_2, CO_2, and N_2. Unit A has an inspired $\dot{V}_A/\dot{Q}$ of 0.0494. This is very low but within the range found in the older normal subject of Figure 5. Note that although the inspired ventilation was 49.4 units (the actual value will depend on the blood flow), the expired ventilation was only 2.5 units. The reason for this

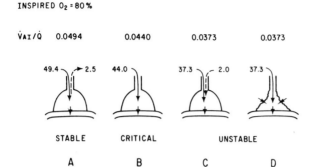

INSPIRED O_2 = 80%

$\dot{V}_{AI}/\dot{Q}$ 0.0494   0.0440   0.0373   0.0373

49.4 ⟋ ⟶ 2.5   44.0 ⟍   37.3 ⟍ ⟋ 2.0   37.3 ⟍

STABLE   CRITICAL   UNSTABLE

A   B   C   D

Figure 7. Behavior of lung units with low ventilation-perfusion ratios during 80% oxygen breathing. A has an inspired ventilation-perfusion ratio of 0.0494 and, as a result, a very small expired ventilation. In B, the expired ventilation is zero, and so the unit is said to be critical. In C and D, more gas enters the blood than is taken in during inspiration and these units may be unstable.

remarkable disparity is the large proportion of the inspired gas which is removed by the blood. One consequence of this is a marked concentration of N_2 in the alveoli. In unit A, the inspired P_{N_2} is 143 Torr, but the alveolar P_{N_2} is 535 Torr under steady state conditions!

If the inspired $\dot{V}_A/\dot{Q}$ is reduced slightly to 0.044 as in unit B, the calculated expired ventilation falls to zero. Now all the inspired gas is being removed by the blood. This has been called the "critical inspired ventilation-perfusion ratio" (42). If the inspired ventilation is reduced even further, two alternatives seem possible. One shown in unit C allows gas to enter the lung unit during the expiratory phase of ventilation. If this is prevented as in D, the unit may gradually collapse. This seems the likely course if the low ventilation is caused by intermittent airway closure which apparently occurs at the bases of the upright, elderly normal lung during normal breathing (43).

Thus, lung units can be divided into two groups—those that have an inspired ventilation-perfusion ratio above the critical value and are, therefore, stable and those with ratios which are below and which are, therefore, potentially unstable. The actual value of the critical inspired ventilation-perfusion ratio depends strongly on the inspired O_2 concentration as shown in Figure 8. Note that the healthy subject of Figure 5 apparently has lung units which would become unstable if the inspired O_2 concentration were raised above about 50%. Other variables that determine the value of the critical inspired ventilation-perfusion ratio are the P_{O_2} and P_{N_2} in mixed venous blood.

The gas exchange of unit C in Figure 7 is notable. Such a unit will absorb O_2 and thus not be detected as a shunt by measuring the arterial P_{O_2} during 100% O_2 breathing. On the other hand, this unit will not eliminate CO_2 or any of the infused inert gases. Lenfant (44) obtained evidence for the existence of such units in the normal lung during 90% O_2 breathing.

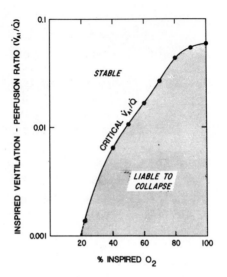

Figure 8. Relationship between the critical inspired ventilation-perfusion ratio and the concentration of inspired oxygen. Note that the normal subject of Figure 4 had lung units which would be expected to become unstable if the inspired oxygen was raised above 50%. Reprinted with permission of J. Appl. Physiol. 38:886 (1975).

GAS EXCHANGE IN PRESENCE OF HIGHLY SOLUBLE INERT GASES

An important variable in the behavior of lung units with low ventilation-perfusion ratios is the solubility of the inert gas, normally N_2, which accompanies the O_2 and CO_2. Farhi and Olszowka (45) have explored the consequences of replacing N_2 with a more soluble carrier gas such as nitrous oxide. An important situation in which this occurs in practice is N_2O anesthesia.

It has been known for some time that during the induction of N_2O anesthesia, when high concentrations of this very soluble gas are administered, the arterial P_{O_2} may be appreciably higher than that expected from the concentration of inspired O_2 (46, 47). This can be explained by the increased concentration of alveolar O_2, which occurs as a result of rapid uptake of nitrous oxide from the alveoli into the blood. Under conditions of fixed inspired ventilation, as may occur with a respirator, the arterial P_{CO_2} may also rise. Opposite changes may occur during the elimination of N_2O at the conclusion of the anesthesia when the large volumes of this gas which are evolved into the alveoli reduce the P_{O_2} and P_{CO_2} (48, 49).

Farhi and Olszowka (45) have analyzed the changes in P_{O_2} and P_{CO_2} in lung units with various ventilation-perfusion ratios as an inert gas is either taken up or eliminated. They chose to concentrate on N_2O as the inert gas because it has a high solubility and is inhaled at high concentration during anesthesia. Calculations were made of the alveolar P_{O_2} and P_{CO_2} at various times during the intake and elimination of N_2O as the partial pressure of this gas in the mixed venous blood changed.

Figure 9 shows the alveolar P_{O_2} plotted against the inspired ventilation-perfusion ratio for various inspired fractions of N_2O. For this graph, the inspired O_2 was 21% and the remainder of the inspired gas was N_2O. Inspired, as opposed to expired, ventilation-perfusion ratio was plotted because this is normally determined by the respirator setting. Expired ventilation will be appreciably less than inspired because of the uptake of N_2O. For this figure, the mixed venous blood was assumed to contain no N_2O so that the situation corresponds to that at the onset of breathing the gas. The topographical range of ventilation-perfusion ratios in the upright lung (50) is shown by the *vertical, broken lines*.

It can be seen that, when no N_2O was present, the P_{O_2} varied from about 60–130 Torr from base to apex (50). However, as the inspired concentration of N_2O was increased, the regional differences in P_{O_2} were reduced. Indeed, when the inspired gas was 79% N_2O and 21% O_2 with no N_2 present, the P_{O_2} at the base of the lung exceeded that at the apex. This can be explained by the fact that the uptake of N_2O at the base was so fast that the concentration of O_2 was doubled.

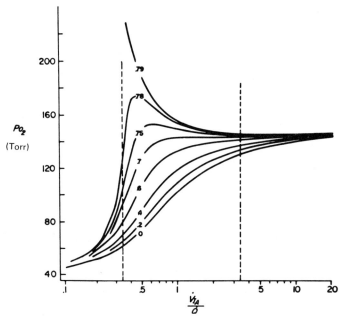

Figure 9. Alveolar P_{O_2} plotted against the inspired ventilation-perfusion ratio in lung units which are inspiring various fractions of N_2O (shown by the numbers on the lines). The range of ventilation-perfusion ratios in the normal upright human lung is shown by the two *vertical broken lines*. Note that when the inspired concentration of N_2O is very high, the P_{O_2} at the base (*left vertical broken line*) exceeds that at the apex. Reprinted with permission of Respir. Physiol. 5:53 (1968).

It should be noted that Figure 9 is drawn for the situation in which the N_2O partial pressure in mixed venous blood is zero. However, as N_2O is taken up, its partial pressure in the venous blood will gradually rise, and thus the rate of absorption of the gas will decrease. As a consequence, the rise in P_{O_2} in units with low ventilation-perfusion ratios will become less marked.

An interesting feature of Figure 9 is that it predicts a higher P_{O_2} in arterial blood than mixed alveolar gas (negative $A - a$ difference for P_{O_2}) during the inspiration of 79% nitrous oxide. This is because the base of the lung with its low ventilation-perfusion ratios and high blood flow has a higher P_{O_2} than the apex with its high ventilation-perfusion ratio and low blood flow. However, the depression of the arterial P_{O_2} by bronchial and Thebesian venous blood will tend to override this distribution effect.

During N_2O elimination, when the gas is present in the mixed venous blood but not in the inspired gas, the direction of the changes shown in Figure 9 will be reversed. However, Farhi and Olszowka (45) showed that the depression of P_{O_2} in units with low ventilation-perfusion ratios is only some 10 Torr in magnitude as opposed to the much larger rise in P_{O_2} during N_2O uptake. The modest decrease in P_{O_2} can be ascribed to two causes. First, because the subject is breathing air, the changes caused by dilution of alveolar gas will chiefly affect N_2. Second, the fact that the P_{O_2} in units with low ventilation-perfusion ratios is on the steep part of the O_2 dissociation curve means that the blood serves as an O_2 reservoir by liberating substantial amounts of this gas. The changes in P_{CO_2} are relatively small during both the uptake and elimination of N_2O for the same reason, namely that the CO_2 dissociation curve is steep and the absorption or liberation of this gas buffers its change in partial pressure.

GAS EXCHANGE WITH SERIES INEQUALITY

So far, this chapter has been concerned with the traditional model of ventilation-perfusion inequality in which the gas exchanging units are assumed to be ventilated in parallel. This is generally a reasonable assumption in that the bronchi form a multiple branching system with the alveoli situated near the ends of the airways.

However, it is important to consider the consequences of having one lung region inspire alveolar gas from another region, so-called "series inequality of ventilation." There are two chief mechanisms for this in the normal lung. First, some alveoli are more proximally located on the airways than others, with the result that the latter inspire some gas exhaled from the former. This situation, in which the composition of the inspired dead space gas is varied, has been analyzed by Ross and Farhi (51). Second, the lung has communications between adjacent regions both at the respiratory bronchiole and alveolar levels which presumably allow gas exchange. In the diseased lung, additional mechanisms, such as "pendulluft" caused by unequal time constants, and dilatation of the terminal bronchioles as in centrilobular emphysema, are supposedly responsible for movement of gas between lung units.

Gas exchange in the presence of series inequality has been studied in lung models by numerical analysis (52). The subject is complicated by the fact that the gas composition of one compartment affects that of the other, but solutions can be obtained by iterative techniques. Figure 10 shows an example of calculated gas transfer in a simple two-compartment model in which the distal (so-called "parasitic") compartment receives all its inspired gas from a proximal compartment. Both compartments are perfused and have independent ventilation-perfusion ratios.

It can be seen that as the ventilation and blood flow to the parasitic compartment were increased (keeping the ventilation-perfusion ratio constant at 0.85), both the O_2 uptake and CO_2 output of the model fell, compared with the homogeneous lung. All the other variables, such as the composition of the inspired gas and mixed venous blood, and the total ventilation and blood flow were held constant. It is of interest that the CO_2 output was reduced much more than the O_2 uptake; this is the reverse of the situation seen in most parallel models of ventilation-perfusion inequality (53).

When the O_2 uptake and CO_2 output are kept constant, series inequality causes both a fall in arterial P_{O_2} and a rise in P_{CO_2}. However, an interesting feature of this situation is that an increase in overall ventilation results in a marked rise in arterial P_{O_2}. By contrast, in most parallel models the rise in P_{O_2} tends to be small when the degree of ventilation-perfusion inequality is severe.

Recently, Wagner and Evans (54) have examined the exchange of inert gases in models with series inequality. They sought to determine whether there was a

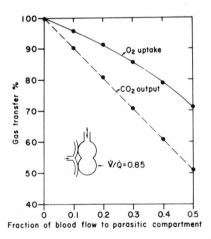

Figure 10. O_2 uptake and CO_2 output in a lung model with series inequality. Note that as the proportion of the ventilation and blood flow going to the parasitic compartment increased, both O_2 uptake and CO_2 output were reduced, especially the latter. Reprinted with permission of J. Appl. Physiol. 30:479 (1971).

specific pattern of uptake or elimination of the gases which could not be represented by an equivalent parallel model. Their general conclusion was that there was not; that is, there is always a parallel model in which gas exchange behavior is equivalent to that of a series model. The only exception in principle occurred when a lung was eliminating inert gas but the inspired gas contained some of the gas in question. However, in this situation, the difference between the series model and the near-equivalent parallel model was so minor that it would be impossible to detect the difference in practice. Thus, the inert gas method outlined above cannot be used to distinguish between series and parallel inequality.

TIME COURSE OF P_{CO_2} IN PULMONARY CAPILLARIES

Since the early calculations of the time course of P_{O_2} in pulmonary capillaries by Bohr (55), it has generally been assumed that equilibration between alveolar and capillary P_{CO_2} must be very fast. This assumption was based on the more rapid diffusion rate of carbon dioxide than oxygen through tissue slices (56). However, the elimination of carbon dioxide from blood involves several processes, including the dehydration of bicarbonate, chloride shift, and the carbarmino reaction. These processes are not necessarily fast. Thus, predicting the carbon dioxide diffusing capacity from the oxygen value by multiplying by 20 is a gross oversimplification.

Recently, calculations of the time course of P_{CO_2} have been made which take account of the chemical reactions (57–59). A meticulous analysis by Hill and her colleagues (58) showed that the rate of equilibration between the P_{CO_2} in alveolar gas and the capillary red blood cell is somewhat slower than that for P_{O_2} (Figure 11). Moreover, the chemical reactions are not complete by the time the red cell has reached the end of the capillary, with the result that the P_{CO_2} in the blood subsequently increases slightly (Figure 11). Plasma pH apparently continues to fall for some 15 s after the blood has left the capillary because the dehydration of bicarbonate is very slow in the absence of carbonic anhydrase. Forster and Crandall (59) have confirmed the slow change in plasma pH in a stopped-flow rapid reaction apparatus using human red cell suspensions.

FORMAL ANALYSIS OF GAS
EXCHANGE IN NONHOMOGENEOUS LUNGS

The preceding sections have dealt with numerical analysis of pulmonary gas exchange, which has become a powerful tool but suffers from the disadvantage that it does not allow general statements which hold true under a wide variety of physiological conditions. Recently, a new approach for dealing with nonhomogeneous lungs has emerged, that of formal mathematical analysis. With this, it is possible to make broad statements which can be shown to be true for all possible distributions of ventilation and bloodflow.

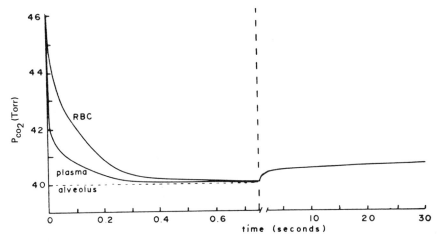

Figure 11. Calculated time course for P_{CO_2} in a pulmonary capillary. Note that equilibration for both the plasma and particularly the red blood cell are relatively slow. In addition, the P_{CO_2} rises after the blood leaves the capillary, as indicated by the *vertical broken line*. Reprinted with permission of Am. J. Physiol. 224:904 (1973).

One question which has been tackled in this way is a fundamental one: does ventilation-perfusion inequality always interfere with gas exchange, or can conditions be found under which gas exchange is actually enhanced by ventilation-perfusion inequality? Evans and his coworkers (25) compared gas exchange in two theoretical lung models which had the same overall ventilation and blood flow. One was homogeneous, whereas the other consisted of a variable number of compartments having different ventilation-perfusion ratios. Only one gas was permitted to exchange, the other being assumed to have a vanishingly low solubility in blood, an assumption which greatly simplifies the analysis.

It was found that the homogeneous lung always eliminated (or took up) more gas than the nonhomogeneous lung in the same time if, and only if, the relationship between the alveolar partial pressure and the ratio of perfusion to ventilation (sic) was everywhere concave. This in turn led to a condition on the dissociation curve such that, for gas uptake in the homogeneous lung to exceed that in the nonhomogeneous lung, the plot of the inverse of blood gas content against blood gas partial pressure had to be convex everywhere. This was shown always to be the case for O_2, CO_2, and CO, and also for the inert gases. Thus, under the assumptions of the analysis, the imposition of ventilation-perfusion inequality always reduces the uptake of all gases of physiological interest. This strong, comprehensive statement is true of all possible parallel distributions of ventilation-perfusion ratios.

A corresponding finding was that gas elimination is reduced by ventilation-perfusion inequality if, and only if, there is a convex relationship between blood gas content and the inverse of blood gas partial pressure. All inert gases and CO_2

show this relationship. However, it is of interest that both CO and O_2 have an area of concavity. It is thus theoretically possible to have a situation in which the elimination of O_2 or CO is actually enhanced by the imposition of ventilation-perfusion inequality. However, it was demonstrated that this could only occur under clearly unphysiological conditions in which the partial pressure of O_2 and CO in mixed venous blood exceeded 800 and 50 Torr, respectively.

REFERENCES

1. Krogh, A., and Lindhard, J. (1917). The volume of the dead space in breathing and the mixing of gases in the lungs of man. J. Physiol. (London) 51:59.
2. Haldane, J. S. (1922). Respiration. Yale University Press, New Haven.
3. Rahn, H., and Fenn, W. O. (1955). A Graphical Analysis of the Respiratory Gas Exchange. American Physiol. Society, Washington, D.C.
4. Riley, R. L., and Cournand, A. (1949). "Ideal" alveolar air and the analysis of ventilation-perfusion relationships in the lungs. J. Appl. Physiol. 1:825.
5. Kelman, G. R. (1966). Digital computer subroutine for the conversion of oxygen tension into saturation. J. Appl. Physiol. 21:1375.
6. Kelman, G. R. (1967). Digital computer procedure for the conversion of P_{CO_2} into blood CO_2 content. Respir. Physiol. 3:111.
7. Olszowka, A. J., and Farhi, L. E. (1968). A system of digital computer subroutines for blood gas calculation. Respir. Physiol. 4:270.
8. Olszowka, A. J., and Farhi, L. E. (1969). A digital computer program for constructing ventilation-perfusion lines. J. Appl. Physiol. 26:141.
9. West, J. B. (1969). Ventilation-perfusion inequality and overall gas exchange in computer models of the lung. Respir. Physiol. 7:88.
10. West, J. B., and Wagner, P. D. Pulmonary gas exchange. In J. B. West (ed.), Bioengineering Aspects of the Lung Biology.   Marcell Dekker, Inc., New York, in press.
11. Severinghaus, J. W. (1966). Blood gas calculator. J. Appl. Physiol. 21:1108.
12. Adair, G. S. (1925). The oxygen dissociation curve of hemoglobin. J. Biol. Chem. 83:529.
13. Kelman, G. R. (1968). Computer program for the production of O_2-CO_2 diagrams. Respir. Physiol. 4:260.
14. Gomez, D. M. (1961). Considerations of oxygen-hemoglobin equilibrium in the physiological state. Am. J. Physiol. 200:135.
15. Austin, W. H., Lacombe, E., Rand, P. W., and Chatterjee, M. (1963). Solubility of carbon dioxide in serum from 15 to $38°C$. J. Appl. Physiol. 18:301.
16. van Slyke, D. D., and Sendroy, J., Jr. (1928). Studies of gas electrolyte equilibria in blood. XV. Line charts for graphic calculation by the Henderson-Hasselbalch equation, and for calculating plasma carbon dioxide content from whole blood content. J. Biol. Chem. 79:781.
17. Singer, R. B., and Hastings, A. B. (1948). An improved clinical method for the estimation of disturbances of the acid base balance of human blood. Medicine 27:223.
18. Lloyd, B. B., and Michel, C. C. (1966). A theoretical treatment of the carbon dioxide dissociation curve of true plasma in vitro. Respir. Physiol. 1:107.
19. Rahn, H. (1949). A concept of mean alveolar air and the ventilation-blood-

flow relationships during pulmonary gas exchange. Am. J. Physiol. 158:21.

20. West, J. B. (1976). Ventilation Bloodflow and Gas Exchange, Ed. 3. Blackwell Scientific Publications, Edinburgh.

21. Farhi, L. E., and Rahn, H. (1955). A theoretical analysis of the alveolararterial oxygen difference with special reference to the distribution effect. J. Appl. Physiol. 7:699.

22. Lenfant, C., and Okuba, T. (1968). Distribution function of pulmonary blood flow and ventilation-perfusion ratio in man. J. Appl. Physiol. 24:668.

23. West, J. B. (1969-70). Effect of slope and shape of dissociation curve on pulmonary gas exchange. Respir. Physiol. 8:66.

24. Colburn, W. E., Evans, J. W., and West, J. B. (1974). Analysis of the effect of solubility on gas exchange in nonhomogeneous lungs. J. Appl. Physiol. 37:547.

25. Evans, J. W., Wagner, P. D., and West, J. B. (1974). Conditions for reduction of pulmonary gas transfer by ventilation-perfusion inequality. J. Appl. Physiol. 36:533.

26. Kety, S. S. (1951). The theory and applications of the exchange of inert gas at the lungs and tissues. Pharmacol. Rev. 3:1.

27. Farhi, L. E. (1967). Elimination of inert gas by the lung. Respir. Physiol. 3:1.

28. Wagner, P. D., Naumann, P. F., and Laravuso, R. B. (1974). Analysis of foreign gas mixtures in gas or blood by gas chromatography. J. Appl. Physiol. 36:600.

29. West, J. B., Wagner, P. D., and Derks, C. M. W. (1974). Gas exchange in distributions of $\dot{V}_A/\dot{Q}$ ratios: the partial pressure-solubility diagram. J. Appl. Physiol. 37:533.

30. Wagner, P. D., Saltzman, H. A., and West, J. B. (1974). Measurement of continuous distributions of ventilation-perfusion ratios: theory. J. Appl. Physiol. 36:585.

31. Evans, J. W., and Wagner, P. D. Limits on $\dot{V}_A/\dot{Q}$ distributions from analysis of experimental inert gas elimination. J. Appl. Physiol., in press.

32. Jaliwala, S. A., Mates, R. E., and Klocke, F. J. (1975). Constrained optimization technique for determination of $\dot{V}_A/\dot{Q}$ distributions from inert gas eliminations. J. Clin. Invest. 55:188.

33. Olszowka, J. A. (1975). Does inert gas exchange data provide enough information to recover $\dot{V}_A/\dot{Q}$ distributions present in the lung? Respir. Physiol. 25:191.

34. Wagner, P. D. A general approach to the evaluation of ventilation-perfusion ratios in normal and abnormal lungs. In press.

35. Wagner, P. D., Laravuso, R. B., Uhl, R. R., and West, J. B. (1974). Continuous distributions of ventilation-perfusion ratios in normal subjects breathing air and 100% O_2. J. Clin. Invest. 54:54.

36. Raine, J. M., and Bishop, J. M. (1963). A − a difference in O_2 tension and physiological dead space in normal man. J. Appl. Physiol. 18:284.

37. Mellemgaard, K. (1966). The alveolar-arterial oxygen difference: its size and components in normal man. Acta Physiol. Scand. 67:10.

38. Wagner, P. D., Laravuso, R. B., Goldzimmer, E., Naumann, P. F., and West, J. B. (1975). Distributions of ventilation-perfusion ratios in dogs with normal and abnormal lungs. J. Appl. Physiol. 38:1099.

39. Ashbaugh, D. G., and Uzawa, T. (1968). Respiratory and hemodynamic changes after injection of free fatty acids. J. Surg. Res. 8:417.

40. West, J. B. (1974). Pulmonary gas exchange in the acutely ill patient. Critical Care Med. 2:171.
41. Briscoe, W. A., Cree, E. M., Filler, J., Houssay, H. E., and Cournand, A. (1960). Lung volume, alveolar ventilation and perfusion interrelationships in chronic pulmonary emphysema. J. Appl. Physiol. 15:785.
42. Dantzker, D. R., Wagner, P. D., and West, J. B. (1975). Instability of lung units with low $\dot{V}_A/\dot{Q}$ ratios during O_2 breathing. J. Appl. Physiol. 38:886.
43. Holland, J., Milic-Emili, J., Macklem, P. T., and Bates, D. V. (1968). Regional distribution of pulmonary ventilation and perfusion in elderly subjects. J. Clin. Invest. 47:81.
44. Lenfant, C. (1965). Effect of high F_{IO_2} on measurement of ventilation-perfusion distribution in man at sea level. Ann. N. Y. Acad. Sci. 121:797.
45. Farhi, L. E., and Olszowka, A. J. (1968). Analysis of alveolar gas exchange in the presence of soluble inert gases. Respir. Physiol. 5:53.
46. Epstein, R. M. (1964). Uptake and execution of nitrous oxide; a prototype of inert gas exchange. Br. J. Anaesth. 36:172.
47. Heller, M. L., Watson, T. R., and Imredy, D. S. (1967). Effects of nitrous oxide uptake on arterial oxygenation. Anesthesiology 28:904.
48. Fink, B. R. (1955). Diffusion anoxia. Anesthesiology 16:511.
49. Rackow, H., Salanitre, E., and Frumin, J. J. (1961). Dilution of alveolar gases during nitrous oxide excretion in man. J. Appl. Physiol. 16:723.
50. West, J. B. (1962). Regional differences in gas exchange in the lung of erect man. J. Appl. Physiol. 17:893.
51. Ross, B. B., and Farhi, L. E. (1960). Dead space ventilation as a determinant in the ventilation-perfusion concept. J. Appl. Physiol. 15:363.
52. West, J. B. (1971). Gas exchange when one lung region inspires from another. J. Appl. Physiol. 30:479.
53. West, J. B. (1969). Ventilation-perfusion inequality and overall gas exchange in computer models of the lung. Respir. Physiol. 7:88.
54. Wagner, P. D., and Evans, J. W. (1975). Comparison of inert gas exchange in series and parallel models of the lung. Physiologist 18:435.
55. Bohr, C. (1909). Uber die spezifische Tätigkeit der Lungen bei der respiratorischen Gasaufnahme und ihr Verhalten zu der durch die Alveolarwand Stattfinden Gasdiffusion. Scand. Arch. Physiol. 22:221.
56. Krogh, A. (1920). The rate of diffusion of gas through animal tissues, with some remarks on the coefficient of invasion. J. Physiol. (London) 52:391.
57. Wagner, P. D., and West, J. B. (1972). Effects of diffusion impairment on O_2 and CO_2 time courses in pulmonary capillaries. J. Appl. Physiol. 33:62.
58. Hill, E. P., Power, G. G., and Longo, L. D. (1973). Mathematical simulation of pulmonary O_2 and CO_2 exchange. Am. J. Physiol. 224:904.
59. Forster, R. E., and Crandall, E. D. (1975). Time course of exchanges between red cells and extracellular fluid during CO_2 uptake. J. Appl. Physiol. 38:710.

International Review of Physiology
Respiratory Physiology II, Volume 14
Edited by John G. Widdicombe
Copyright 1977   University Park Press   Baltimore

4
Respiratory Function
of Hemoglobin

H. BARTELS AND R. BAUMANN

Physiologisches Institut der Medizinischen, Hochschule, Hannover, Germany

MOLECULAR BASIS OF HEMOGLOBIN FUNCTION   108
   Chemical Structure   108
   Molecular Basis for Cooperative Ligand Binding   110
   Oxygen Equilibrium of Hemoglobin   111

CONTROL OF HEMOGLOBIN FUNCTION
  BY ALLOSTERIC EFFECTOR MOLECULES   112
   Protons   112
   Carbon Dioxide   114
   Organic Phosphates   115
   Other Ions   116

SPECIAL ASPECTS OF HEMOGLOBIN FUNCTION   117
   Ontogenetic Aspects   117
     Structure and Function of Embryonic Hemoglobin   117
     Structure and Function of Fetal Hemoglobin   122
   High Altitude   124
     Animals   124
     Human Natives   125
     Human Sojourners   125
   Pathological Hemoglobins   126

Recent years have seen considerable progress in the understanding of the control of hemoglobin function under physiological conditions. The results show a clear

Reviews of special aspects of hemoglobin structure and function are found in references 1, 7, 8, 13, 53, 54, 99, and 100.

pattern, despite the complexity one encounters with respect to comparative data. Through an intricate interplay between metabolites of the red cell and the individual hemoglobin, the functional properties are adjusted to meet the specific physiological demands.

MOLECULAR BASIS OF HEMOGLOBIN FUNCTION

Chemical Structure

Mammalian hemoglobins are chromoproteins with an average molecular weight of around 64,000, consisting of a protein moiety, the globin, and the prosthetic group attached to the globin, i.e., the heme group. The globin part is tetrameric, due to combination of two pairs of dissimilar polypeptide chains which in the case of adult hemoglobins are referred to as α and β chains, respectively. To each chain a hemegroup is attached, consisting of protoporphyrin with a ferrous iron atom in the center which reversibly associates oxygen. Thus, 1 mol of hemoglobin can combine with 4 mol of oxygen.

The primary structure of hemoglobin (i.e., the amino acid sequence of α and β chains) has been elucidated for a number of hemoglobins (1). Comparison of these sequences has led to the proposition that natural selection played a dominant role in the evolution of hemoglobin (2).

The use of x-ray crystallography (3, 4) could resolve the three-dimensional structure of the hemoglobin molecule, that is, a) the degree of helix content of the individual chain (the secondary structure), b) the spatial folding of the chains (their tertiary structure), and c) the relative orientation of the chains toward each other in the tetramer (quaternary structure).

In regard to the secondary structure (Figure 1), all chains have a large amount of α helix (around 80%), helical segments being named with the letters A to H, starting at the α-amino end of the chain. So-called nonhelical segments are designated by the adjoining helical segments (FG, for example). The amino acids are numbered starting from the α-amino end. The tertiary structures of the α and β chains show a high degree of similarity despite the fact that their primary structures are different.

There are two types of contacts between the α and β chains, the first being called $\alpha_1 \beta_1$, the second $\alpha_1 \beta_2$. The $\alpha_1 \beta_2$ contact shows large structural changes upon ligand binding and seems to be important for the cooperativity of oxygen binding to hemoglobin (5).

The most important result of the crystallographic work has been the finding that the quaternary and tertiary structure of the hemoglobin molecule is dependent upon the presence or absence of ligand (5). Thus, the three-dimensional structure of deoxyhemoglobin is different from that of oxygenated hemoglobin, and this is the key to the peculiar functional characteristics of the hemoglobin molecule.

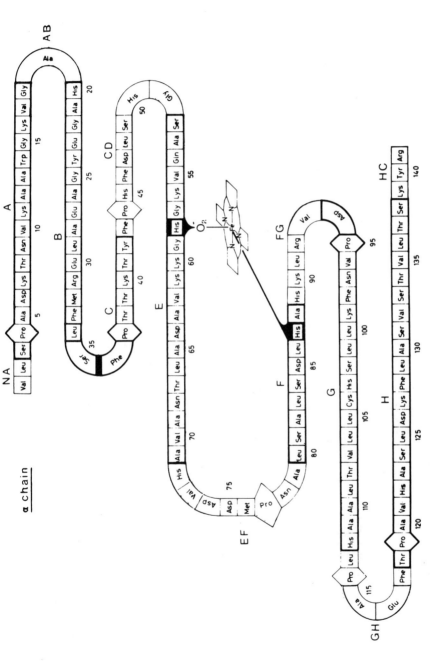

Figure 1. The α chain of human hemoglobin. Reprinted with permission of North-Holland Publishing Company, The Red Blood Cell, Vol. II, pp. 909–934. (1974).

The heme group is embedded in a hydrophobic pocket between helices F and G. This site serves as a protection against auto-oxidation of the iron atom, which readily occurs when the heme group is exposed to a polar environment; Fe^{3+} is, however, incapable of oxygen binding. There are about 60 contacts between the heme protoporphyrin and the globin. The iron atom is linked covalently to the 4 nitrogen atoms of the protoporphyrin pyrrole rings and with one coordination site to His FG8 of the globin. The sixth site is free to bind oxygen. The characteristic spectra of hemoglobin which arise from the heme group are dependent upon the type of ligand bound to position 6 of the iron atom.

The high concentration of hemoglobin (5 mM) found in the red cells of higher vertebrates demands a high solubility. This is achieved because polar side chains of the amino acids are found in abundance on the surface of the molecule, whereas hydrophobic side chains are oriented toward the interior of the molecule. Both the tertiary structure of the individual chain and the quaternary structure of the tetramer are largely dependent upon hydrophobic bonds.

Molecular Basis for Cooperative Ligand Binding

Cooperative ligand binding is characterized by a change in affinity for the ligand during the course of ligation. A positive cooperative process, as in the case of hemoglobin, is characterized by an increase of the affinity of the hemoglobin molecule for oxygen after the first molecule of oxygen has been bound. This type of cooperative binding leads to the typical sigmoidally shaped oxygen equilibrium curve (Figure 2).

Although knowledge about the structures of oxygenated and deoxygenated hemoglobin has reached a high degree of refinement, there is much less information about the dynamics of the structural changes that occur during binding or

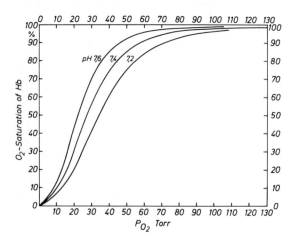

Figure 2. The oxygen dissociation curve of human blood and its dependence on pH (Bohr effect). The position of the normal oxygen dissociation curve corresponds to that at pH 7.4.

release of oxygen. It is well documented that binding of oxygen changes the geometry of the heme, and this in turn alters the tertiary structure of the respective globin chain (5). It is also known that cooperativity in hemoglobin apparently requires the presence of α and β chains, as best illustrated by the fact the human HbH (β_4) lacks cooperativity and shows no structural changes upon ligand binding. The $\alpha_1\beta_2$ contact region in particular is of major importance. Substitutions in this region, as encountered in a number of human hemoglobino-pathies, are invariably associated with decreased cooperativity (6–8).

Because there exist at least two distinct quaternary conformations in hemo-globin corresponding to the liganded and unliganded state, repeated attempts have been made to explain the behavior of the hemoglobin molecule in terms of either the allosteric model of Monod et al. (9) (MWC model) or the "induced fit" model of Koshland et al. (10) (KNF model). The MWC model demands two quaternary states, designated T and R, where T stands for tense (a term used to describe quaternary constraints) and characterizes the low affinity conformation (corresponding in the case of Hb to the deoxy quaternary confirmation) and R denotes the "relaxed state" characterized by a high affinity for the ligand and in this case corresponding to oxyhemoglobin. The main feature of the model is that it demands the switch from one conformation to another to take place con-certedly; that is, all subunits change simultaneously toward the T or R confor-mation. The KNF model, on the other hand, supposes that ligand binding to 1 subunit induces changes in the tertiary structure of the neighboring subunit that alter ligand affinity, and the conformational transition occurs in a sequential manner. Both models have been found to accomodate experimental data with sufficient precision, but that does not prove the validity of either model in respect to hemoglobin function.

For the present discussion, it is sufficient to know that hemoglobin exists in at least two different quaternary structures which are characterized by their different affinities for oxygen and are in equilibrium with each other. The molecules controlling hemoglobin oxygen affinity under physiological condi-tions—namely protons, carbon dioxide, organic phosphates, and other small anions—bind preferentially to the low affinity form, deoxyhemoglobin; there-fore, in their presence the conformation equilibrium is shifted toward the low oxygen affinity conformation.

Oxygen Equilibrium of Hemoglobin

In terms of physiological significance, the sigmoidally shaped oxygen equilib-rium curve warrants sufficient oxygen saturation at the oxygen pressure (P_{O_2}) present normally in the lung and sufficient release of oxygen to tissue at a relatively high P_{O_2}, thus improving conditions for diffusion (see Figure 2).

Hill's number n can be derived from his equation

$$\frac{Y}{100} = \frac{K(P_{O_2})^n}{1 + K(P_{O_2})^n}$$

where Y is the percentage of oxygen saturation, K is the dissociation constant, and, n is the commonly used index of cooperativity. The linearized form of the equation which holds for the saturation range between 20–80% is

$$\frac{\log Y}{100 - Y} = \log K + n \log P_{O_2}$$

This equation permits both evaluation of the oxygen half-saturation pressure (P_{50}) and n. Although Hill's equation proved to be incorrect for description of oxygen binding to hemoglobin, it still remains a useful tool to describe the oxygen equilibrium in the range between 20 and 80%.

For nearly all hemoglobins, n lies between 2.6 and 3.0 in the physiological pH range and is, therefore, the most stable characteristic, whereas other functional properties, such as affinity for oxygen and allosteric effector molecules, are largely different even in closely related species.

The oxygen affinity of hemoglobin is strongly influenced by temperature. Due to the exothermic character of oxygen binding, a rise in temperature leads to a decrease of oxygen affinity. This relationship is described by the temperature coefficient $\Delta\log P_{50}/\Delta T$ which is of the order 0.020 for human hemoglobin. Physiologically, an increase in temperature occurs during muscular work (11) where it augments oxygen delivery. Seasonal changes in oxygen affinity caused by the temperature-dependence of hemoglobin oxygen affinity occur in hibernating animals, in which central body temperature may drop to +1°C.

CONTROL OF HEMOGLOBIN FUNCTION
BY ALLOSTERIC EFFECTOR MOLECULES

The most important step in the evolution of the hemoglobin molecule was the development toward a protein with pronounced positive cooperativity of ligand binding. However, it is also clear that the benefits of cooperative behavior can be fully realized only within a certain range of oxygen affinity (Figure 3). The in vivo half-saturation pressures (P_{50}) for mammalian hemoglobins with normal cooperativity (i.e., n values between 2.6 and 3.0) range between 20 and 50 Torr. It is evident that the limits recorded for P_{50} values of warm blooded animals are not accidental. With P_{50} values higher than 50 Torr, arterial oxygenation is progressively impaired and tolerance to hypoxia diminished. On the other hand, P_{50} values lower than 20 Torr reduce the diffusion gradient for oxygen from blood to tissue and, therefore, hamper oxygen extraction.

The following sections deal with those factors that determine the in vivo oxygen affinity of hemoglobins.

Protons

The classical Bohr effect (12) describes the decrease of hemoglobin oxygen affinity when the hydrogen ion activity is increased by changes in P_{CO_2}. The physiological importance of this effect lies in the facilitation of oxygen release

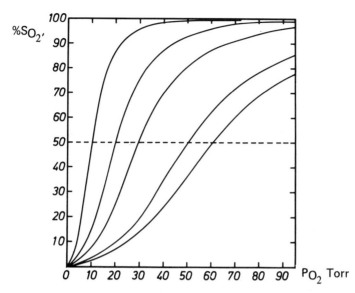

Figure 3. Hemoglobin-oxygen dissociation curves for P_{50} values of 10, 20, 30, 50, 60 Torr. For explanation, see text.

to tissue, because the pH of the blood passing through the capillaries drops continuously due to uptake of carbon dioxide and other acids. Thus, the Bohr effect is particularly important under conditions of heavy muscular exercise (11).

To describe the Bohr effect, the Bohr coefficient $\Delta \log P_{50} / \Delta pH$, which for mammalian blood is of the order of -0.5, is usually used. Wyman (13), using the linked function principle, was the first to show that under certain conditions the Bohr coefficient adequately describes the proton release due to oxygenation.

$$\left(\frac{\Delta \log P_{O_2}}{\Delta pH} \right) S_{O_2} = \left(\frac{\Delta HbH^+}{\Delta HbO_2} \right) P_{O_2}$$

The right-hand term of the equation is referred to as the "Haldane coefficient." This equation implies that hydrogen ion release is linearly related to oxygen uptake. Furthermore, the shape of the oxygen equilibrium curve should not vary with pH, and the activity of other factors interacting with hemoglobin must remain constant during the process of oxygenation. Because differential titration of purified hemoglobin solutions yielded the same value for $\Delta \log P_{O_2} / \Delta pH$ compared to the one obtained by measuring oxygen affinity in dependence of pH, the validity of Wyman's approach was proved (14). Kinetic data showed that hydrogen release was linearly related to ligand binding (15, 16). The molecular basis for the Bohr effect has been clarified in part through the results obtained from crystallographic studies of deoxy- and oxyhemoglobin. In deoxyhemoglobin, certain so-called "salt bridges" are found—namely between the guanidi-nium group of Arg 141 α_1 and the γ-COOH group of Asp 126 α_2, between the terminal COOH group of the β chain and the ϵ-NH$_2$ group of Lys 40 α_1, and between the imidazole of His 146 β_1 and the γ-COOH group of Asp 94 β_1 (5). These residues are invariant in all mammalian hemoglobins so far analyzed in their primary structure (1). The formation of these salt bridges in deoxyhemo-globin raises the pK of the proton binding groups (17) and hence leads to a net uptake of protons upon deoxygenation. Upon ligand binding, these salt bridges are broken and protons are released. Aside from the differential affinity of protons for the purified hemoglobin molecule, the in vivo Bohr effect is also dependent upon the interaction between hemoglobin and carbon dioxide (see under "Carbon Dioxide") as well as on the interaction between hemoglobin and 2,3-diphosphoglycerate (2,3-DPG) (see under "Organic Phosphates"). In addi-tion, it has become evident that oxygen-linked binding of chloride contributes to about 25% of the Bohr effect measured in purified hemoglobin solutions (18) at physiological concentrations of Cl$^-$. Although studies of hemoglobin solutions in vitro help to analyze the various sources that contribute to the Bohr effect, only the determination of the in vivo Bohr effect allows an assessment of the role it plays under physiological conditions.

In recent years, a pronounced dependence of $\Delta \log P_{O_2}/\Delta pH$ on oxygen saturation has been reported for human whole blood (19–21), and the conclu-sion has been drawn that proton release from human hemoglobin is not linearly related to oxygen saturation. This reasoning, however, is not valid because the divergence of the Bohr coefficient and the Haldane coefficient has to be expected since the activity of the main allosteric effector (i.e., 2,3-DPG in mammalian blood) does not remain constant when hemoglobin is liganded. Furthermore, the binding of 2,3-DPG is strongly pH-dependent (22). Both factors preclude that $\Delta \log P_{O_2}/\Delta pH = HbH^+/HbO_2$, and the divergence between both coefficients is in fact a measure of the degree of interaction between other factors and hemoglobin.

Carbon Dioxide

The combination of carbon dioxide with hemoglobin, leading to the formation of carbamate compounds of hemoglobin, occurs according to the following reaction scheme.

$$RNH_3 \overset{K_z}{\rightleftharpoons} RNH_2 + H^+$$

$$RNH_2 + CO_2 \overset{K_c}{\rightleftharpoons} RNHCOO^- + H^+$$

Although the combination of carbon dioxide with hemoglobin was established more than 40 years ago (23), the unequivocal demonstration of oxygen-linked carbamino compounds resulted from the work of Rossi-Bernardi and Roughton (24), who showed that at constant pH and P_{CO_2} more carbon dioxide is bound to deoxyhemoglobin than to oxyhemoglobin. Their results also showed that the Bohr effect $\Delta H^+/\Delta HbO_2$ is reduced in the presence of carbon dioxide, because a substantial number of protons are released when oxygen-linked carbon dioxide is bound to deoxyhemoglobin. Because carbon dioxide combines preferentially with uncharged NH_2 groups, it was long suspected and finally experimentally verified (25) that the α-NH_2 groups of the α and β chain NH_2 termini are the sites involved in the binding of carbon dioxide. On the relative contribution of these groups to oxygen-linked carbamate formation, there has been some controversy, but it now seems clear that the β chain NH_2 termini are the predominant sites (26, 27) in human hemoglobin, as originally suggested by the experiments of Bauer (28). For human adult hemoglobin, the role of oxygen-linked carbamate formation, both with respect to the regulation of oxygen affinity and carbon dioxide transport, is much less important than originally inferred (29). This is because the other allosteric effector molecule (namely, 2,3-DPG), which plays a dominant role in the regulation of the oxygen affinity, competes with carbon dioxide for the β chain NH_2 termini as binding sites. Therefore, in the presence of physiological concentrations of 2,3-DPG, oxygen-linked carbon dioxide formation of human hemoglobin is reduced by about 60%.

The contribution of oxygen-linked carbamate to total carbon dioxide exchange in the lung is thus only 10% (29).

Organic Phosphates

Following the original demonstration of Benesch and Benesch (30) and Chanutin and Curnish (31) that 2,3-DPG greatly reduces human hemoglobin oxygen affinity, numerous subsequent studies have confirmed this finding.

2,3-DPG is the major organic phosphate constituent of most mammalian red cells. In human blood, it is present in a concentration of about 5 mM/liter of red cells. It is bound to human deoxyhemoglobin in a stoichiometric ratio of 1 mol of 2,3-DPG/mol of Hb_4 (32). From chemical as well as crystallographic analyses the binding sites of the molecule have been identified (33–35). 2,3-DPG is bound to the internal cavity of the deoxyhemoglobin molecule, which is lined with polar residues.

The residues involved in the binding of 2,3-DPG are NA β1 (that is the NH_2-terminal amino group of the β chains), His NA β2, His β 143, and Lys β 82. Of major importance in the electrostatic binding of 2,3-DPG are the NH_2-terminal α-NH_2 groups and His β2. The binding of 2,3-DPG leads to changes in the quaternary and tertiary structures of human deoxyhemoglobin, which stabilizes the low affinity conformation (35). The main importance of the organophosphates seems to be an adaption of the intrinsically high hemoglobin oxygen affinity of, for example, human hemoglobin (P_{50} = 11 Torr at physiological pH and temperature in the absence of 2,3-DPG) to physiological demands. Thus, in the presence of 1 mol of 2,3-DPG/mol of hemoglobin, the P_{50} is increased by about 100% to 24 Torr (36).

Comparative studies have shown that the oxygen affinities of a large number of mammalian hemoglobins are rather high in the absence of organic phosphates (37, 38) and that these hemoglobins obviously need to adapt via a potent allosteric effector molecule.

This reasoning is supported by the finding that those groups of mammalian hemoglobins which have a low oxygen affinity in the absence of organic phosphates also have low concentrations of this compound in their erythrocytes and only minimal or no interaction at all with 2,3-DPG under physiological conditions. The best investigated species in this respect are the Artiodactyla hemoglobins in sheep, goat, and cattle and the Felidae hemoglobins.

All of these hemoglobins lack His $\beta 2$, which is deleted in the Artiodactyla hemoglobins (1) and replaced by phenylalanine in cat hemoglobins (39). Felidae hemoglobins of type B have, in addition, an acetylated β chain NH_2 terminus (39), which also interferes with the binding of 2,3-DPG as first demonstrated for human hemoglobin A_{Ic} and F_{Ic} (33). Recently it has been proven (40) that another low affinity hemoglobin belonging to the prosimian primate *Lemur fulvus fulvus* has a substitution at NA B2 and also shows reduced interaction with 2,3-DPG, as well as low concentrations of organic phosphates in the erythrocyte, which also holds for other Lemuroidae (41) so far investigated.

In other classes of animals, there are also organic phosphates involved in the regulation of hemoglobin oxygen affinity. In birds, inositol phosphates take the place of 2,3-DPG (42). In fish, ATP and GTP are the most important organic phosphates (43). All three compounds seem to share the same binding sites and differ only in their affinity for oxy- and deoxyhemoglobin.

In addition to the discovery of the effect on oxygen affinity, it has been established that binding of organic phosphates increases the proton affinity of deoxyhemoglobin (44–46). The binding of 2,3-DPG to deoxyhemoglobin raises the pK of the imidazolinium groups of His $\beta 2$ and His β 143 and of the NH_2-terminal α-NH_2 groups of the β chains, which leads to a net uptake of protons (that is, an increase of $\Delta H^+/\Delta HbO_2$). The Bohr coefficient $\Delta \log P_{O_2}/\Delta pH$ is also increased in the presence of physiological amounts of 2,3-DPG (47); this is, however, an expression of the pH dependence of the binding constants for 2,3-DPG (46).

Finally, there is a further effect of 2,3-DPG on hemoglobin oxygen affinity, which is not dependent upon any specific interaction between 2,3-DPG and the hemoglobin. Because 2,3-DPG is an impermeable anion, an increase of the red cell concentration of this compound leads to a decrease of red cell pH at constant plasma pH (36) due to the Gibbs-Donnan equilibrium. This results in a decrease of hemoglobin oxygen affinity as a consequence of the Bohr effect.

Other Ions

The effect of small anions such as chloride or inorganic phosphate on hemoglobin oxygen affinity is long established (48). Although the binding of these ions is much weaker than that of the organic phosphates, it cannot be neglected in the case of chloride, which is present in a concentration of about 0.1 M in the erythrocyte. This effect is especially obvious in the case of those hemoglobins in which in vivo oxygen affinity is not controlled by 2,3-DPG (40, 49, 50).

There seem to be at least two classes of sites involved in the oxygen-linked binding of chloride (49, 51); they are also responsible for the enhancement of the Bohr effect (18). From x-ray studies it was concluded that small anions bind between the NH_2-terminal α-NH_2 group of the β chains and Lys β 82 (35), sites which are also involved in the binding of organic phosphates. Whereas Lys β 82 seems a likely candidate for chloride binding (52), the NH_2-terminal α-NH_2 groups do not participate in chloride binding (49, 52). There is evidence for other chloride binding sites which are not shared by organic phosphates (51) and remain to be identified.

SPECIAL ASPECTS OF HEMOGLOBIN FUNCTION

Ontogenetic Aspects

During embryonic and fetal development, conditions for oxygen uptake are less favorable than those during lung breathing because of the smaller diffusion gradient for oxygen, the smaller exhange area, and the large diffusion distance in the placenta. A fairly high oxygen affinity of hemoglobin during development would, therefore, be advantageous for oxygen uptake (see under "Oxygen Equilibrium of Hemoglobin"), and, as a matter of fact, all experimental data support this idea because the oxygen affinity of blood during this period is higher than that of the corresponding adult blood.

During the various ontogenetic stages, different hemoglobin types are synthesized, designated as embryonic, fetal, and adult hemoglobin. Synthesis of embryonic hemoglobin starts in isolated blood islands in the yolk sac before a closed circulatory system is established. After the termination of yolk sac erythropoiesis in mammals, the liver and spleen become the most important hemoglobin-synthesizing organs. This change coincides in most species with the onset of the fetal stages of development. Principally, there are two types of hemoglobin that can be synthesized during this period, namely fetal and adult hemoglobin.

Although in some species (e.g., man) embryonic hemoglobin is replaced first by fetal and later by adult hemoglobin (Figure 4), in other species (e.g., pig), there is a direct switch from emybronic to adult hemoglobin (53, 54).

Structure and Function of Embryonic Hemoglobin Embryonic hemoglobin was discovered (55) in human embryos 7–12 weeks old. During the last few years, embryonic hemoglobins have been demonstrated in many species. Because of the difficulties of sampling sufficient amounts of embryonic hemoglobin, functional studies are still rather incomplete.

In man, embryonic hemoglobin consists of three fractions: Gower I ($\epsilon 4$), Gower II ($\alpha_2 \epsilon_2$), and Portland ($\gamma_2 \xi_2$). Until now, only the Portland frac-

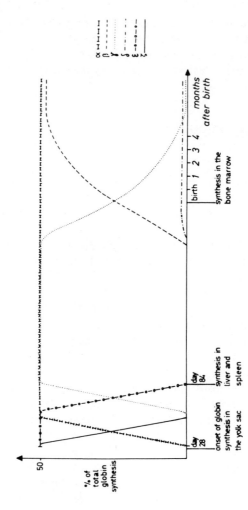

Figure 4. Globin chain synthesis during ontogeny (man). ε and ζ chains are embryonic; γ chains contribute to fetal hemoglobin. Reprinted with permission of University of Göttingen, H. Melderis, doctoral dissertation.

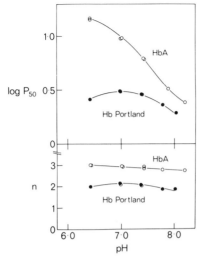

Figure 5. Bohr effect (log P_{50}) and n values of human embryonic hemoglobin (Portland) compared with adult hemoglobin (HbA). Reprinted with permission of FEBS Lett. 49:390 (1975).

tion has been investigated (56) (Figure 5). The oxygen affinity is much higher (P_{50} = 3 Torr at pH 7.2 and 25°C) than for adult hemoglobin (P_{50} = 6.3 Torr). Hill's number is 2, signifying a lower cooperativity, and the Bohr effect reverses at pH 7 compared to pH 6 for adult hemoglobin. This behavior might be explained by a possible lack of His 122 in the δ chain (57). Data on nuclear erythroblasts (58) containing around 30% embryonic hemoglobins showed no significant differences compared with the oxygen binding properties of fetal red cells.

In mice (strain BALB/c), there are also three fractions: E_1 (x_2y_2), E_2 (α_2y_2), and E_3 (α_2z_2). The globin synthesis during ontogeny (59) is shown in Figure 6. The amino acid sequences have been partially elucidated (60). Hemoglobin solutions of embryos (12½ days gestational age) were investigated (61). Figure 7 shows the high affinity of embryonic blood compared to that of adult blood. The Bohr effect (Figure 8) is slightly smaller and reverses at around pH 7.2 instead of at pH 5.8 as for the adult hemoglobin. These characteristics are very similar to hemoglobin Portland (see above paragraph). The influence of 2,3-DPG on oxygen binding is less pronounced in embryonic blood and of minor importance at this stage of development, because only 1.4 mM/liter of red cells (adult 8.1 mM/liter of red cells) were found. The E_2 (x_2y_2) fraction was isolated and showed an even higher oxygen affinity (P_{50} = 7 Torr) than did the three fractions together (62).

The E_1 fraction is the first to appear in mouse embryos. The primary structure of its x chain shows remarkable homology to the ζ chain of human hemoglobin Portland and the x chain of rabbit embryonic hemoglobin, leading to

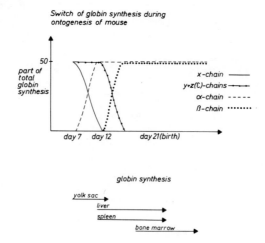

Figure 6. Globin synthesis during ontogeny of mouse (BALB/c). Reprinted with permission of University of Göttingen, H. Melderis, doctoral dissertation.

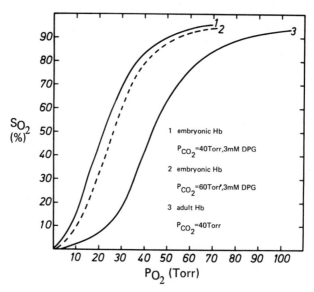

Figure 7. Oxygen dissociation curves of embryonic mouse hemoglobin (12½ days after conception) at 37°C and 40 Torr P_{CO_2} (1) and at 60 Torr P_{CO_2} (2) compared to that of adult mouse hemoglobin (3) (62).

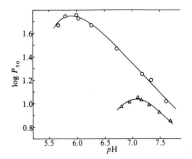

Figure 8. The Bohr effect of embryonic mouse hemoglobin (12½ days after conception) at 37°C (△) compared to that of adult mouse hemoglobin (○). Reprinted with permission of Nature 257:333 (1975).

the conclusion that the x chains represent precursors of the α type hemoglobin chains (60).

In chicken, up to six fractions of embryonic hemoglobin have been identified (63–66). Because of easier availability of embryonic blood, the functions of embryonic chicken hemoglobin have been studied in greater detail. The sequence of globin chain synthesis until hatching is shown in Figure 9. Chicken

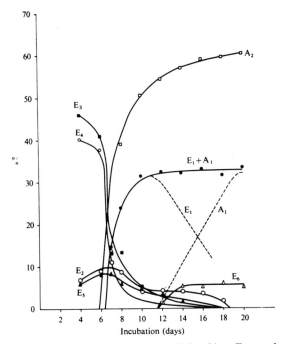

Figure 9. Hemoglobin synthesis in the chicken until hatching. For explanation, see text. Reprinted with permission of J. Embryol. Exp. Med. 28:681 (1972).

embryonic development ends 8½ days after incubation, but embryonic hemo-globin synthesis is continued because of the persistence of the yolk sac in birds until hatching. Yolk sac erythropoiesis is maximum between the 12th and 14th day after incubation (64).

At the 5th day after incubation, Manwell et al. (67) found a very high oxygen affinity of embryonic hemoglobin (as did others (68) at the 6th day) and a smaller Bohr effect (−0.4 instead of −0.67 for adult hemoglobin). The effect of the major allosteric effector inositol hexaphosphate (IHP) on hemoglobins E_3 and E_4 is much less than on the respective adult hemoglobins A_2 and A_1 (68). In blood from the 9th day after incubation until 3 days after hatching, very pronounced changes in the affinity were observed (69–71), showing the highest affinity some days before hatching (Figure 10). During this period, adult hemoglobins A_2 and A_1 account for more than 80% of total hemoglobin (Figure 9). At the 14th day, a high ATP concentration was found which decreased rapidly until day 18 with a concomitant fall of P_{50} (70, 72) (Figure 11). Although the concentration of 2,3-DPG increases during this period, the oxygen affinity has to increase because the effect of 2,3-DPG on hemoglobins A_1 and A_2 is much less than the effect of ATP (73).

Structure and Function of Fetal Hemoglobin The demonstration of a higher alkali resistance of human fetal hemoglobin as compared to adult hemo-globin was the first indication that these hemoglobins are different in their structure (74). Fetal hemoglobins consist generally of two α and two γ chains. The amino acid sequences of several γ chains are known (1).

In all mammals so far investigated, the oxygen affinity of fetal blood was found to be higher than that of adult blood. After birth, the oxygen affinity decreases to the adult level. The time course of this change and the underlying mechanisms are different in different species. The principal factors controlling oxygen affinity during the perinatal period are discussed in the subsequent sections.

In man, the synthesis of β chains leading to the appearance of adult hemoglobin ($α_2β_2$) starts around 6 weeks before birth (Figure 4). At 4 months

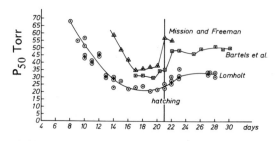

Figure 10. Oxygen half-saturation pressure (P_{50}) of chicken blood during chicken develop-ment (69–71).

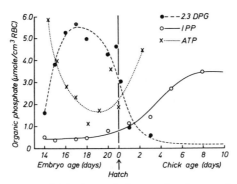

Figure 11. Concentrations of 2,3-DPG, inositol pentaphosphate, and ATP in chicken red cells during development (71, 72).

after birth, adult hemoglobin has almost completely replaced fetal hemoglobin. A small residual synthesis of γ chains persists for the rest of the life.

The higher oxygen affinity of human fetal blood has been known since 1931 (75), but the mechanism responsible has been clarified only recently (76–78). In the absence of 2,3-DPG, both fetal and adult hemoglobin have almost identical oxygen affinities, but the response of fetal hemoglobin to 2,3-DPG is reduced because the γ chains (which correspond to the β chains of adult hemoglobin) lack one binding site for 2,3-DPG. In the β chains, histidine is found at position 143, whereas serine takes this place in the γ chains. Thus, although the concentration of 2,3-DPG is the same in human fetal and adult blood, the oxygen affinity of fetal blood is higher.

In sheep and goats, fetal hemoglobin of both species has a much higher oxygen affinity than has adult hemoglobin, so that replacement of fetal by adult hemoglobin (which starts at birth) automatically decreases oxygen affinity. A high concentration of 2,3-DPG is found during the first 2 weeks after birth. Although 2,3-DPG has no direct influence on the oxygen affinity of either fetal or adult hemoglobin (79), it may contribute to the pronounced fall in red cell pH which occurs after birth (80, 81). This decrease in cell pH is the second mechanism contributing to the postnatal decrease of oxygen affinity in sheep and goats.

During the fetal periods, the dog (82), horse (83), and pig (84–87) synthesize only adult types of hemoglobin which are strongly influenced by 2,3-DPG. Before birth, the red cell concentration of this cofactor is low. Consequently, the oxygen affinity is higher than after birth, when a rapid increase in 2,3-DPG toward adult levels is found, with a concomitant decrease of oxygen affinity.

To arrive at an understanding of the role a high fetal oxygen affinity plays with respect to oxygen transfer in the placenta, P_{O_2}, P_{CO_2}, and pH must be measured in the uterine and umbilical vessels without disturbing placental circulation. This requirement, however, presents considerable experimental difficulties. With the use of indwelling vascular catheters, it has been possible to obtain appropriate samples from conscious pregnant ewes (88), mares, and cows (83). Table 1 gives data from four species in which maternal oxygen affinity differs widely. It is clear that fetal oxygen affinity reflects to some extent the P_{O_2} in the umbilical vein (fetal arterialized blood). Species with the lowest P_{O_2} values have the highest oxygen affinities. The advantage of the higher oxygen affinity becomes obvious particularly in the case of sheep if the oxygen saturation of fetal blood (S_{O_2}) is compared with the value (S_{O_2}') that would be obtained if fetal blood possessed maternal oxygen affinity.

Finally, it should be mentioned that, although considered in some detail here, fetal oxygen affinity is only one part of the complicated gas exchange system in the placenta and certainly not the limiting factor (89).

High Altitude

Sufficient oxygen uptake is the main problem for animals living at high altitude, where oxygen pressure is decreased.

Animals   Species living higher than 3,000 m, presumably for millions of years, have comparatively high blood oxygen affinities. This holds for the Camelidae, which includes the different llamas (*L. glama* (90, 91), vicuña (90), and guanaco (92)) living in the Andes and the camels (bactrians (90) and dromedaries (93)), some of which are living at altitudes above 4,000 m (in Afghanistan). All of these species have a rather high oxygen affinity, with P_{50} values of 20–22 Torr. Two small rodents, the viscacha and the guinea pig of South America, have a higher oxygen affinity than comparable lowland species (90, 94). The same is true for birds living at high altitudes (e.g., the Bolivian goose (90) and the Indian goose (92)) (Table 2).

Table 1. Oxygen saturation (S_{O_2}) of fetal blood at oxygen pressures and pH in the umbilical vein[a]

	Fetal					Maternal
	P_{O_2} (Torr)	pH	P_{50} (Torr)	S_{O_2} (%)	S_{O_2}' (%)	P_{50} (Torr)
Man[b]	35	7.35	22	77.8	69.0	26
Horse	48	7.39	27	82.5	76.5	31
Cattle	38	7.40	25	75.6	53.6	36
Sheep	35	7.40	20	81.9	41.1	40[c]

[a]S_{O_2}, oxygen saturation at which fetal blood arrives with the oxygen half-saturation (P_{50}) of maternal blood. The effectiveness of a higher fetal oxygen affinity is obvious, especially in cattle and sheep.
[b]Newborn, before first breath.
[c]Sheep hemoglobin type B.

Table 2. Oxygen half-saturation pressure (P_{50}) of hemoglobin solutions of the blood of lowland and high alitutude mammals and birds in the presence and absence of organic phosphates

	P_{50} (Torr)				
	Hb, pH 7.2, without cofactors	Hb, pH 7.2, with cofactor	Blood, pH 7.4 (P_{CO_2} = 40 Torr)	(2,3-DPG) (Hb)	(IPP)[a] (Hb)
Man	11.8	24.7	26.6	1.2	
L. guanaco	14.8	20.7	22.5	0.57	
Ansa ansa	6.0	43.1	42.0		0.80
Ansa indiaca	4.6	33.4	29.7		0.87

[a]Inositol pentaphosphate.

A comparison of hemoglobins from lowland species with hemoglobins from high altitude species shows that different mechanisms can be responsible for the higher in vivo oxygen affinity of high altitude species (Table 2). Guanaco hemoglobin has a lower oxygen affinity then human hemoglobin in the absence of 2,3-DPG. However, the interaction with this cofactor and the red cell concentration of 2,3-DPG are reduced in the guanaco and, consequently, the whole blood oxygen affinity is higher in the guanaco than in man. The hemoglobin of *Ansa indiaca* has a higher oxygen affinity than that of *Ansa ansa*. This is also the reason for the higher in vivo oxygen affinity, because both the concentration of inositol phosphate and the response toward it are the same for the two hemoglobins.

Human Natives Residents living in the Andes at high altitudes (95) up to 5,000 m have a slightly lower oxygen affinity (P_{50} = 30 Torr, 4,500 m) compared to residents at sea level (P_{50} = 27 Torr). The 2,3-DPG concentration is significantly higher in the blood of such natives, which explains the lower oxygen affinity. However, the small decrease of oxygen affinity is not the main adaptive mechanism with respect to gas transport in blood. The oxygen capacity is increased from 22 to 28 ml of O_2/100 ml of blood, and thus the arterial oxygen concentration can be kept fairly high (20.5 ml of O_2/100 ml of blood). With an arteriovenous oxygen concentration difference of 5 ml/100 ml, the mixed venous oxygen pressure drops by only 6 Torr (39−33 Torr).

Human Sojourners The oxygen affinity of sojourners at high altitude decreases (P_{50} = 30 Torr (96, 97)) within the first 24 h of exposure. The main cause for this decrease in oxygen affinity is the rapid increase of the concentration of 2,3-DPG, which is caused chiefly by the increase of pH due to hyperventilation. This explains also why the decrease of oxygen affinity is partially cancelled after a few days because of the metabolic compensation of the respiratory alkalosis.

It should be remembered that the in vitro results described above do not represent the in vivo conditions. Taking into account the pH changes during acclimatization, it is found that the in vivo oxygen affinity is practically unchanged in sojourners. The same observations were made in guinea pigs and rats during acute and chronic hypoxia (98).

If one compares the biological significance of changes in the oxygen affinity and oxygen capacity of blood for the acclimatization to high altitude, it is obvious that the increase of oxygen capacity represents by far the most efficient adaptive process.

Pathological Hemoglobins

Whereas impairment of the synthesis of one or more of the globin chains is the cause for the thalassaemia syndromes (for reviews see 99 and 100), hemoglobinopathies are characterized by a qualitative structural change, usually due to substitution of one amino acid. Because human fetal hemoglobin has the structure $\alpha_2 \gamma_2$, many more β chain variants than γ chain variants have been reported, as serious abnormalities of the α chain can be expected to cause early fetal death.

Up to now, about 200 mutant hemoglobins have been detected (8, 100). A great number of them do not affect hemoglobin function or red cell stability. To some extent, the consequences of a substitution can be predicted, and the hemoglobins can be classified according to their molecular pathology, because the structure of normal human hemoglobin is known.

Substitutions at the surface of the molecule do not usually alter hemoglobin function or stability, because they are unlikely to change heme environment tertiary structure or interchain contacts. In a few instances (most notably hemoglobin S), substitution at the surface results in an increased tendency of the molecule to form aggregates, a behavior that is also found in some normally occurring animal hemoglobins (101–103). Hemoglobin S was the first mutant to be discovered and is also the most prevalent. The main characteristic of sickle cell disease is that deoxygenation leads to gelling with subsequent cell damage, and it is assumed that substitution of valine for glutamic acid at position β 6 creates a site in the deoxygenated molecule which can link with another site of an adjacent normal hemoglobin molecule (6, 104). The approach toward possible therapy of hemoglobin S disease is based on the reasoning that, if at any given degree of oxygen saturation the population of molecules in the deoxy conformation can be decreased, the sickling tendency is also reduced. Carbamylation of the end terminal α-NH_2 groups with cyanate (105–107), which impairs binding of 2,3-DPG and also increases intrinsic hemoglobin oxygen affinity (108), has experimentally proven the validity of the concepts. However, limited knowledge of possible harmful side effects of cyanate precludes the clinical use of the drug at the moment.

As mentioned before (under "Chemical Structure"), the structure of the hemoglobin molecule largely depends on nonpolar internal bonds; therefore, uncharged substitutions of internal nonpolar residues usually reduce the stability of the hemoglobin molecule and in some instances lead to gross conformational changes (109). The unstable hemoglobins have an increased tendency to precipitate inside the cell, especially if a heme contact is affected, reducing heme-globin bonding. Globin devoid of heme or with heme only on two chains is particularly unstable.

Most M hemoglobinopathies are caused by substitution of tyrosine for either the proximal or distal histidine in α or β chains. An ionic bond is formed between the phenolic oxygen of tyrosine and the heme iron, which is stabilized in the ferric state and is thus incapable of oxygen binding.

Substitutions at the $\alpha_1\beta_2$ subunit contact usually lead to a reduction of cooperativity, often accompanied by increased oxygen affinity. Increased oxygen affinity is also observed if substitutions occur at positions that are involved in the binding of 2,3-DPG (110) or the alkaline Bohr (111) effect.

From the physiological point of view, those hemoglobin variants with markedly increased or decreased oxygen affinity are perhaps the most interesting in so far as they allow some estimation of the limits within which hemoglobin oxygen affinity can be varied without the need for compensatory mechanisms that ensure oxygen transport and delivery. High affinity variants such as Hb Yakima (112) and Hb Rainier (113) (P_{50} = 12 Torr) both show an increased oxygen capacity (24 ml of O_2/100 ml of blood), and a slight increase in oxygen capacity (22.6 ml of O_2/100 ml of blood) is also found in Hb Chesapeake (114) (P_{50} = 18.6 Torr). Hemoglobin Seattle (115), on the other hand, has a rather low oxygen affinity (P_{50} = 40.5 Torr) and a reduced oxygen capacity (13.2 ml of O_2/100 ml of blood). Thus, within the range of P_{50} values discussed so far, there is an inverse relation between oxygen half-saturation pressure and oxygen capacity. This relation does not extend to Hb Kansas (116) in which oxygen affinity is so low (P_{50} = 70 Torr) that arterial oxygen saturation is greatly reduced (to about 60%). Subjects with Hb Kansas were found to have a nearly normal oxygen capacity. The adjustment of oxygen capacity in these subjects keeps the arteriovenous oxygen concentration difference within normal limits (117) in the resting state. Likewise, cardiac output is normal in this condition. It can be assumed, however, that tolerance of hypoxia or exercise is reduced for carriers of Hb Seattle and Kansas because of a decrease of oxygen reserves.

The fact that hemoglobin oxygen affinity and capacity are interrelated implies that oxygen affinity is a factor involved in the control of erythropoiesis, and measurements of erythropoietin excretion support this view (118).

REFERENCES

1. Dayhoff, M. O. (1972). Atlas of Protein Sequence and Structure. National Biochemical Research Foundation, Washington, D. C.
2. Goodman, M., Moore, G. W., and Matsuda, G. (1975). Darwinian evolution in the genealogy of hemoglobin. Nature 253:603.

3. Perutz, M. F., Muirhead, H., Cox, J. M., and Goamann, L. C. G. (1968). Three dimensional Fourier synthesis of horse oxyhaemoglobin at 2.89 Å resolution: the atomic model. Nature 219:131.
4. Muirhead, H., and Greer, J. (1970). The three dimensional Fourier synthesis of human deoxy haemoglobin at 3.5 Å resolution. Nature 228:516.
5. Perutz, M. F. (1970). Stereochemistry of cooperative effects in haemoglobin. Nature 228:726.
6. Perutz, M. F., and Lehmann, H. (1968). Molecular pathology of human haemoglobin. Nature 219:902.
7. Huisman, T. H. J. (1972). Normal and abnormal human hemoglobins. Adv. Clin. Chem. 15:149.
8. Ranney, H. M., and Lehmann, H. (1975). The hemoglobinopathies. In The Red Blood Cell, Vol. II, pp. 874–908. D. MacN-Surgenor (ed.), Academic Press, New York.
9. Monod, J., Wyman, J., and Changeux, J. P. (1965). On the nature of allosteric transitions: a plausible model. J. Mol. Biol. 12:88.
10. Koshland, D. E., Nemethy, G., and Filmer, D. (1966). Comparison of experimental binding data and theoretical models in proteins containing subunits. Biochemistry 5:365.
11. Thompson, J. M., Dempsey, J. A., Chosy, L. W., Shahadi, N. T., and Reddan, W. G. (1974). Oxygen transport and oxyhemoglobin dissociation during prolonged muscular work. J. Appl. Physiol. 37:658.
12. Bohr, C., Hasselbalch, K., and Krogh, A. (1904). Über einen in biologischer Beziehung wichtigen Einfluss, den die Kohlensäurespannung des Blutes auf dessen Sauerstoffspannung ausübt. Scand. Arch. Physiol. 16:402.
13. Wyman, J. (1948). Heme proteins. Adv. Protein Chem. 4:407.
14. Antonini, E., Wyman, J., Brunori, M., Bucci, E., Fronticelli, C., and Rossi-Fanelli, A. (1963). Studies on the relations between molecular and functional properties of hemoglobin. IV. The Bohr effect in human hemoglobin measured by proton binding. J. Biol. Chem. 238:2950.
15. Antonini, E., Schuster, T. M., Brunori, M., and Wyman, J. (1965). The kinetics of the Bohr effect in the reaction of human hemoglobin with carbon monoxide. J. Biol. Chem. 240:PC 2262.
16. Gray, R. D. (1970). The kinetics of the alkaline Bohr effect of human hemoglobin. J. Biol. Chem. 245:2914.
17. Kilmartin, J. V., Breen, J. J., Roberts, G. C. K., and Ho, C. (1973). Direct measurements of the pK values of an alkaline Bohr group in human hemoglobin. Proc. Natl. Acad. Sci. U.S.A. 70:1246.
18. Rollemaa, H. S., de Bruin, S. H., Janssen, L. H. M., and van Os, G. A. J. (1975). The effect of potassium chloride on the Bohr effect of human haemoglobin. J. Biol. Chem. 250:1333.
19. Siggaard-Andersen, O., and Salling, N. (1971). Oxygen-linked hydrogen binding of human hemoglobin. Effect of carbon dioxide and 2,3-diphosphoglycerate. II. Studies on whole blood. Scand. J. Clin. Lab. Invest. 27:361.
20. Siggaard-Andersen, O., Salling, N., Nörgaard, B., and Rørth, M. (1972). Oxygen-linked hydrogen binding of human hemoglobin. Effects of carbon dioxide and 2,3-diphosphoglycerate. III. Comparison of the Bohr effect and the Haldane effect. Scand. J. Clin. Lab. Invest. 29:185.
21. Garby, L., Robert, M., and Zaar, B. (1972). Proton and carbamino-linked oxygen affinity of normal human blood. Acta Physiol. Scand. 84:482.
22. Benesch, R. E., Benesch, B., and Yu, C. F. (1969). The oxygenation of

hemoglobin in the presence of 2,3-diphosphoglycerate: effect of temperature, pH, ionic strength and hemoglobin concentration. Biochemistry 8:2567.

23. Henriques, O. M. (1929). Über Carb Hämoglobin. Ergeb. Physiol. 28:625.
24. Rossi-Bernardi, L., and Roughton, F. J. W. (1967). The specific influence of carbon dioxide and carbamate compounds on the buffer power and Bohr effect in human haemoglobin solutions. J. Physiol. (Lond.) 189:1.
25. Kilmartin, J. V., and Rossi-Bernardi, L. (1969). Inhibition of CO_2 combination and reduction of the Bohr effect in human haemoglobin chemically modified at its α-amino groups. Nature 222:1243.
26. Perella, M., Kilmartin, J. V., Fogg, J., and Rossi-Bernardi, L. (1975). Identification of the high and low affinity CO_2-binding sites of human haemoglobin. Nature 256:759.
27. Bauer, C., Baumann, R., Engels, U., and Pacyna, B. (1975). The carbon dioxide affinity of various human hemoglobins. J. Biol. Chem. 250:2173.
28. Bauer, C. (1970). Reduction of the carbon dioxide affinity of human haemoglobin solutions by 2,3-diphosphoglycerate. Respir. Physiol. 10:10.
29. Bauer, C., and Schröder, E. (1972). Carbamino compounds of haemoglobin in human adult and fetal blood. J. Physiol. (Lond.), 227:457.
30. Benesch, R., and Benesch, R. E. (1967). The effect of organic phosphates from the human erythrocyte on the allosteric properties of human hemoglobin. Biochem. Biophys. Res. Commun. 26:162.
31. Chanutin, A., and Curnish, R. R. (1967). Effect of organic and inorganic phosphate on the oxygen equilibrium of human erythrocytes. Arch. Biochem. Biophys. 121:96.
32. Benesch, R., Benesch, R. E., and Yu, C. I. (1968). Reciprocal binding of oxygen and diphosphoglycerate by human hemoglobin. Proc. Natl. Acad. Sci. U.S.A. 59:526.
33. Bunn, H. F., and Briehl, R. W. (1970). The interaction of 2,3-diphosphoglycerate with various human hemoglobins. J. Clin. Invest. 49:1088.
34. Benesch, R. E., Benesch, R., Renthal, R., and Maeda, N. (1972). Affinity labeling of the polyphosphate binding site of hemoglobin. Biochemistry 11:3576.
35. Arnone, A. (1972). X-ray diffraction study of binding of 2,3-diphosphoglycerate to human deoxyhaemoglobin. Nature 237:146.
36. Duhm, J. (1971). Effects of 2,3-diphosphoglycerate and other organic phosphate compounds on oxygen affinity and intracellular pH of human erythrocytes. Pfluegers Arch. 326:341.
37. Bunn, H. F. (1971). Differences in the interaction of 2,3-DPG with certain mammalian hemoglobins. Science 172:1049.
38. Bunn, H. F., Seal, U. S., and Scott, A. F. (1974). The role of 2,3-diphosphoglycerate in mediating hemoglobin function of mammalian red cells. Ann. N. Y. Acad. Sci. 241:498.
39. Taketa, F. (1974). Organic phosphates and hemoglobin: structure-function relationships in the feline. Ann. N. Y. Acad. Sci. 241:524.
40. Bonaventura, C., Sullivan, B., and Bonaventura, J. (1974). Effects of pH and anions on functional properties of hemoglobin from Lemur fulvus fulvus. J. Biol. Chem. 249:7039.
41. Dhindsa, D. S., Metcalfe, J., and Hoversland, A. S. (1972). Comparative studies of the respiratory functions of mammalian blood. IX. Ring-tailed

lemur (*Lemur catta*) and black lemur (*Lemur macaco*). Respir. Physiol. 15:331.

42. Vandecasserie, C., Schnek, A. G., and Leonis, J. (1971). Oxygen affinity studies of avian hemoglobin. Eur. J. Biochem. 24:284.

43. Powers, D. A. (1974). Structure, function and molecular ecology of fish hemoglobin. Ann. N. Y. Acad. Sci. 241:472.

44. Riggs, A. (1971). Mechanism of the enhancement of the Bohr effect in mammalian hemoglobins by diphosphoglycerate. Proc. Natl. Acad. Sci. U.S.A. 68:2062.

45. de Bruin, S. H., Janssen, L. H. M., and van Os, G. A. J. (1973). The interaction of 2,3-diphosphoglycerate with human deoxy- and oxy-hemoglobin. Biochem. Biophys. Res. Commun. 55:193.

46. Benesch, R. E., and Rubin, H. (1975). Interaction of hemoglobin with three ligands: organic phosphates and the Bohr effect. Proc. Natl. Acad. Sci. U.S.A. 72:2465.

47. Tomita, S., and Riggs, A. (1971). Studies of the interaction of 2,3-diphosphoglycerate and carbon dioxide with hemoglobin from mouse, man and elephant. J. Biol. Chem. 246:547.

48. Rossi-Fannelli, A., Antonini, E., and Caputo, A. (1961). Studies on the relations between molecular and functional properties of human hemoglobin. II. The effect of salts on the oxygen equilibrium of human hemoglobin. J. Biol. Chem. 236:397.

49. Baumann, R., and Haller, E. A. (1975). Cat haemoglobin A and B: differences in the interaction with Cl⁻, phosphate and CO_2. Biochem. Biophys. Res. Commun. 65:220.

50. Bauer, C., and Jung, H. D. (1975). A comparison of respiratory properties of sheep haemoglobin A and B. J. Comp. Physiol. 102:167.

51. Chiancone, E., Norne, P. E., Forsen, S., Bonaventura, J., Brunori, M., Antonini, E., and Wyman, J. (1975). Identification of chloride binding sites in hemoglobin by nuclear-magnetic resonance quadrupole-relaxation studies of hemoglobin digests. Eur. J. Biochem. 55:385.

52. Nigen, A. M., and Manning, J. M. (1975). The interaction of anions with hemoglobin carbamylated on specific NH_2-terminal residues. J. Biol. Chem. 250:8248.

53. Kleihauer, E., and Stöffler, G. (1968). Embryonic hemoglobins of different animal species: quantitative and qualitative data about production and properties of hemoglobins during early developmental stages of pig, cattle and sheep. Mol. Gen. Genet. 101:59.

54. Kitchen, H., and Brett, I. (1974). Embryonic and fetal hemoglobin in animals. Ann. N. Y. Acad. Sci. 241:653.

55. Drescher, H., and Künzer, W. (1954). Der Blutfarbstoff des menschlichen Feten. Klin. Wochenschr. 32:92.

56. Tuchinda, S., Nagai, K., and Lehmann, H. (1975). Oxygen dissociation curve of haemoglobin Portland. FEBS Lett. 49:390.

57. Kamuzora, H., Jones, R. T., and Lehmann, H. (1974). The ζ-chain, an α-like chain of human embryonic haemoglobin. FEBS Lett. 46:195.

58. Huehns, E. R., and Farooqui, A. M. (1975). Oxygen dissociation properties of human embryonic red cells. Nature 254:335.

59. Melderis, H. (1974). Synthese und Struktur der embryonalen Hämoglobine der Maus: Implikationen für die frühe Erythropoiese des Menschen. Doctoral dissertation, University of Göttingen.

60. Melderis, H., Steinheider, G., and Ostertag, W. (1974). Evidence for a

unique kind of α-type globin chain in early mammalian embryos. Nature 250:774.

61. Bauer, C., Tamm, R., Bartels, R., and Bartels, H. (1975). Oxygen affinity and allosteric effects of embryonic mouse haemoglobin. Nature 257:333.

62. Petschow, D., Bauer, C., and Bartels, H. unpublished results.

63. Fraser, R., Horton, B., Dupourque, D., and Chernoff, A. (1972). The multiple hemoglobins of the chick embryo. J. Cell Physiol. 80:79.

64. Schalekamp, M., Schalekamp, M., van Goor, D., and Slingerland, R. (1972). Re-evaluation of the presence of multiple haemoglobins during the ontogenesis of the chicken. J. Embryol. Exp. Med. 28:681.

65. Bruns, G. A. P., and Ingram, V. M. (1973). Erythropoiesis in the developing chick embryo. Dev. Biol. 30:455.

66. Brown, J. L., and Ingram, V. M. (1974). Structural studies on chick embryonic hemoglobins. J. Biol. Chem. 249:3960.

67. Manwell, C., Baker, C. M. A., and Betz, T. W. (1966). Ontogeny of haemoglobin in the chicken. J. Embryol. Exp. Morphol. 16:65.

68. Cirotto, C., and Geraci, G. (1975). Embryonic chicken hemoglobins: studies on the oxygen equilibrium of two pure components. Comp. Biochem. Physiol. 51A:159.

69. Bartels, H., Hiller, G., and Reinhardt, W. (1966). Oxygen affinity of chicken blood before and after hatching. Respir. Physiol. 1:345.

70. Mission, B. H., and Freeman, B. M. (1972). Organic phosphates and oxygen affinity of chick blood before and after hatching. Respir. Physiol. 14:343.

71. Lomholt, J. P. (1975). Oxygen affinity of bird embryo blood. J. Comp. Physiol. 99:339.

72. Isaacks, R. E., and Harkness, D. R. (1975). 2,3-Diphosphoglycerate in erythrocytes of chick embryos. Science 189:393.

73. Baumann, R., Haller, E. A., and Bartels, H., unpublished results.

74. Körber, E. (1866). Über Differenzen des Blutfarbstoffes. Inaugural dissertation, Dorpat.

75. Haselhorst, G., and Stromberger, K. (1931). Über den Gasgehalt des Nabelschnurblutes vor und nach der Geburt des Kindes und über den Gasaustausch in der Placenta. Z. Geburtshilfe Gynaekol. 100:48.

76. Bauer, C., Ludwig, I., and Ludwig, M. (1968). Different effects of 2,3-DPG and adenosine triphosphate on the oxygen affinity of adult and foetal human haemoglobin. Life Sci. 7:1339.

77. de Verdier, C. H., and Garby, L. (1969). Low binding of 2,3-diphosphoglycerate to haemoglobin F: a contribution to the knowledge of the binding site and an explanation for the high oxygen affinity of fetal blood. Scand. J. Clin. Lab. Invest. 23:149.

78. Tyuma, I., and Shimizu, K. (1969). Different response to organic phosphates of human fetal and adult hemoglobins. Arch. Biochem. Biophys. 129:405.

79. Baumann, R., Bauer, C., and Rathschlag-Schaefer, A. M. (1972). Causes of the postnatal decrease of blood oxygen affinity in lambs. Respir. Physiol. 15:151.

80. Hilpert, P., Fleischmann, R. G., Kempe, D., and Bartels, H. (1963). The Bohr effect related to blood and erythrocyte pH. Am. J. Physiol. 205:337.

81. Battaglia, F. C., McGaughey, H., Makowski, E. L., and Meschia, G. (1970).

Postnatal changes in the oxygen affinity of sheep red cells: a dual role of diphosphoglyceric acid. Am. J. Physiol. 219:217.

82. Dhindsa, D. S., Hoversland, A. S., and Templeton, J. W. (1972). Postnatal changes in oxygen affinity and concentration of 2,3-DPG in dog blood. Biol. Neonate 20:226.

83. Comline, R. S., and Silver, M. (1974). A comparative study of blood gas tensions, oxygen affinity and red cell 2,3-DPG concentrations in foetal and maternal blood in the mare, cow and sow. J. Physiol. (Lond.) 242:805.

84. Duhm, K., and Kim, H. D. (1972). Effect of the rapid postnatal increase of 2,3-diphosphoglycerate concentration in erythrocytes on the oxygen affinity of pig blood. Second International Symposium of Erythrocites, Thrombocytes and Leucocytes. Thieme, Stuttgart.

85. Baumann, R., Teischel, F., Zoch, R., and Bartels, H. (1973). Changes in red cell 2,3-diphosphoglycerate concentration as cause of the postnatal decrease of pig blood oxygen affinity. Respir. Physiol. 19:153.

86. Tweedale, P. M. (1973). DPG and the oxygen affinity of maternal and foetal pig blood and haemoglobins. Respir. Physiol. 19:12.

87. Novy, M. J., Hoversland, A. S., Dhindsa, D. S., and Metcalfe, J. (1973). Blood oxygen affinity and hemoglobin type in adult, new born, and fetal pigs. Respir. Physiol. 19:1.

88. Meschia, G., Makowski, E. L., and Battaglia, F. C. (1970). The use of indwelling catheters in the uterine and umbilical veins of sheep for a description of fetal acid-base balance and oxygenation. Yale J. Biol. Med. 42:154.

89. Longo, L. D., and Bartels, H. (1973). Respiratory gas exchange and blood flow in the placenta. Department of Health, Education, and Welfare, Publication No. NIH 73-361. Washington, D.C.

90. Hall, F. G., Dill, D. B., and Barron, G. (1936). Comparative physiology in high altitudes. J. Cell Comp. Physiol. 8:301.

91. Bartels, H., Hilpert, P., Barbey, K., Betke, K., Riegel, K., Lang, E. M., and Metcalfe, J. (1963). Respiratory functions of blood of the yak, llama, camel, dybowsky deer and African elephant. Am. J. Physiol. 205:331.

92. Petschow, D., Baumann, R., Würdinger, I., and Bauer, C. (1975). Comparative studies of hemoglobin from lowland and highland mammals and birds. Pfluegers Arch. Suppl. 359:R3.

93. Riegel, K., Bartels, H., El Yassin, D., Oufi, J., Kleihauer, E., Parer, J. T., and Metcalfe, J. (1967). Comparative studies of the respiratory functions of mammalian blood. III. Fetal and adult dromedary camel blood. Respir. Physiol. 2:173.

94. Bartels, H., and Harms, H. (1959). Sauerstoffdissoziationskurven des Blutes von Säugetieren. Pflügers Arch. 268:334.

95. Torrance, J. D., Lenfant, C., Cruz, J., and Marticorena, E. (1970/71). Oxygen transport mechanisms in residents at high altitude. Respir. Physiol. 11:1.

96. Lenfant, C., Torrance, J., English, E. Finch, C. A., Reynafarje, C., Ramos, J., and Faura, J. (1968). Effect of altitude on oxygen binding by hemoglobin and on organic phosphate levels. J. Clin. Invest. 47:2652.

97. Mulhausen, R. O., Astrup, P., and Mellemgaard, K. (1968). Oxygen affinity and acid-base status of human blood during exposure to hypoxia and carbon monoxide. Scand. J. Clin. Lab. Invest. Suppl. 103, 22:9.

98. Baumann, R., Bauer, C., and Bartels, H. (1971). Influence of chronic and

acute hypoxia on oxygen affinity and red cell 2,3-diphosphoglycerate of rats and guinea pigs. Respir. Physiol. 11:135.
99. Bank, A., Rifkind, R. A., and Marks, P. A. (1975). The Thalassemia syndromes. *In* The Red Blood Cell, Ed. 2, Vol. II, pp. 909–934. D. MacN-Surgenor (ed.), Academic Press, New York.
100. Lehman, H., and Huntsman, R. G. (1974). Man's Haemoglobins. North-Holland Publishing Company, Oxford.
101. Moon, J. H. (1960). Tactoid formation in deer haemoglobin. Am. J. Physiol. 199:190.
102. Morrow, J. S., Wittebort, R. J., and Gurd, F. R. N. (1974). Ligand-dependent aggregation of chicken hemoglobin A_I. Biochem. Biophys. Res. Commun. 60:1058.
103. Mauk, A. G., Whelan, H. T., and Taketa, F. (1974). "Holly wreath" morphology of feline erythrocytes: the effects of cyanate and 4,4'-dipyridyldisulfide. Proc. Soc. Exp. Biol. Med. 145:578.
104. Murayama, M. (1966). Molecular mechanism of red cell sickling. Science 153:145.
105. Cerami, A., and Manning, J. M. (1971). Potassium cyanate as an inhibitor of the sickling of erythrocytes in vitro. Proc. Natl. Acad. Sci. U.S.A. 68:1180.
106. de Furia, F. G., Miller, D. R., Cerami, A., and Manning, J. M. (1972). The effects of cyanate in vitro on red blood cell metabolism and function in sickle cell anemia. J. Clin. Invest. 51:566.
107. Jensen, M., Bunn, H. F., Halikas, G., Kan, Y. W., and Nathan, D. G. (1973). Effects of cyanate and 2,3-DPG on sickling. J. Clin. Invest. 52:2542.
108. Kilmartin, J. V., Fogg, J., Luzzana, M., and Rossi-Bernardi, L. (1973). Role of the amino groups of the α and β chains of human hemoglobin in oxygen-linked binding of carbon dioxide. J. Biol. Chem. 248:7039.
109. Pulsinelli, P. D. (1973). Structure of deoxyhaemoglobin Yakima: a high affinity mutant form exhibiting oxy-like $\alpha_1\beta_2$ subunit interactions. J. Mol. Biol. 74:57.
110. Bromberg, P. A., Alben, J. O., Bare, G. H., Balcerzak, S. P., Jones, R. T., Brimhall, B., and Padilla, F. (1973). High oxygen affinity variant of haemoglobin (Little Rock) with unique properties. Nature (New Biol.) 243:177.
111. Perutz, M. F., Pulsinelli, P., TenEyck, L., Kilmartin, J. V., Shibata, S., Iduchi, I., Miyaji, T., and Hamilton, H. B. (1971). Haemoglobin Hiroshima and the mechanism of the alkaline Bohr effect. Nature (New Biol.) 232:147.
112. Novy, M. J., Edwards, M. J., and Metcalfe, J. (1967). Hemoglobin Yakima. II. High blood oxygen affinity associated with compensatory erythrocytosis and normal hemodynamics. J. Clin. Invest. 46:1848.
113. Adamson, J. W., Parer, J. T., and Stamatoyannopoulos, G. (1969). Erythrocytosis associated with hemoglobin Rainier: oxygen equilibria and marrow regulation. J. Clin. Invest. 48:1376.
114. Charache, S., Weatherall, D. J., and Clegg, J. B. (1966). Polycythemia associated with a hemoglobinopathy. J. Clin. Invest. 45:813.
115. Stamatoyannopoulos, G., Parer, J. T., and Finch, C. A. (1969). Physiologic implications of a hemoglobin with decreased oxygen affinity (hemoglobin Seattle). N. Engl. J. Med. 281:915.
116. Reissmann, K. R., Ruth, W. E., and Namura, T. (1961). A human hemo-

globin with lowered oxygen affinity and impaired heme-heme interactions. J. Clin. Invest. 40:1826.

117. Parer, J. T. (1970). Oxygen transport in human subjects with hemoglobin
variants having altered oxygen affinity. Respir. Physiol. 9:43.

118. Adamson, J. W. (1968). The erythropoietin/hematocrit relationship in
normal and polycythemic man: implications of marrow regulation.
Blood 32:597.

International Review of Physiology
Respiratory Physiology II, Volume 14
Edited by John G. Widdicombe
Copyright 1977   University Park Press   Baltimore

5
Pulmonary
Circulation
and Fluid Balance

J. M. B. HUGHES

Royal Postgraduate Medical School, Hammersmith Hospital, London, England

FUNCTIONAL ANATOMY OF PULMONARY VESSELS   136
     Morphometry   136
     Extrapulmonary Vessels   138
     Intrapulmonary Noncapillary Vessels   139
     Alveolar Vessels   140

PULMONARY CAPILLARY BED   140
     Vascular Waterfall   140
     Three-zone Model of Distribution of Blood Flow   144
     Effect of Surface Tension   146
     Lung Inflation   148
     Distension   149
     Recruitment   151
     Pulsatile Blood Flow   153

EXTRA-ALVEOLAR VESSELS   154
     Definition   154
     Perivascular Space   154
     Interstitial Pressure   155
     Effect of Lung Inflation: Zone 4   157

HYPOXIC VASOCONSTRICTION   159
     Oxygen Sensitivity of Pulmonary Vessels   159
     Hypoxia and Local $\dot{V}_A/\dot{Q}$ 161
     Possible Mechanisms   164

WATER BALANCE IN LUNG   167
     Ultrastructure of Alveolar Capillary Membranes   167
     Physiological Basis for Protein Transport   170
     Lymphatic Transport   171

Measurement of Lung Water   172
Distribution of Lung Water   175

Up to about 1961, research into the pulmonary circulation in general (1) and hypoxic vasoconstriction in particular (2) was excellently reviewed by Fishman. In the subsequent decade, symposiums on pulmonary vascular smooth muscle and other features of the pulmonary circulation (3) and on the measurement of lung water (4) and pulmonary edema (5) were published.

The last 15 years have seen an expansion of interest and knowledge in certain areas, notably in the effects of gravity on the pulmonary circulation, in the correlation between vascular structure and function, and in the measurement of pulmonary edema. The effect of hypoxia on pulmonary blood vessels has continued to attract much attention. Rather than attempt a comprehensive review, this chapter considers in more detail a few topics of current interest.

FUNCTIONAL ANATOMY OF PULMONARY VESSELS

Morphometry

Morphometric techniques, especially the description of branching systems, were reviewed by Cumming (6), but since then data on the pulmonary circulation from Horsfield and Cummings's laboratory have been published in full by Singhal et al. (7), and it seems pertinent to summarize their findings. From a cast of a human pulmonary arterial tree, the diameter, length, order, and end branches down to 0.8 mm in diameter were measured, together with a sample of structures smaller than this (0.8–0.1 mm diameter). Some of these measurements and some computed values are shown in Table 1. The cast was made from the lungs of a 32-year-old woman free from respiratory disease. The lungs were fixed at a fairly high lung volume (5 liters), and the pulmonary arterial pressure was maintained at 25 cm H_2O during the casting process. The branches were numbered according to the Strahler system of ordering, with the precapillary vessel, one for each alveolus, being number 1 and the main pulmonary artery number 17. Data for orders 1–5 were obtained by extrapolation. Several interesting facts emerge from Table 1. The cross-sectional area of each order increases in a "thumbtack" fashion with a sudden expansion at the precapillary level (order 1), whereas the bronchial tree expands more like a "trumpet." For a pulmonary blood flow of 5 liters min^{-1}, Cumming et al. (8) computed a pressure drop of 0.8 cm H_2O from order 10–1. This calculation of pressure drop was made with the use of Poiseuille's equation for laminar flow. Apart from orders 15–17, Reynolds numbers in the pulmonary arteries are low (<200), well away from the range for turbulent flow (>2,000); nevertheless, the frequent branching

Table 1. Morphometric measurements of human pulmonary arterial tree from pulmonary artery (order 17) to precapillary vessels with computed values for arterial volumes and velocity

Order	No. of branches	Diameter (mm)	Total cross-sectional[a] area (cm^2)	Cumulative volume[b] (ml)	Velocity[c] (cm/s)
17	1.000	30.000	7.07	63.97	11.32
16	3.000	14.830	5.18	80.55	15.44
15	8.000	8.060	4.08	85.00	15.79
14	2.000×10	5.820	5.32	96.01	13.80
13	6.600×10	3.650	6.91	108.37	10.16
12	2.030×10^2	2.090	6.96	115.68	9.01
11	6.750×10^2	1.330	9.38	121.87	6.66
10	2.290×10^3	0.850	12.99	127.96	4.19
9	5.861×10^3	0.525	12.69	131.97	5.92
8	1.756×10^4	0.351	16.99	135.54	4.50
7	5.255×10^4	0.224	20.71	138.40	3.63
6	1.574×10^5	0.138	23.54	140.54	3.19
5	4.713×10^5	0.086	27.38	142.32	2.74
4	1.411×10^6	0.054	32.31	143.74	2.32
3	4.226×10^6	0.034	38.37	144.85	1.96
2	1.266×10^7	0.021	43.85	145.73	1.82
1	3.000×10^8	0.013	398.20	150.92	0.20

From Singhal et al. (1973).
[a]Summed area for all branches in each order.
[b]Total volume added cumulatively from higher to lower orders.
[c]Mean velocity assuming pulmonary blood flow 80 ml s^{-1}.

prevents the establishment of pure laminar flow (9) and pressure drop calculations underestimate the actual impedance. Most of the pulmonary arterial volume is taken up in larger vessels (87% in arteries > 0.8 mm diameter). The volume of the whole cast was 400–500 ml, and it seemed to be equally distributed between arteries, capillaries (vessels < 13 μm diameter), and veins. A capillary volume of 150 ml is about double that calculated by the single breath carbon monoxide technique, perhaps reflecting fuller recruitment and distension of the capillary bed postmorten. There are interesting linear relationships between order number and log diameter, length, and number of branches. This pattern appears to be a common property of naturally occurring branching systems in animals (bile ducts, bronchi, cerebellar dendrites, hepatic arteries, and veins) and nature (rivers, glaciers, and trees).

The intravenous injection of albumin microspheres labeled with radioactive technesium or indium is frequently used to measure regional pulmonary blood flow for physiological experiments and in clinical situations. The microspheres are manufactured to a size ranging from 20–80 μm diameter. Calculations from Singhal's data (7) show that the proportion of the vascular bed obstructed by the microspheres, assuming that 75×10^3 are administered, would be 0.6% for 20-μm spheres, rising to 1.8, 5, and 16% for 35-, 50-, and 80-μm spheres respectively. The smallest microspheres measure the peripheral distribution of blood flow more accurately and are safer.

Extrapulmonary Vessels

At birth, the main pulmonary artery is indistinguishable in its structure from that of the aorta (10). This is not surprising, because in fetal life the pressure within the two vessels is similar. After birth, there is a rapid fall in pulmonary vascular resistance and pulmonary arterial pressure (11) associated with atrophy of the elastic layers. The adult pulmonary artery is a predominantly elastic vessel with a thin medial coat of muscle with about eight layers of elastic tissue interspersed (12); its thickness is only one-fifth of that of the aorta. Changes in caliber of blood vessels are dependent upon the ratio between extensibility and transmural pressure (intravascular minus perivascular pressure). Extensibility may be modified by changes in vascular smooth muscle tone. For extrapulmonary vessels, perivascular pressure is pleural or intrathoracic pressure. Increases of intrathoracic pressure may occur transiently during coughing or continuously during ventilation with a positive end-expiratory pressure; circulatory adjustments usually occur which raise the intravascular pressure to the same extent as for intrathoracic pressure to maintain the caliber and volume of these vessels. Whereas the intravascular and extravascular (pleural or esophageal) pressures can be measured in extrapulmonary vessels with reasonable accuracy, the transmural pressures of vessels within the lung cannot, for technical reasons, be defined very precisely (see under "Effect of Surface Tension" and "Perivascular Space").

Intrapulmonary Noncapillary Vessels

After entering the lung, pulmonary arteries gradually become less elastic and more muscular. The elastic laminae within the medial coat become progressively more fragmented and at about the 9th generation down from the main pulmonary artery (vessels of 2 mm diameter), at the level where bronchial cartilage ceases, the vessels are generally considered to be "muscular" as opposed to "elastic" (12). Nevertheless, elastic laminae within the medial coat do not completely disappear until the bronchiolar level (vessel diameter < 1 mm). The thickness of the medial coat remains fairly constant at 2% of the external diameter for vessels down to 200 μm, but within the acinus the muscular coat increases its thickness to 10% of the external diameter (12). Maximum muscularity appears to occur within the acinus itself, at or peripheral to the alveolar ducts, in vessels of 100–200 μm diameter; between 100 and 30 μm diameter, vessels rapidly lose their muscular coat (12).

The development of the pulmonary arterial tree is of some interest. At birth, the muscularity of vessels greater than 200 μm is twice (4% wall thickness) that of equivalent vessels from the age of 4 months onward (13). In the fetus, muscular arteries extend into the lobule, but not as far as respiratory bronchioles; not until 3 years of age are muscular arteries found in association with alveolar ducts, and full penetration of muscular vessels into the acinus is not found until growth is complete (more than 14 years) (13). The development of muscle in the wall of pulmonary veins starts at 28 weeks' gestation, but unlike the arterial tree, the muscularity of veins remains fairly constant from birth until adult life is achieved. The percentage of wall thickness is about half of that of arteries of equivalent size. A muscular coat is seen in all veins down to 100 μm diameter (14).

There is abundant evidence linking the muscularity of intrapulmonary vessels with local vascular pressure. The changes in muscularity of pulmonary arteries after birth is accompanied by a 5-fold drop in pressure over the first 2 weeks of life as the lungs expand and alveolar oxygen tension rises. Changes in the smaller vessels up to 250 μm have been observed as early as 3 days after birth (13). There are no pressure changes in the venous system during this period and no changes in muscularity (14). Nevertheless, reversal of the direction of pulmonary blood flow in dogs produces venous medial hypertrophy (15). In rats exposed to a low barometric pressure (380 Torr), the muscle coat extends peripherally into the smallest arterial vessels—called by Reid and Meyrick "transfer vessels" (16)—which are normally poorly muscularized or not muscularized. New muscle forms from other vessel wall constituents, possibly the pericyte. Peripheral extension of the arterial muscular coat has also been described in normal human subjects who were born in and lived permanently in Andean villages of Peru above altitudes of 11,300 ft (17). In rats which were removed from a decompression chamber after 37 days and killed after a 37-day recovery period at 760 Torr barometric pressure, the pulmonary hypertensive changes regressed (18). Heath et al. (19) examined the muscularity of pulmonary arteries less than 150 μm diameter in a llama, two dogs, two cats, two bulls, and a cow, all of which were born at and had lived at high altitude. All except the llama had thick-walled pulmonary arteries. This lack of thickness may represent a special adaptation to high altitudes in the case of the llama.

In summary, the pulmonary arterial tree contains a large volume of elastic vessels, which act as a capacitance for the right ventricular stroke volume, in series with a smaller volume of muscular vessels (arteries less than 1 mm diameter) serving as the potential resistive element. The low pulmonary vascular resistance, in relation to the systemic circulation, is associated with a scarcity of muscle in pulmonary vessels less than 100 μm diameter. When these vessels are well muscularized, as with exposure to hypoxia or in fetal life, pulmonary vascular resistance rises significantly.

Alveolar Vessels

Figure 1 is an en face view of part of an alveolar wall from a cat lung perfused with silicone elastomer. This appearance suggested to Fung and Sobin (20) that the capillary bed could be analyzed as if it were two endothelial sheets of tissue held apart by "stays" or "posts" of septal tissue. In contrast, the conventional view of the capillaries, as portrayed in Figure 7 and 8, for example, is that of a series of tubes or tunnels branching repeatedly from feeding arteriole to collecting venule. The capillary bed in the "sheet-flow" concept, as shown schematically in Figure 2 (21), appears to a red cell as an underground parking garage with floor, ceiling, and intervening support posts. The capillary vessels in the alveoli are so short and communicate so frequently with one another that the concept of a "sheet" is more helpful than the usual notion of a series of tubes. Each alveolar capillary membrane consists of a layer of epithelial lining cells and a layer of endothelial cells with an interstitium in between; the total thickness varies from less than 0.2 to 1.2 μm. The interstitium which is gathered together at the posts is composed of basement membranes, collagen fibers, and a gel-like ground substance, mainly hyaluronic acid. In the cat, the volume occupied by the posts in each sheet is about 10% of the volume occupied by the blood (22). The thickness of the vascular sheet varies with the transcapillary pressure (the difference between the capillary vascular pressure and alveolar gas pressure) as is discussed under "Distension."

PULMONARY CAPILLARY BED

Vascular Waterfall

Banister and Torrance (23) in 1960 first showed the importance of alveolar pressure to the pressure-flow relationships of the pulmonary circulation. They perfused isolated cat lungs with steady flows and a constant tracheal pressure.

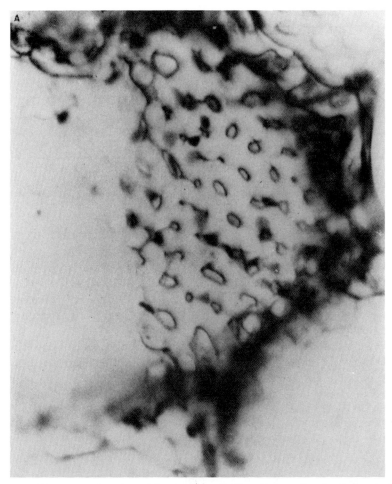

Figure 1. Planar or en face view of the alveolar wall of a cat's lung, showing that part within the depth of focus of the microscope. The lung is perfused with a silicone elastomer. Note the posts in the alveolar wall. Reprinted with permission of J. Appl. Physiol. 26:472 (1969).

Because there was no ventilation, tracheal pressure was the same as alveolar pressure. Figure 3 shows the relationship between blood flow and pulmonary arterial pressure (P_A) at different levels of tracheal (P_T) and venous (P_V) pressure. For the same P_A, flow is strikingly reduced at the higher tracheal pressure (P_T 12, *right*). With P_V at zero, for example, flow at P_A of 8 cm H_2O is about 40 ml min^{-1} at P_T 4 cm H_2O, but falls to zero when P_T is raised to 12 cm H_2O. This happens because the thin-walled vessels in the alveolar septa collapse when the pressure in the alveoli exeeds the intravascular pressure, as shown in Figure 4; consequently, there will be no flow when P_T exceeds P_A. What is less

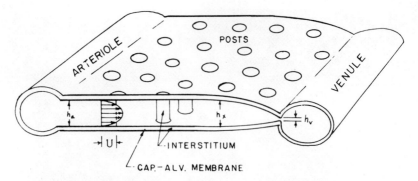

Figure 2. Diagram of the sheet-flow concept of the pulmonary capillary bed. U represents mean flow velocity with a profile as indicated, and h the thickness of the sheet at the arterial (a), mean capillary (x), and venous (v) ends of the alveolar sheet. Reprinted with permission of Microvosc. Res. 7:89 (1974).

obvious, but clearly shown in Figure 3 (*right*), is that P_V has no influence on the pressure-flow relationship when it is itself less than P_T. The pressure-flow lines at P_T 12 for $P_V 0$ and $P_V 8$ are virtually superimposed. Banister and Torrance (23) drew an analogy with the Starling resistor method of controlling extracorporeal blood flow (Figure 5). Generally, the driving pressure for flow through a tube is the pressure difference between inlet and outlet (upstream minus downstream pressure), but, if the tubing is collapsible and enclosed within a chamber, the driving pressure for flow depends upon the level of the downstream pressure relative to chamber pressure. When the latter exceeds downstream pressure, a

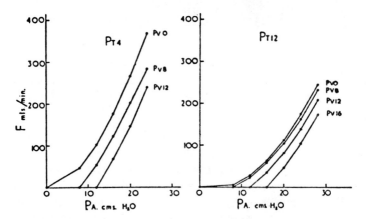

Figure 3. Relationship between blood flow (F) and pulmonary arterial pressure (P_A) at different levels of venous pressure (P_v). Airway or tracheal (P_T) pressure was changed from 4 cm H_2O (*left*) to 12 cm H_2O (*right*). Reprinted with permission of Q. J. Exp. Physiol. 45:352 (1960).

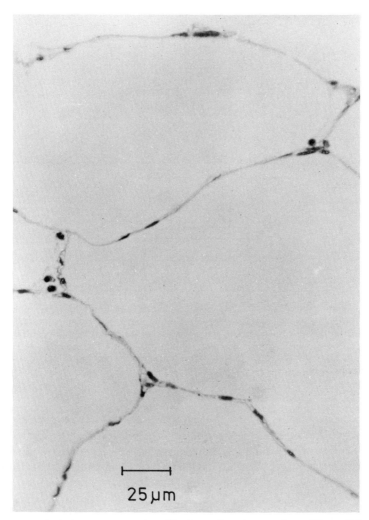

Figure 4. Histological appearance of rapidly frozen lung in zone 1 conditions. Pulmonary arterial pressure was 24 cm H_2O less than alveolar pressure. Note complete collapse of lung capillaries except at the junctions of two or three alveolar walls. Reprinted with permission of J. Appl. Physiol. 26:65 (1969).

constriction develops at the downstream end of the tube. The pressure at the collapse point equals chamber pressure because the tube does not resist collapse, and the driving pressure becomes upstream minus chamber pressure. Under these conditions, downstream pressure no longer influences the pressure-flow relationships, just as the height of a waterfall (or sluice) is irrelevant to the flow of water over it. In models, instability develops and the collapse may extend upstream but the first point of closure is at the downstream end.

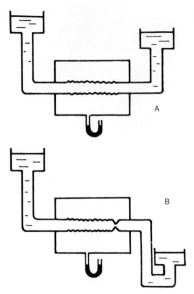

Figure 5. Model to illustrate a Starling resistor with a thin wall collapsible rubber tube enclosed within a chamber. When outflow pressure is higher than chamber pressure, flow is determined by inflow minus outflow pressure in the ordinary way (*A*). By contrast, when downstream pressure is less then chamber pressure, the rubber tube collapses at its downstream end and flow is determined by the difference between upstream pressure and chamber pressure (*B*).

The characteristics of flow through a Starling resistor were set out more formally by Permutt et al. (24), and this model enabled them to account for a number of experimental findings of their own and of previous workers. The notion of the Starling resistor has many applications in circulatory and respiratory physiology.

Three-zone Model of Distribution of Blood Flow

It is convenient to introduce here the well known model of West et al. (25) of pulmonary blood flow distribution, because the terms zone 1, 2, and 3 describe, in a shorthand way, relationships between pulmonary arterial, alveolar, and venous pressures which will be referred to frequently.

In general, the behavior of pulmonary blood flow in relation to arterial, alveolar, and venous pressures can be predicted from the experiments of Banister and Torrance (23) and Permutt et al. (24). Nevertheless, it was West and his colleagues who linked the concept of the vascular waterfall with the influence of gravity on the distribution of blood flow. They perfused an isolated left lung of a greyhound dog (in the vertical position these lungs are 30–35 cm in height) at known pulmonary arterial, alveolar, and venous pressures. The distribution of blood flow was measured by injecting ^{133}Xe in solution into the main pulmonary artery and scanning the lung for radioactivity with a pair of moving counters during an apneic period.

Figure 6 sets out in diagrammatic form a typical distribution of blood flow in the vertical lung in relation to vascular and alveolar pressures. Zone 1 is that part of the lung where alveolar pressure exceeds arterial pressure. Alveolar pressure in Figure 6 is shown as atmospheric (during quiet breathing, alveolar pressure does not depart by more than 1 cm H_2O from that level). Measurements of blood flow with ^{133}Xe show no perfusion in this zone, and histological sections confirm that most of the small vessels up to 30 μm in diameter are collapsed (Figure 4).

In zone 2, pulmonary arterial pressure exceeds alveolar pressure, but alveolar exceeds venous. As with the Starling resistor (Figure 5), the driving pressure for flow is arterial minus alveolar pressure. Because the former increases by 1 cm H_2O/cm of distance because of gravity, whereas alveolar pressure remains constant, the driving pressure and flow increase down this zone. Histological examination of the lung in zone 2 in Figure 7 shows that many capillaries are open and filled with red cells; in other parts of the septum capillaries remain collapsed as they are in zone 1. The gradual opening up of new capillary channels with distance down zone 2 is discussed later (see under "Recruitment").

Zone 3 is that part of the lung where venous pressure exceeds alveolar pressure. The driving pressure for flow remains fixed in this zone because arterial and venous pressures are increasing equally per cm of distance. Nevertheless, vascular resistance steadily decreases with distance down zone 3 and flow increases. The reason for this is capillary distension and recruitment (see under "Distension" and "Recruitment"), which can be clearly seen if the histological appearance of the lung in zone 3 (Figure 8) is compared with that in zone 2 (Figure 7). Early measurements, from which Figure 6 was drawn, suggested a slower increase in flow in zone 3 than in zone 2, but a later study under carefully controlled conditions showed that the rate of increase of blood

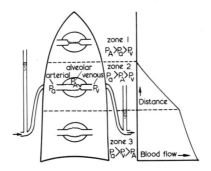

Figure 6. Diagram to explain the influence of pulmonary arterial, venous, and alveolar pressures on the distribution of blood flow. Reprinted with permission of J. Appl. Physiol. 19:713 (1964).

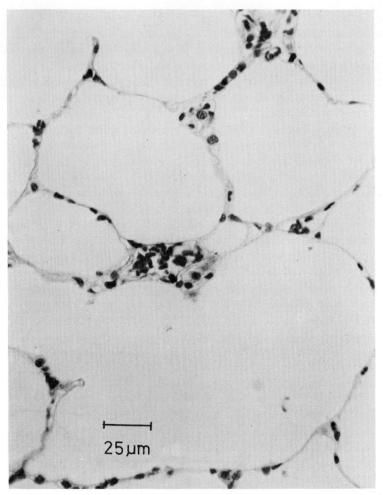

Figure 7. Histological appearance of rapidly frozen lung in zone 2 conditions. Note capillaries in the alveolar septa contain red cells, but the filling is patchy. Reprinted with permission of J. Appl. Physiol. 26:65 (1969).

flow/cm was the same in zone 2 and zone 3 (26). According to sheet-flow theory most of the pressure drop in the alveolar vessels occurs at the downstream end in both zones 2 and 3 so that the hemodynamic conditions may be the same whether or not venous exceeds alveolar pressure (20).

Note that the three-zone model examines the influence of only those vessels exposed to alveolar pressure, i.e., capillaries. The contribution of extra-alveolar vessels to the distribution of blood flow is examined under "Perivascular Space."

Effect of Surface Tension

The pressure surrounding alveolar septal vessels is strictly the pericapillary or septal interstitial pressure, and this may or may not be the equivalent of alveolar

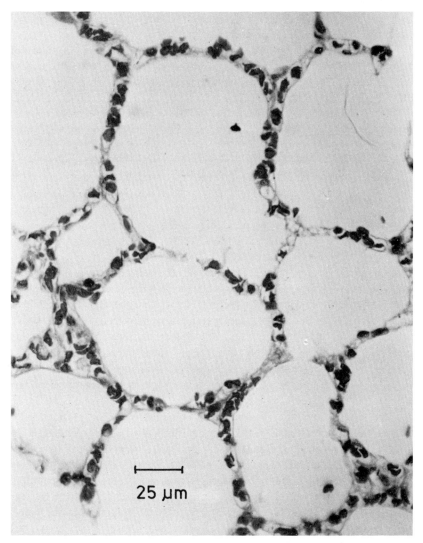

Figure 8. Histological appearance of rapidly frozen lung in zone 3 conditions. Pulmonary venous pressure exceeded alveolar pressure by 44 cm H_2O. Note capillary distension compared with Figures 5 and 8. Reprinted with permission of J. Appl. Physiol. 26:65 (1969).

pressure. The curved surface of the alveolar epithelial membrane supports a pressure difference across itself by virtue of the air-liquid interface between alveolar gas and the lining layer of pulmonary surfactant. This pressure difference, which is due to surface tension, is less than one would predict from the surface tension of water or saline solution and the radius of curvature of the surface (law of Laplace), because the lining layer (dipalmitoyl lecithin) has a very low surface tension. Nevertheless, for a spherical airspace, surface tension, however feeble, lowers the pressure on the capillary side of the epithelial membrane relative to that in alveolar gas.

The consequences of surface tension are 2-fold. First, some flow occurs in those parts of air-filled lungs in which alveolar pressure is equal to or greater than arterial pressure, but not in saline-filled lungs in which the air-liquid interface has been abolished (27). Secondly, surfactant exhibits hysteresis, having a much lower tension when the surface is being compressed than during expansion. For the same alveolar pressure, flow ceased when arterial pressure equaled alveolar pressure on deflation, but not until arterial pressure fell to about 3 cm H_2O below alveolar pressure on inflation (28). Similarly, Pain and West (29), by measuring regional blood flow with radioactive xenon, found that blood flow rose an average of 4 cm higher up the lung (for the same vascular and alveolar pressures) on inflation than at the same volume on deflation. The effect of surface forces is to make pericapillary pressure up to 6 cm H_2O less than alveolar pressure after large inflations. During tidal breathing, the effect is smaller.

It is unlikely that surface tension affects pericapillary pressure equally throughout the capillary bed. The alveolar sac is more hexagonal than spherical in shape, and videomicroscopic pictures show that the alveolar walls at the pleural surface fold and unfold during respiratory movements (30). Most of the capillaries along the alveolar septum lie flush with the alveolar wall or even bulge into it (Figure 8). The radius of curvature and the effect of surface tension here must be minimal, or even reversed. Nevertheless, for capillaries which lie at the junction of two alveolar septa, so-called "corner vessles," the radius of curvature may be greater, and pericapillary pressure may become as much as 10 cm H_2O less than alveolar pressure. Histological examination of rapidly frozen dog lungs showed that corner vessels contained significantly more red cells even when alveolar pressure exceeded arterial by 24 cm H_2O, although the capillaries in the remainder of the septum were collapsed (31). Rosenzweig et al. (32) showed that blood could flow from the arterial to venous sides of the circulation in excised dog lungs when alveolar pressure exceeded vascular pressure by 10–15 cm H_2O. India ink injections demonstrated that the communications were the corner vessels. For the same vascular and alveolar pressures, the corner vessel flow was greater at high lung volumes and transpulmonary pressures. At high lung volumes, corner vessels are probably exposed to radial forces arising from the expansion of the lung (see under "Extra-alveolar Vessels"), in addition to purely surface forces.

Lung Inflation

When lung volume and transpulmonary pressure are increased from 10–25 cm H_2O and the relationship between vascular and alveolar pressures is held constant, the volume of blood in alveolar vessels decreases and mean capillary width diminishes to half its previous value (31). Because the capillaries are the major constituent of the alveolar septum and share in the increase in septal length which occurs with inflation, a simultaneous decrease in width would be expected if Poisson's ratio was less than 1. Poisson's ratio for lung tissue has recently been measured and found to be 0.3 (33). Narrowing of the pulmonary capillary bed is probably the major cause of the rise in pulmonary vascular resistance which occurs with negative pressure inflation of the lungs (i.e., at constant alveolar pressure) (34). The behavior of alveolar vessels at lower levels of inflation (<10 cm H_2O transpulmonary pressure) is not known.

Distension

Figure 9, redrawn from Glazier et al. (31), shows changes in capillary width at right angles to the alveolar septum under conditions of low (zone 2) and high (zone 3) venous pressure. The surface of perfused dog lungs was frozen instantaneously by pouring on liquid freon cooled to $-150°C$ by liquid nitrogen. For zone 2 measurements, the abscissa is the equivalent (in cm H_2O) of pulmonary arterial pressure, alveolar pressure being the zero point. In zone 3, distance is equivalent to the venous pressure (in cm H_2O), because both arterial and venous pressures are increasing by 1 cm H_2O/cm of distance. Under both conditions, a 50% increase in capillary width takes place for an increase of arterial pressure of 30 cm H_2O. In zone 3, it was possible to increase venous pressure to 100 cm H_2O, but no significant increase in capillary width was seen after 50 cm H_2O and comparatively little after 20 cm H_2O.

Because the measurements in Figure 9 were made at the same lung volume and alveolar pressure, the mean capillary pressures in zones 2 and 3 must have been the same at the same capillary width. For example, capillary pressure 10 cm down zone 3 was equivalent to that 20 cm down zone 2. Because the

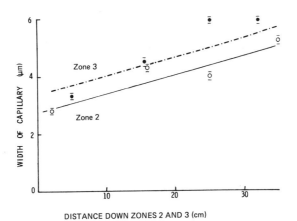

Figure 9. Mean capillary width measured in rapidly frozen lungs plotted against distance under zone 2 and 3 conditions. Note extensibility (Δ width/cm of distance) is the same in both zones. On the *abscissa*, capillary pressure increases by 1 cm H_2O/cm of distance, but see text for details of absolute levels. Redrawn and reprinted with permission of J. Appl. Physiol. 26:65 (1969).

arterial-venous pressure difference in zone 3 experiments of Glazier et al. (31) was kept low ($<$4 cm H_2O), the capillary pressure in zone 3 in the example must have been 12 ± 2 cm H_2O; at that capillary pressure in zone 2, the arterial pressure was 20 cm H_2O and the alveolar pressure 0 cm H_2O. Thus, in zone 2, mean capillary pressure appeared to be a little closer to upstream (arterial) than downstream (alveolar) pressure. Fung and Sobin (20), on the other hand, predicted from sheet-flow theory that mean capillary pressure would be much closer to the upstream pressure.

Measurements of the thickness of the alveolar sheet in the cat lung with the use of silicone elastomer injections by Sobin et al. (35) showed a linear relationship between width and capillary pressure up to 30 cm H_2O (Figure 10). At 10 cm H_2O distending pressure, the rate of increase of sheet thickness in the cat was 0.234 μm cm H_2O^{-1} compared to 0.122 in the dog. Measurements by Glazier et al. (31) in the dog refer to mean capillary width, whereas those of Sobin et al. (35) represent the maximum width. At 30 cm H_2O distending pressure in the dog lung, the compliance of the capillaries drops to 0.079 μm cm H_2O^{-1}, but it increases to 0.173 at 5 cm H_2O.

Pulmonary capillaries appear to be more distensible than some systemic capillaries, for example, those in the mesentery of the frog which show insignificant distension up to 100 Torr intracapillary pressure (36). This rigidity may be caused by the supporting structures, but in the lung, pulmonary capillaries are relatively unsupported by connective tissue in the direction of the alveolar space.

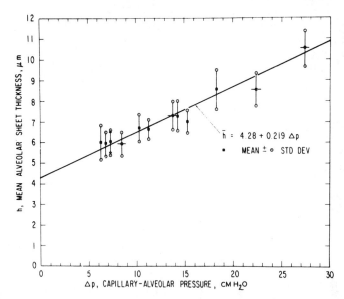

Figure 10. Thickness of alveolar sheet in the cat lung plotted against capillary pressure. Note the linear increase in thickness with a slope greater than that in the dog in Figure 9. Reprinted with permission of Circ. Res. 30:440 (1972).

Recruitment

Figure 7 shows the appearance of the alveolar septum in a dog lung rapidly frozen while being perfused under zone 2 conditions. The filling of the septa is patchy, some parts containing no red cells, whereas others contain many erythrocytes. As perfusion pressure increased in zone 2 and in zone 3, there was a pronounced increase in septal filling. Glazier et al. (31) measured mean capillary width and counted the number of red cells per unit of septal length at different levels in the lung corresponding to different perfusing pressures in zones 2 and 3. The number of red cells in the alveolar septum is a function of the number of open capillaries (recruitment) and their width (distension). From these measurements, the relative roles of recruitment and distension in zones 2 and 3 could be computed (Figure 11). Warrell et al. (37), using a similar freezing technique, measured the number of open capillaries/mm of septal length as shown in Figure 12. The percentage of the septum occupied by open capillaries was 17% for a perfusion pressure of 1 cm H_2O and 88% at 87 cm H_2O. Note the rapid increase in the number of open capillaries at low perfusion pressures. This corresponds to the situation in the upper third of the upright lung in vivo, a region in which there is a rapid increase in blood flow.

Analysis of the phenomena of recruitment and distensibility requires knowledge of the distribution of vascular pressures through the capillary network. For example, in zone 3, is mean capillary pressure closer to upstream (arterial) or downstream (venous) pressure? The assumption that capillary pressure reflects

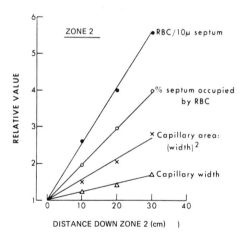

Figure 11. Number of red blood cells (*RBC*)/10 μm septum (*upper line*) and capillary width (*lower line*) plotted against distance down zone 2. Capillary width has been squared, showing increase in capillary area due to expansion of already open vessels, i.e., distension. The difference between the line for capillary area and for the number of red blood cells per unit of septal length (*uppermost line*), i.e., total blood content of septum, represents recruitment of new vessels. In zone 2, approximately one-half the increase in red cell volume per unit of septal length is due to recruitment of new vessels and one-half to distension. Reprinted with permission of J. Appl. Physiol. 26:65 (1969).

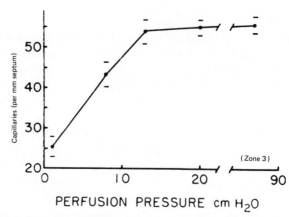

Figure 12. Number of open capillaries per unit of septal length in rapidly frozen lungs at different perfusion pressures in zone 2 and zone 3 conditions. Note rapid increase in capillary recruitment in the first 15 cm of zone 2. Reprinted with permission of J. Appl. Physiol. 32:346 (1972).

changes in venous pressure has led to some arguments about the relative roles of recruitment and distensibility. Permutt et al. (38) found that most of the changes in capillary blood volume, as reflected by the diffusing capacity for carbon monoxide, were closely related to changes in pulmonary arterial pressure, but not to pulmonary venous pressure. In the frozen lung preparation, Glazier et al. (31) found that septal filling in zone 3 reflected arterial (upstream) pressure more closely then venous pressure. They compared a small arterial-venous (A-V) pressure difference (3 cm H_2O) with a large one (17 cm H_2O) and found that the number of red cells in the septum at the high A-V difference was equivalent to that 17 cm H_2O higher with a low A-V difference for equivalent levels of venous pressure. With reverse perfusion, the capillaries again appeared to "see" upstream pressure. The lack of influence of venous pressure on the filling of the capillary bed seemed to argue in favor of recruitment as the determinant of septal filling and against distensibility, although this conflicted with the histological evidence.

Fung and Sobin (20), on the other hand, attributed changes in capillary blood volume principally to distensibility. Because of the large compliance of pulmonary capillaries (Figure 9) and the alveolar sheet (Figure 10), they predicted that most of the pressure drop must occur at the downstream end of the capillary bed in zones 2 and 3. If this were so, then recruitment and distensibility would both depend on upstream rather than downstream pressure, and some of the difficulties in interpretation would be removed. Fung and Sobin (20) do not consider capillary recruitment in their sheet-flow analysis, but there is abundant morphological (Figures 10 and 11) and physiological (see under "Measurement of Lung Water") evidence that it occurs.

As regards the mechanism of recruitment, it was originally suggested that as pulmonary arterial pressure rises the critical opening pressures of muscular pulmonary arterioles are exceeded and more of the capillary bed opens up. With the rapid freezing technique, Warrell et al. (37) compared capillary filling in adjacent septa with those more widely separated. They found no evidence that recruitment occurred on the basis of arteriolar domains, because unevenness of filling was as great within as between adjacent septa. Recently, West et al. (39) examined a model network of the pulmonary capillary bed. The capillary opening pressures and resistance were chosen. Figure 13 shows an example of the flow pattern in such a network as arterial pressure is increased in steps. Initially, a preferential channel of elements with low critical pressures opens up. More channels are recruited as arterial pressure increases, so that vascular resistance decreases even if there is no distension. In the channel marked by the asterisk (Figure 13), flow reversal occurs between B and D, because of the changing relationship between the pressure difference across the segment and its critical pressure. It is not known whether the microcirculation behaves in this way, but West et al. (39) have calculated that critical pressures of less than 0.02 cm H_2O would be required.

Pulsatile Blood Flow

Acceleration of the blood with each systole was observed by Stephen Hales (40) in 1731 in the course of his studies on the capillary circulation of the frog lung. Lee and Dubois (41) showed in human subjects in a plethysmograph pulsatile uptake of nitrous oxide by the lung during breathholding. Pulsatile flow

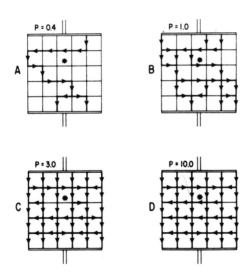

Figure 13. Examples of flow patterns in a network of channels simulating a part of the pulmonary capillary bed as upstream pressure was raised in steps. *P*, the input pressure in arbitrary units. In *A*, a low resistance channel has opened up, and in *B*, *C*, and *D*, further recruitment has occurred. Note that the element marked by the *asterisk* shows reversal of flow between *B* and *D*. Reprinted with permission of J. Appl. Physiol. 39:976 (1975).

has been seen on the surface of the lung by direct microscopy (42). In the main pulmonary artery, the systolic-diastolic pressure difference (pulse pressure) may be as much as 16 cm H_2O recumbent and 11.5 cm H_2O sitting (43). Maloney and his colleagues (44) examined the transmission of the pulmonary artery pressure wave down to the pulmonary capillaries. At 0.1 Hz, about 50% of the incident pressure wave was transmitted to the collapsible vessels. At 1 Hz, this was reduced to 30%. The mean-to-peak pulmonary arterial pressure in the vertical lung in man is about 7 cm H_2O. About one-third of this is transmitted to the capillaries; thus, there would be a 2-cm difference in the height to which the blood flow rises during the cardiac cycle.

EXTRA-ALVEOLAR VESSELS

Definition

The previous section dealt with the small vessels of the lung lying in and around the alveolar septa, often referred to as "alveolar vessels." Extra-alveolar vessels include most arteries and veins larger than about 30 μm diameter and although the anatomical boundary between the two types of vessels is not precise, the operational definition, in terms of function, is quite strict. Macklin (45) and Howell et al. (46) filled the vessels of excised lungs with latex or kerosene, neither of which was able to penetrate into capillaries because of surface tension effects. When the lungs were inflated with positive pressure, further filling of the vessels occurred, although alveolar pressure had risen relative to vascular pressure. On the other hand, if continuity had been established between all vessels, with saline solution filling for example, the same maneuver caused fluid to move out of the lungs. Thus arose the concept of the "expanded" and "compressed" parts of the vascular bed. It was clear that the expanded compartment containing all the larger vessels was not exposed to alveolar pressure but to a pressure lower than this. Because lung expansion is roughly isotropic, with alveolar width and depth increasing proportionately, structures embedded in the parenchyma, such as vessels and bronchi, will increase their dimensions in roughly similar fashion. In brief, the forces expanding the lung operate similarly on the vessels and bronchi. Thus, at a first approximation, extra-alveolar vessels are exposed to lung-distending pressure; in other words, their perivascular pressure equals pleural pressure. This is discussed further under "Interstitial Pressure."

Perivascular Space

Figure 14 shows a small pulmonary venule surrounded by lung parenchyma. The interstitial space separating the vessel wall from alveolar structures is in places extremely thin, less than 5 μm thick; elsewhere it has probably been disturbed by the fixation process. Its outer (alveolar) aspect is bounded by a limiting membrane which is continuous with the adjacent alveolar wall. The perivascular compartment is essentially a potential space; it is the main pathway for lym-

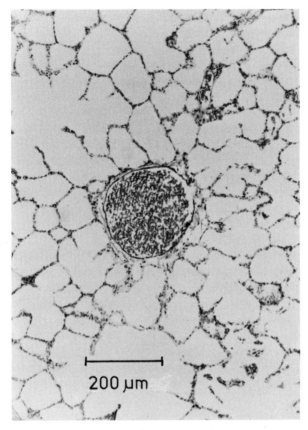

Figure 14. Histological section from a dog lung showing a pulmonary venule and its thin perivascular space surrounded by alveolar tissue.

phatic clearance and it becomes swollen and engorged in pulmonary edema. Interstitial ground substance (hyaluronic acid), lymph vessels, nerves, vasa vasorum, collagen fibers, and a variety of cells including mast cells are found throughout this space. The perivascular space surrounding pulmonary arteries is continuous with that belonging to the neighboring bronchus or bronchiole. Several authors have demonstrated that dye can track along these spaces from small vessels to the hilum of the lung (47, 48).

Interstitial Pressure

It is easy to see from Figure 14 how the parenchyma of the lung can distend extra-alveolar vessels by virtue of radial traction. If vessels (or bronchi) make a perfect fit within the lung so that the distending pressure of the adjacent alveoli is the same as for all other alveoli (i.e., no local distortion), the pressure in the perivascular space (interstitial pressure) will equal pleural pressure. But if these structures do not expand sufficiently to fill the space left for them by the parenchyma, the pressures exerted on them by the surrounding alveolar structures may be considerable. Permutt (49), for example, showed that the pressure surrounding extra-alveolar vessels could fall until it was 17 cm H_2O below pleural pressure. In these experiments, excised lungs were kept in zone 1 conditions with burettes attached to the main artery and vein. As the lungs were inflated, the level of the burettes was lowered to keep the volume of the extra-alveolar vessels constant. Of course, if the vessels were allowed to fill as the lung expanded, as would happen in life, the perivascular pressures would not become so negative. Others have shown that peribronchial pressure behaves similarly if intrabronchial expansion is restricted when the lungs are inflated. Hughes et al. (50) showed that peribronchial pressure could fall by at least 15 cm H_2O relative to pleural pressure. Mead et al. (51) have proposed a theory of lung elasticity which explains how mechanical interdependence between neighboring structures acts as an important stabilizing factor against local collapse or overexpansion.

With excised lobes, Benjamin et al. (52) measured extra-alveolar arterial and venous dimensions after insufflating tantalum dust into the vessels. As the lung expanded from the undistended state to 7 cm H_2O transpulmonary pressure (P_{TP}), at a constant vessel diameter, the change of perivascular pressure was about 2 cm H_2O/cm H_2O change of P_{TP}, but at higher lung volumes this fell to 0.5 cm H_2O/cm H_2O P_{TP} (see their Figure 9). At first sight, this result appears to conflict with theory and previous experiments which suggest that at high lung volumes the mechanical linkage between vessels and parenchyma would be greater, not less, as suggested by these results. In fact, the relationship between perivascular pressure and pleural pressure will depend upon the matching of vascular volume to local parenchymal volume. (The compliance of the limiting membrane in relation to that of the lung should also be taken into account.) The introduction of mismatching of one relative to the other alters perivascular pressure for two reasons: 1) the recoil pressure of the surrounding alveolar tissue now operates on a different surface area, and the distending force (pressure X area) alters, and 2) local tissue stress changes in proportion to the distortion brought about by the change of vessel dimensions. In the case of bronchi, the contribution of these two factors has been analyzed (50). In the experiments of Benjamin et al. (52), the vessels in the undistended state had intravascular pressures of 15 cm H_2O or more and were close to maximum size. At low lung volumes, they may have been too large for the lung, causing considerable distortion of the adjacent alveoli; hence, the large change in perivascular pressure relative to pleural pressure. At larger lung volumes, the matching between vascular and alveolar volumes may have improved so that perivascular pressure began to approach pleural pressure.

Thus, there is no easy answer to the question: what is interstitial pressure? For extra-alveolar vessels, the perivascular interstitial pressure is related to pleural pressure, but it may be profoundly modified by local geometrical factors such as the diameter of the vessel, the characteristics of the limiting membrane, and the stress-strain characteristics of the adjacent alveoli, particularly when they are distorted.

Effect of Lung Inflation: Zone 4

Careful measurements of the distribution of blood flow in vertical lungs obtained by scanning the lungs with a pair of scintillation counters after intravenous administration of [133] Xe generally show a reduction of blood flow in the most dependent part of the lung (26). This is somewhat surprising in view of the three-zone model of the lung (Figure 6), because vascular pressures are highest at the base of the lung. Figure 15 shows the distribution of blood flow in an isolated lung as transpulmonary pressure was increased stepwise from 10 to 20 cm H_2O. Note the reduction of blood flow over the most dependent part of the lung at P_{TP} 10 cm H_2O and its gradual elimination at higher lung volumes. The increase of resistance at the base is located in extra-alveolar vessels, not alveolar vessels, for the following reasons. There was no evidence that gas trapping gave a high alveolar pressure locally, nor can surface tension effects (see under "Effect of Surface Tension") explain these changes. Inflation expands extra-alveolar vessels but narrows alveolar ones (see under "Lung Inflation"). Lastly, the extent of the zone of reduced blood flow, which was apparent at low and intermediate lung volumes, could be increased and decreased by infusions of vasoconstrictor (5-hydroxytryptamine) and vasodilatator (isoprenaline) drugs.

It was of interest that a similar reduction of blood flow was found in the dependent part of the lung when measurements of blood flow distribution were made in the upright man (53), as shown in Figure 16. As in the excised lung, the zone of reduced flow was eliminated at high lung volumes. Early measurements of the distribution of blood flow in man, showing a steep gradient from base to apex as at total lung capacity (TLC) in Figure 16, were invariably made during

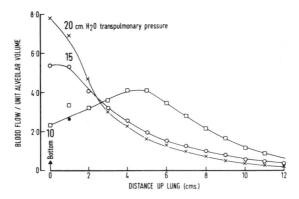

Figure 15. Effect of change of lung volume on the zone of reduced blood flow caused by interstitial pressure in an isolated dog lung. Note that as transpulmonary pressure is raised the zone becomes less marked until it disappears at a transpulmonary pressure of 20 cm H_2O. Reprinted with permission of J. Appl. Physiol. 25:701 (1968).

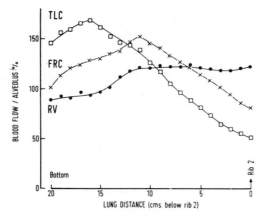

Figure 16. Distribution of blood flow plotted against lung distance at three lung volumes—total lung capacity (*TLC*), functional residual capacity (*FRC*), and residual volume (*RV*). *Points* represent the mean values of the right and left lungs of eight normal subjects. Note the reduction of flow over the lowermost 10 cm of the lung which is marked at low lung volumes but is reduced at full inflation. Reprinted with permission of Respir. Physiol. 4:58 (1968).

breathholding close to full inflation (54); in fact, the distribution of blood flow in erect man during normal breathing is more accurately represented by the functional residual capacity (FRC) line in Figure 16. The reduction in blood flow which extends over the bottom third of the lung at the end-expiratory volume (FRC) becomes so marked at low lung volumes that apical blood flow actually exceeds that at the base. When the change of blood flow/cm of distance is running counter to that expected on the basis of gravity, the extra-alveolar vessels must be exerting the dominant influence over local vascular resistance. At residual volume (RV), extra-alveolar vessels are responsible for the distribution of flow throughout the entire lung. As a result of these findings, the three-zone model of the lung (Figure 6) has been modified to take account of the effect of changes in interstitial pressure on the extra-alveolar vessels. The decrease in blood flow at the base of the lung was designated zone 4 (Figure 17).

How does the perivascular pressure rise sufficiently in the dependent parts of the lung to narrow the caliber of the extra-alveolar vessels? It is known that the dependent parts of the lung are less well expanded than the upper zones, both from direct estimation of alveolar size in dog lungs frozen in situ (55) and from measurements with radioactive gases in man (56). Nevertheless, the gradient of pleural surface pressure of 0.25–0.3 cm H_2O/cm of distance (57) is scarcely sufficient to explain the abrupt change from zone 3 to zone 4 in the face of a 1 cm H_2O/cm of distance increase of intravascular pressure due to gravity, even though pleural and perivascular pressures may differ significantly. Some more complicated geometrical factors must be involved. In Figure 16, intravenous ^{133}Xe arrived in the lung at the appropriate lung volume, but radioactive counting was carried out at full inflation. Therefore, zone 4 at FRC was

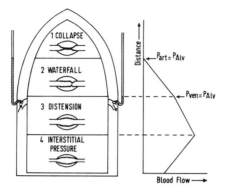

Figure 17. Modification of the three-zone diagram, shown in Figure 6, to include the effects of increased interstitial pressure in the dependent zone. Because of an increase in vascular resistance of the extra-alveolar vessels in this zone, blood flow is reduced. Reprinted with permission of Respir. Physiol. 4:58 (1968).

probably only 6–8 cm in height, about half being above the dome of the diaphragm and half below. It is possible that there is some mechanical distortion of extra-alveolar vessels just above and below the dome of the diaphragm which disappears (though not completely) when the lung is expanded. The pattern of blood flow at low volumes (RV) is similar to that at FRC for the lower 10 cm, but flow remains uniform over the middle and upper zones instead of declining. Again, it is unlikely that the gradient of perivascular pressure matches that for intravascular pressure. Anthonisen and Milic-Emili (58), who made measurements similar to those in Figure 16 without looking low enough in the lung to see zone 4, found (in one subject) an increase of pulmonary wedge pressure of more than 20 Torr at residual volume with an open glottis. A rise of pulmonary arterial pressure of this amount (or more) might explain a relatively uniform distribution of blood flow over the upper two-thirds of the lung at residual volume. The cause of zone 4 in the isolated lung remains unexplained; there was no correlation with edema.

HYPOXIC VASOCONSTRICTION

Oxygen Sensitivity of Pulmonary Vessels

Hypoxic pulmonary vasoconstriction, a well known phenomenon in mammals, was not extensively investigated until 1945 when von Euler and Liljestrand (59) published their classic paper "Observations on the pulmonary arterial blood pressure in the cat." They observed a rise in pulmonary arterial pressure when cats were given hypoxic of hypercapnic mixtures to breathe, and they speculated that local vasoconstriction would allow blood flow to be adjusted according to the efficiency of aeration. Unilateral hypoxia has been used often as a model for the effects of hypoxia on the pulmonary circulation (60), and many studies have shown a redistribution of pulmonary blood flow in man breathing 5–10% oxygen in one lung (61–63). Without pulmonary venous sampling from both lungs, the application of the Fick principle is indirect; Arborelius (64) neatly overcame this problem by injecting an insoluble isotope (^{85} Kr) intravenously and collecting the radioactivity from each lung in Douglas bags. His research (65) represents the most extensive study of unilateral hypoxia in man. The relationship between the change in relative perfusion in the hypoxic lung and inhaled oxygen concentration is plotted in Figure 18.

Stimulus-response curves of pulmonary vessels to changes of oxygen tension were first published by Barer and her colleagues (66). In anesthetized open-chest cats and dogs, blood flow and gas tensions were measured in a pulmonary vein while ventilating the lobe it drained with different gas mixtures. The effect of lowering alveolar oxygen tension on lobar flow in the cat is shown in Figure 19. Some ingenious experiments were carried out by Grant et al. (67) to test the oxygen sensitivity of pulmonary vessels at a lobular or local level in a spontaneously breathing preparation. They chose a small South American mammal, the coatimundi (*Nasua nasua*), because in this species the interlobular fibrous septa are unusually well developed to the exclusion of collateral air flow between subsegments of a lobe. A bronchial catheter with a 3 mm diameter tip was wedged in an airway subtending a group of lobules whose tidal volume was <1% of the tidal volume of the lung as a whole. Figure 20 shows changes of lobule blood flow and ventilation-perfusion ratio ($\dot{V}_A/\dot{Q}$) as the inspired gas composition was altered from 30% to 5% oxygen. With alveolar hypoxia, there was marked vasoconstriction, but no changes in ventilation, hence the high

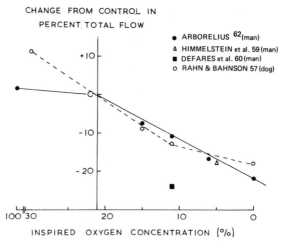

Figure 18. Unilateral hypoxia in awake man and anesthetized dog, showing relationship between inspired oxygen concentration to one lung and its share of the total blood flow. Redrawn and reprinted with permission of M. Arborelius, Ph.D. thesis, Falkmens Bokhandel, Malmo.

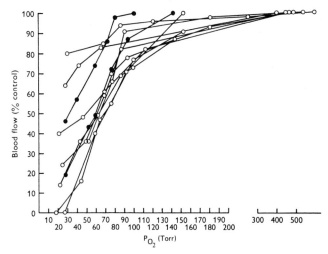

Figure 19. Relationship between left lower lobe blood flow in open-chest anesthetized cats and P_{O_2} of pulmonary venous blood draining the lobe. The lobe was ventilated with different inspired gas mixtures, while the rest of the lung was breathing air (*closed circles*) or 100% oxygen (*open circles*). Reprinted with permission of J. Physiol. (Lond. 211:139 (1970).

$\dot{V}_A/\dot{Q}$ ratios. The subsegmental response to oxygen tension was linear over a wide range of $P_{A_{O_2}}$ (40–150 Torr) with a 1 Torr change of alveolar P_{O_2} leading to a 2% change in local perfusion. Differences between the response in coatis and that in cats, dogs, and man (Figures 18, 19, and 20) may represent a species difference, because the pulmonary arterial vessels in coatis are unusually well muscularized. On the other hand, the responsiveness of pulmonary vessels at a subsegmental level in vivo has yet to be tested in other species.

Hypoxia and Local $\dot{V}_A/\dot{Q}$

The role played by the local pulmonary circulation in maintaining constant local alveolar gas tensions is shown in Figure 21. The response of a lobule in terms of its perfusion, ventilation-perfusion ratio, and alveolar P_{O_2} is shown as local alveolar ventilation was increased and decreased stepwise at 1.5 and 9.5 min by altering the lobule instrumental dead space. Total and alveolar ventilation of the rest of the lung did not change. Continuous monitoring of $\dot{V}_A/\dot{Q}$ and $P_{A_{O_2}}$ shows that changes of $P_{A_{O_2}}$ in response to increases or decreases in $\dot{V}_A$ were accompanied by substantial and rapid changes in blood flow. Had there been no change of perfusion from the control value (3.0 ml min^{-1}), the $\dot{V}_A/\dot{Q}$ ratio would have risen to 1.4 and later decreased to 0.19, as marked by *horizontal bars*; as a consequence, $P_{A_{O_2}}$ would have increased to 122 Torr (instead of 109.5) and fallen to 66 Torr (instead of 83.5). Remarkably, alveolar $P_{A_{CO_2}}$ throughout this period only changed from 31.7 to 33.8 Torr, suggesting that the stimulus was provided by alterations in P_{O_2}.

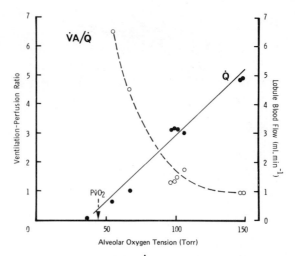

Figure 20. Ventilation-perfusion ratio ($\dot{V}_A/\dot{Q}$) and blood flow of a group of lobules in right lower lobe of coatimundi lung (closed-chest preparation) plotted against lobule alveolar oxygen tension (P_{AO_2}) as the oxygen concentration of inspired gas to the lobule was varied between 30 and 5%. *Arrow* marks the level of mixed venous oxygen tension. Reprinted with permission of J. Appl. Physiol. 40:216 (1976).

The response of $\dot{V}_A/\dot{Q}$ and P_{AO_2} locally with an initial overshoot settling down to a steady level has the hallmark of a negative feedback system in which a primary decrease of P_{AO_2} causes a secondary decrease in $\dot{Q}$, and a primary decrease in $\dot{Q}$ causes a secondary increase in P_{AO_2}. Grant et al. (67) have used control system theory to analyze the gain or efficiency of local pulmonary hypoxic vasoconstriction. As a measure of homeostasis, they used "open loop gain" (OLG), defined as

$$\text{OLG} = \frac{(dP_{AO_2}/d\dot{V}_A) \text{ open}}{(dP_{AO_2}/d\dot{V}_A) \text{ closed}}$$

where $(dP_{AO_2}/d\dot{V}_A)$ open is the change of P_{AO_2}/unit of change of alveolar ventilation if hypoxic vasoconstriction did not exist and $(dP_{AO_2}/d\dot{V}_A)$ closed is the smaller change of P_{AO_2}/unit of change of $\dot{V}_A$ in the presence of hypoxic vasoconstriction. The open loop level of P_{AO_2} is reflected in the *horizontal bars* in Figure 21, whereas the *experimental points* reflect the closed loop condition. Grant et al. (67) should be consulted for further details.

The relationship between OLG at different levels of local P_{AO_2} and $\dot{V}_A/\dot{Q}$ is shown in Figure 22. The bell-shaped curve is caused by the interaction of the sigmoid-shaped oxygen dissociation curve with the linear relationship between local flow and P_{AO_2} (Figure 20). From OLG, a minification ratio (M) can be obtained; $M = 1/(1 + \text{OLG})$, where M as a percentage is the diminution of P_{AO_2}

or $\dot{V}_A/\dot{Q}$ compared with a passive system. For example, an open loop gain of 0.8, corresponding to the highest level in Figure 22, means that only 55% of the change expected from a passive (open loop) system actually occurred; with near-perfect control, less than 1% change would occur. The highest values of OLG were found in the P_{AO_2} range 70–90 Torr and outside these limits the gain due to feedback declined markedly. At best, the system has only a 45% efficiency. Ross et al. (68) examined the efficiency of local vasodilatation in maintaining a constant oxygen supply to the hind limb of the dog. As arterial oxygen saturation (SA_{O_2}) was lowered, local blood flow increased. OLG was greater than 10 as SA_{O_2} was lowered from 100 to 70% giving an efficiency of more than 90%; but when SA_{O_2} was 30%, OLG had fallen 1.0. Although measurements of oxygen supply to systemic tissues cannot be compared directly

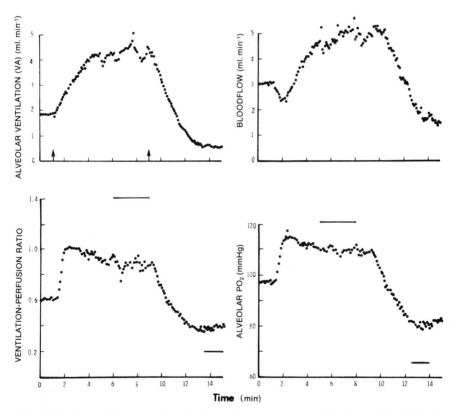

Figure 21. Analysis in a coatimundi lung of changes over a 15-min period of lobule perfusion, ventilation-perfusion ratio $(\dot{V}_A/\dot{Q})$, and alveolar oxygen tension (P_{AO_2}), as alveolar ventilation was increased or decreased as indicated by *arrows. Horizontal lines* indicate the steady state values for $\dot{V}_A/\dot{Q}$ and P_{AO_2} which would have occurred had perfusion remained at its initial value (3.0 ml min^{-1}). Reprinted with permission of J. Appl. Physiol. 40:216 (1976).

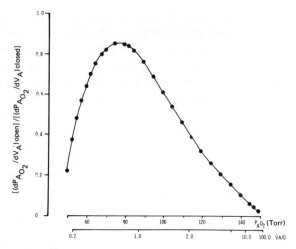

Figure 22. Open loop gain (see text) for hypoxic vasoconstriction plotted against local alveolar oxygen tension and local ventilation-perfusion ratio (log scale). The ability of the local pulmonary circulation to stabilize $P_{A_{O_2}}$ and $\dot{V}_A/\dot{Q}$ is greatest in the physiological range but is relatively poor outside these limits. Reprinted with permission of J. Appl. Physiol. 40:216 (1976).

with the maintenance of a constant alveolar P_{O_2} or local $\dot{V}_A/\dot{Q}$, the systemic circulation appears better equipped to maintain a constant tissue oxygen tension than the pulmonary circulation. Fishman (2) concluded that passive influences were more important than vasomotor activity in the regulation of the pulmonary circulation and that alveolar gas tensions contributed only a fine adjustment.

Possible Mechanisms

The mechanism of hypoxic pulmonary vasoconstriction is by no means settled, and some possibilities are outlined in Figure 23. The situation is confusing, to say the least.

There is extensive parasympathetic and sympathetic innervation of pulmonary arteries and veins down to 30 μm vessels (69). The nervous control of pulmonary blood vessels and reflexes associated with them have been reviewed by Daly and Hebb (70). In general, sympathectomy (71) or α-adrenoceptor blockade (72–74) decreases pulmonary vascular resistance, and β blockade with propranolol or sympathetic stimulation increases it. Nevertheless, the interaction between adrenergic mechanisms and the vasoconstrictor effect of alveolar hypoxia varies from species to species. Cervical sympathectomy appears to reduce the hypoxic vasoconstriction in dogs (75) but not in cats (59), fetal lambs (71), or newborn calves (76). On the other hand, chemical denervation with α-receptor blocking drugs such as phenoxybenzamine or thymoxamine diminishes the hypoxic response in cats (72, 73), but not in dogs (74, 77) or calves (78). In cats, β-blockade enhanced the response to hypoxia (72, 73). Thus,

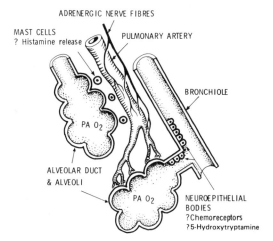

Figure 23. Schematic diagram of small pulmonary artery, bronchiole, alveolar ducts, and alveoli to illustrate some mechanisms which may take part in the hypoxic pressure response. The low alveolar oxygen tension (P_{AO_2}) may be sensed by a) specialized chemoreceptor tissue (neuroepithelial bodies) in terminal airways, b) perivascular mast cells, and c) directly by the pulmonary artery wall. Adrenergic mechanisms may play a role either by direct neural donnections with the central nervous system or by stimulation locally by tissue or humoral mediators. Reprinted with permission of Bull. Physiopathol. Respir. 11:921 (1975).

under certain conditions, adrenergic mechanisms may play a role in modulating hypoxic vasoconstriction.

Because hypoxic vasoconstriction is easily elicited in isolated denervated lungs (79), a possible mechanism is direct diffusion of the low P_{O_2} in mixed venous blood or alveolar gas to the smooth muscle cells in the pulmonary arterial wall. Unfortunately, the behavior of isolated pulmonary arterial strips in response to hypoxia is difficult to assess. After an extensive series of studies, Lloyd (80) concluded that pulmonary arterial strips constricted maximally in the P_{O_2} range 250–100 Torr. This is outside the range at which constriction is seen in vivo. Hypoxic vascular responses are temperature-sensitive (81) and fragile, marked vasoconstriction being obtained with histamine or 5-hydroxytryptamine long after hypoxic vasoconstriction has disappeared. Duke and Killick (79) found that enzyme inhibitors such as sodium monoiodoacetate abolished the hypoxic response in isolated lungs. This suggests that metabolic activity is involved rather than direct smooth muscle membrane depolarization.

There has been considerable interest in the possibility of local synthesis by lung tissue of vasoconstrictors. The mast cell, which is found in abundance in the perivascular and peribronchial spaces, seems well placed for such a role, and for a long time histamine, which is present in mast cells, was the favorite candidate as a mediator of the hypoxic response. Claims have been made for (82) and against

(83) the release of histamine from the hypoxic lung. Similarly, antihistamines may (84) or may not (74) block the hypoxic response in dogs. Mast cells, which contain histamine, proliferate in rats exposed to chronic hypoxia (85, 86), but disodium cromoglycate, which inhibits mast cell degranulation in vitro did not prevent hypoxic vasoconstriction in acute experiments in dogs and cats (74) nor the development of pulmonary hypertension in rats exposed to hypoxia for 3–4 weeks (86). Although histamine is a potent vasoconstrictor in the oxygenated lung, under hypoxic conditions in the neonatal calf (87) and dog lung (74), it acts as a vasodilator. Neither 5-hydroxytryptamine (73) nor prostaglandins of the $F_{2\alpha}$ series (88–90), both potent vasoconstrictors, appear to mediate the hypoxic response. A recent study has shown in rat lungs that the presence of angiotensin II, in amounts insufficient to cause vasoconstriction, was necessary for a significant pressor response to hypoxia to occur (91). Lung tissue contains an endopeptidase enzyme which converts the relatively inactive angiotensin I into the active form (92). Two preliminary reports, in which a specific angiotensin II antagonist, Saralasin (1-sar-8-angiotensin II), was used, failed to find a role for angiotensin as the mediator of the hypoxic response (93, 94).

If a complex tissue response is involved, a specialized sensing mechanism may exist. Collections of cells, called neuroepithelial bodies, have been found in the bronchial, bronchiolar, and alveolar epithelium of many species including man (95). Afferent and efferent nerve endings make synaptic end formations on these cells (96). They contain vesicles and osmiophilic bodies which change their appearance after exposure of the animal to hypoxia (97). These cells are similar in histological characteristics to the chief cells of the carotid body; both types of cell probably form part of the APUD series of cells which produce polypeptide hormones in many different organs (98). Neuroepithelial bodies are more common in newborn and fetal animals, and in the rat they disappear with increasing age. There is a possible link here between the hypoxic environment of the fetal lung, hyperplasia of the carotid bodies in chronic hypoxia (99), and the increased frequency of chemodectomas in high altitude residents (100).

Another feature of interest is the abolition of the hypoxic response by inhalational anesthetics such as halothane and diethylether (101, 102). Intravenously administered narcotics such as thiopentone and pentobarbital, dissociative anesthetic agents (ketamine), and tranquilizing and analgesic drugs have no effect on the response (103). Do inhaled agents depress chemoreceptor function in the alveolar wall? The hypoxic response is also absent in patients with cirrhosis of the liver (104) and in a familial disorder of the autonomic nervous system, dysautonomia (105).

There has been considerable discussion regarding the ability of a low mixed venous (P_{vO_2}), i.e., pulmonary arterial oxygen tension, to initiate vasoconstriction compared to a low alveolar oxygen tension (P_{AO_2}). The problem, which has some bearing on the oxygen-sensitive site in the lung, has been summarized by Hauge (106). A low $P_{\bar{v}O_2}$ increased and a high $P_{\bar{v}O_2}$ diminished the response to alveolar hypoxia, but in the presence of abnormal alveolar oxygen tension the effects of changing $P_{\bar{v}O_2}$ were trivial. For several reasons, alveolar P_{O_2} will be the operative oxygen tension for tissues in the periphery of the lung. First, all tissue, including the wall of vessels up to 100 μm, is within 20 μm of alveolar gas; secondly, pulmonary arteries below 150 μm in diameter are extremely thin-walled and the blood within them probably takes on, or approaches, the oxygen tension of the surrounding alveolar gas. On a teleological basis, the efficiency of pulmonary vasoconstriction in stabilizing alveolar gas tensions at a local level (Figures 20 and 21) would not be met by a system operating on the level of $P_{\bar{v}O_2}$ which is common to all units.

Although some benefits accrue from the ability of the pulmonary circulation to stabilize the alveolar gas environment throughout the lung (especially in the presence of diffuse pulmonary disease (107)), the hypoxic pressure response may represent a special adaptation to fetal life where the lung is not an organ of gas exchange and where alveolar tissue tensions are at systemic level. The persistence of hypoxic vasoconstriction in high altitude residents does not confer any particular advantage, and it is interesting that in one of the best adapted mountain dwellers, the llama, hypoxic vasoconstriction does not persist after birth (19).

WATER BALANCE IN LUNG

Ulstrastructure of Alveolar Capillary Membranes

Figure 24 from Weibel (108) is an electron micrograph of a pulmonary capillary in cross section to show the nonfenestrated endothelial and epithelial cell lining layers with the interstitium between. In places the interstitium widens out to include collagen fibers and fibroblastic cells, but elsewhere it is extremely thin (<0.1 nm), consisting only of the fused basement membranes of the epithelial and endothelial cells. With electron-dense tracers such as horseradish peroxidase (HRP) (molecular weight 40,000, molecular radius 3 nm) and cytochrome c (molecular weight 12,000, molecular radius 1.5 nm), some of the sites of leakage of large molecules from the capillary bed have been defined (109). The molecular radius of HRP is similar to that of albumin (molecular weight 68,000, molecular radius 3.4 nm). The molecular radius of globulin is about 5.4 nm and of fibrinogen 11 nm. Figure 25, from the work of Schneeberger-Keeley and Karnovsky (109), shows penetration of the HRP reaction produce after intravenous injection through the clefts (about 4 nm wide) between capillary endothelial cells and into the basement membrane. The reaction product penetrates the epithelial intercellular clefts with great difficulty, and HRP does not get into the alveolar space. Freeze-fracture studies show a tight "Velcro"-like fit between epithelial cells, compared to the loose and discontinuous junctions between endothelial cells.

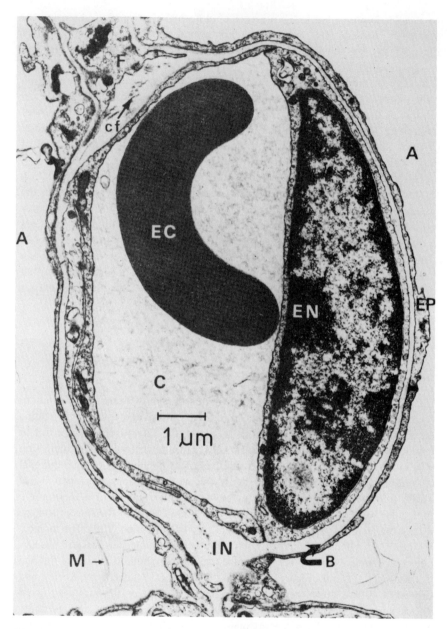

Figure 24. Cross section of capillary from monkey lung to show alveolar epithelium (*EP*), capillary endothelium (*EN*), and interstitium (*IN*), with fibroblast (*F*) and collagen fibrils (*cf*). Basement membranes (*B*) appear as gray lines. Red cell (*EC*) in capillary (*C*). Alveoli (*A*) contain myelin fragments (*M*). × 13,000. Reprinted with permission of University of Chicago Press, The Pulmonary Circulation and Interstitial Space, pp. 9–25 (1969).

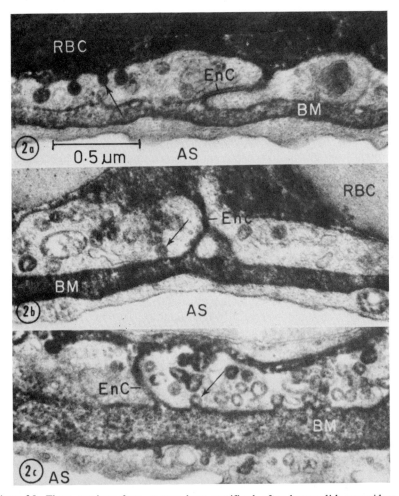

Figure 25. Three sections from mouse lung sacrificed after horseradish peroxidase injection. Reaction product of horseradish peroxidase in capillary lumen extends through endothelial intercellular cleft (*EnC*) into basement membrane (*BM*) and can be seen in endothelial invaginations (*arrowed*) and in unattached (pinocytotic) vesicles. RBC = capillary lumen; AS = alveolar space. × 46,000. Reprinted with permission of J. Cell Biol. 37:781 (1968).

Pinocytotic vesicles (Figure 25) in endothelium and epithelium may play a part in HRP transport, especially in clearance from the alveolar space. Schneeberger (110) has shown more recently that HRP only passes through the endothelial junctions with relatively large volume injections at presumably an elevated pulmonary capillary pressure. At normal pressure, only the smaller tracer, cytochrome *c,* escapes from the capillaries. These findings suggest that the endothelial junctions are stretched at high capillary pressure. Larger molecules such as HRP ferritin and immunoglobulins are thought to be transported by pinocytotic vesicles.

Physiological Basis for Protein Transport

In the absence of definite proof, it is generally assumed that samples of lung lymph reflect the composition of interstitial fluid. In the unanesthetized sheep, the lymph concentration to plasma concentration (L:P) ratios for albumin and globulin range from 0.5 to 0.8 and 0.2 to 0.5, respectively (111). The transport of protein from plasma to interstitium appears to be by "restricted" diffusion, because the L:P ratio for the smaller albumin molecule is greater than that for globulin. Blake and Staub (111) (also see Staub (5), p. 795) have measured L:P ratios for these two proteins over a wide range of pulmonary capillary pressures. Their model of the capillary membrane of the adult sheep postulated a few large leaks (>100 nm radius) and two populations of intercellular junction pores (2 and 12.5 nm radius). By measuring L:P ratios for a variety of marker substances, Boyd et al. (112), in the fetal sheep, arrived at similar conclusions, namely, the presence of intercellular pores of 15 nm radius and some large unrestricted leaks. Large leaks can be attributed to pinocytosis. (To the uninitiated, it is interesting that intercellular junctions of 12–13 nm radius can severely restrict the passage of HRP (3 nm radius) under normal conditions, permitting the passage of cytochrome (1.5 nm radius) only.) In newborn lambs, pore radius was less (9.0 nm), possibly because of the fall in pumonary vascular pressure after birth. Similar studies by Normand et al. (113) on the alveolar epithelium show exclusion of all molecules with radii greater than 0.5 nm. Olver and Strang (114) have shown that the alveolar epithelial pores (0.5–0.6 nm) severely restrict the passage of an electrolyte such as sodium (hydrated radius being about 0.3 nm). Thus, in the absence of net solute movement, net leakage of water through the epithelium is prevented, and relative dryness of the alveolar air spaces is maintained.

The sequence of events in edema is by no means clear. No structural alterations in the alveolar capillary membranes, such as the opening up of large gaps, have been described. Schneeberger (110) and Fishman and Pietra (115) both favor the idea, first suggested by Shirley et al. (116), that an increase in capillary pressure stretches the intercellular junctions and allows larger molecules to diffuse out. On the other hand, the appearance of protein in alveolar liquid has not been satisfactorily explained. The increase in interstitial pressure may in some way unlock the tight intercellular epithelial junctions, or it may enhance pinocytosis through the alveolar lining cell.

The situation at birth in which the liquid-filled fetal lung rapidly accommodates itself to air breathing was covered by Strang (117) in Volume 1 of this series and formed the major topic of a recent Ciba Symposium on lung liquids (118).

Lymphatic Transport

The basis of fluid filtration was discussed by Starling (119) 80 years ago. In modern terminology,

$$\dot{Q}_f = K_f ((P_{mv} - P_{pmv}) - \sigma(\pi_{mv} - \pi_{pmv}))$$

where $\dot{Q}_f$ is the net transvascular flow of fluid, K_f is the fluid filtration coefficient, P_{mv} and P_{pmv} are the microvascular and perimicrovascular hydro-static pressures, π_{mv} and π_{pmv} are the corresponding protein osmotic pressures, and σ is the apparent osmotic reflection coefficient (the "effective" transvascular osmotic difference). A normal water balance in the lung can be maintained only if $\dot{Q}_f$ is matched by an adequate flow of lymph removing excess water from

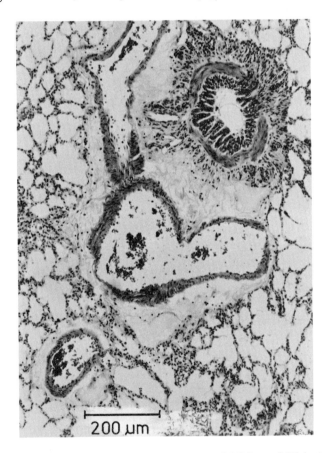

Figure 26. Lower lobe of dog lung after rapid infusion of 1.9 liters of 6% dextran in saline solution. Note the distended perivascular spaces, in the absence of alveolar flooding, with lakes of fluid in dilated lymphatics. Reprinted with permission of J. Appl. Physiol. 25:701 (1968).

the interstitial space. Staub (5), whose comprehensive review on pulmonary edema is the source of information for this section, concluded that there were no lymphatics in the alveolar walls themselves. Nevertheless, they are easily seen in the perivascular spaces surrounding arteries, veins, and bronchi, particularly when these are distended with edema fluid, as shown in Figure 26. During the formation of edema, excess fluid is detected first in these perivascular spaces (120).

There appears to be free communication between the lymphatics on the pleural surface and those deeper in the lung. All drain into a maze of interconnecting paratracheal and mediastinal lymph nodes. It was formerly thought that 80% of lung lymph drained into the right subclavian vein via the right lymphatic duct (RLD). More recent studies (see Staub (5), p. 689) suggest that the RLD accounts for only about 25% of lung lymph, presumably draining from the right upper lobe. The remaining lymph drains into the thoracic duct from the left tracheobronchial duct (left upper lobe) and the common mediastinal duct (CMD) draining the lower lobes. The CMD is not present in dog or man. The collection of so-called "pure lung lymph" is most easily made from the RLD although contributions from the heart, chest wall, diaphragm, etc. must be taken into account, as discussed by Humphreys et al. (121).

The fine structure of lymphatics has been examined by Lauweryns and Boussauw (122). The smallest lymphatic vessels in the perivascular and peribronchial spaces, called lymphatic capillaries, have a thin, irregular endothelium with intercellular gaps which ferritin molecules (molecular weight 600,000; molecular radius 5.5 nm) easily penetrate. They possess a well-established system of valves (123). The endothelial cells contain actin-like filaments, and it is very likely that lymphatics have contractile properties (124).

Measurement of Lung Water

Experimentally, lung water content can be measured by drying specimens to a constant weight and calculating the wet to dry weight ratio (125). Histological examination is a useful adjunct and may be more sensitive in detecting early edema than weighing (126). These methods are not applicable in vivo except when lung biopsies can be taken. Methods for detecting and quantitating pulmonary edema in vivo present certain problems. Radiology is the simplest technique, but is difficult to quantitate and not very sensitive to mild or moderate accumulations of lung water. Pulmonary densitometry and impedance plethysmography do not distinguish intravascular from extravascular liquid. The most widely used method has been the double-indicator dilution technique of Chinard and Enns (127), which uses a diffusible indicator which equilibrates in one passage with the water volume of the lung and a nondiffusible indicator which is confined to the vascular bed. Tritium (^3H_2O), which has been used as a diffusible indicator, suffers from the disadvantage that it requires arterial sampling and tedious laboratory counting procedures because it has no significant γ

energy. On the other hand, ^{15}O emits positrons which annihilate to give 511 k.e.v γ rays. By substituting $H_2^{15}O$ for tritium, the volume of distribution of water following an intravenous injection can be derived from the time-activity curves over the lung fields recorded with scintillation probes. Indium-113m, which binds to the plasma protein transferrin and emits 390 k.e.v. γ rays, forms a suitable vascular indicator. Time-activity curves for these two tracers injected intravenously in man in the supine position are shown in Figure 27.

In anesthetized dogs in the lateral position, there was very good agreement between the mean transit time difference for the diffusible and nondiffusible indicators recorded by external counting over the lung compared with arterial sampling (128). This correlation is shown in Figure 28 where both regional and arterial mean transit time values have been multiplied by the cardiac output to give extravascular lung water volume (ELWV) in milliliters.

As explained diagrammatically in Figure 29, ELWV is proportional to the difference in mean transit time ($\bar{t}$) between the two indicators, multiplied by the

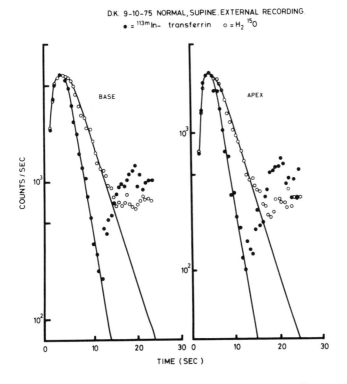

Figure 27. Time-activity curves for a normal subject recorded externally over the right lower and upper zone in the supine posture following intravenous injection of intravascular (^{113m}In) and water ($H_2^{15}O$) tracers. Reprinted with permission of Br. J. Radiol. 49:393 (1976).

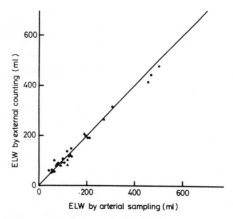

Figure 28. Extravascular lung water (ELW) measured in supine anesthetized dogs in the lateral position using the double-indicator radioisotope method, comparing external counting over the lung with withdrawal of blood from aorta. From F. Fazio et al., to be published.

water flow (blood flow $\times$ 0.8). Fazio et al. (129) devised the ratios, shown in Figure 29, which relate regional ELWV to local blood volume and blood flow. In this way, regional blood flow in absolute terms, determination of which would add considerably to the complexity of the procedure, need not be measured. In addition, with regional information lung water must be normalized to some

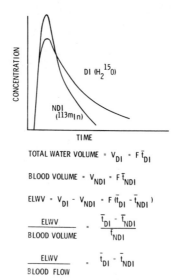

$$\text{TOTAL WATER VOLUME} = V_{DI} = F\,\bar{t}_{DI}$$

$$\text{BLOOD VOLUME} = V_{NDI} = F\,\bar{t}_{NDI}$$

$$\text{ELWV} = V_{DI} - V_{NDI} = F\,(\bar{t}_{DI} - \bar{t}_{NDI})$$

$$\frac{\text{ELWV}}{\text{BLOOD VOLUME}} = \frac{\bar{t}_{DI} - \bar{t}_{NDI}}{\bar{t}_{NDI}}$$

$$\frac{\text{ELWV}}{\text{BLOOD FLOW}} = \bar{t}_{DI} - \bar{t}_{NDI}$$

Figure 29. Representation of time-activity curves for diffusible (*DI*) and nondiffusible (*NDI*) indicators recorded externally from the lung as in Figure 27. Derivation of ratios of regional extravascular water volume (*ELWV*) per unit of blood volume and flow is shown. V is the volume of distribution of indicator; $\bar{t}$, mean transit time, and F, flow.

other measurement, ideally dry lung weight. In normal subjects studied supine, Fazio et al. (129) found that regional ELWV per unit of blood volume and flow was distributed uniformly between the apex and base of the lung; in patients with left heart disease, studied similarly, the ratios were elevated and the value in the lower lobe exceeded that for the upper lobe. Studies in the erect posture have not yet been reported. Of course, the importance of regional variations in local blood volume and flow in the EVLW ratios given in Figure 29 remains to be assessed. Nevertheless, the procedure is attractively simple, requiring only an intravenous injection and may prove the most practical way of assessing lung water in vivo. Although ^{15}O has a half-life of only 2 min, other substances such as antipyrine labeled with ^{123}I or ^{125}I may be substituted, because they appear to be handled similarly to water by the lung (130).

Unfortunately, with an intravenous tracer, extravascular water will only be measured in those parts of the pulmonary capillary bed which are perfused (compare Figures 4, 7, and 8). Inadequate recruitment of capillaries is the accepted explanation for the fact that indicator dilution methods underestimate ELWV by about 35% when compared to a direct estimate of lung water by drying (see Staub (5), Table 7 for references). On the other hand, increases of pulmonary arterial pressure and flow, in exercise for example, should increase the proportion of ELWV seen by indicator dilution measurements. In dogs, Goresky et al. (131) found the measured fraction of water was 0.81 at rest, increasing to 0.94 at near-maximum exercise. Goresky and his colleagues (132) have extended these studies to man. Eleven normal subjects were studied at rest and two levels of exercise (50 and 100 watts) seated on a bicycle ergometer. Cardiac output increased 3.6 times at the high level of exercise. Central blood volume and the single breath diffusing capacity for carbon monoxide increased linearly with cardiac output. Interestingly, ELWV (ml kg^{-1} of body weight) increased from 2.16 ± 0.47 to 2.55 ± 0.47 at the first level of exercise, but did not increase further at the higher exercise level. Recruitment would appear to have reached a maximum at the 50 watts exercise level. Cardiac output increased from 1.06 ± 0.15 ml s^{-1} kg^{-1} at rest to 2.6 ± 0.78 at 50 watts; from other data, mean pulmonary arterial pressure might have increased from 16.5 to 23 cm H_2O at 50 watts exercise (43). Goresky et al. (132) felt the increase in single breath carbon monoxide uptake from 50 to 100 watts without any change in ELWV might be blood flow-dependent. This would be a relatively new concept for carbon monoxide uptake; an alternative explanation would be additional distension of the capillary bed, increasing pulmonary capillary blood volume (see under "Distension" and "Recruitment").

Distribution of Lung Water

In the vertical lung, the distribution of wet to dry weight ratios is uniform in the normal situation and in moderate edema (133), but at the stage of alveolar flooding there is generally an excess in the lower lobes (134). The lower (caudal) lobes also have higher wet to dry weight ratios than the upper lobes in dogs in which edema has been induced in the inverted position (135). Thus, the distribution of lung water in edema is determined more by the rate of filtration and removal at a local level (i.e., local vascular and perivascular pressures and lymph flow rate, etc.) than by passive drainage from superior to dependent regions.

In vertical isolated perfused lungs, Jones et al. (136) measured the distribution of ELWV, blood volume, and flow with radioisotopes just before taking lung biopsies for calculation of wet to dry ratios. Compared to wet to dry ratios, the radioisotopic determination, using $H_2{}^{15}O$, underestimated the water content of the apical regions where flow was low. The ratio of ELWV to blood volume was uniform at all levels, although in absolute terms each was highest at the base and least at the apex. The ratio of extravascular lung water to blood flow increased with distance up the lung from 0.9 in the lower zone to 1.66 at the apex. The dependence of the measurement of lung water on blood flow and capillary recruitment has been discussed in the previous section ("Measurement of Lung Water").

REFERENCES

1. Fishman, A. P. (1963). Dynamics of the pulmonary circulation. In W. F. Hamilton and P. Dow (eds.). Handbook of Physiology, Section 2, Circulation, Vol. 2, pp. 1667–1743. American Physiology Society, Washington, D.C.
2. Fishman, A. P. (1961). Respiratory gases in the regulation of the pulmonary circulation. Physiol. Rev. 41:214.
3. Fishman, A. P., and Hecht, H. E. (1969). The Pulmonary Circulation and the Interstitial Space. University of Chicago Press, Chicago.
4. Giuntini, C. (1971). Central Hemodynamics and Gas Exchange. Minerva Medica, Torino.
5. Staub, N. C. (1974). Pulmonary edema. Physiol. Rev. 54:679.
6. Cumming, G. (1974). Pulmonary circulation. In A. C. Guyton and C. E. Jones (eds.), MTP International Review of Science, Physiology Series I, Vol. 1, Cardiovascular Physiology, pp. 94–122. University Park Press, Baltimore.
7. Singhal, S., Henderson, R., Horsfield, K., Harding, K., and Cumming, G. (1973). Morphometry of the human pulmonary arterial tree. Circ. Res. 33:190.
8. Cumming, G., Henderson, R. Horsfield, K., and Singhal, S. (1969). The functional morphology of the pulmonary circulation. In A. P. Fishman and H. Hecht (eds.), The Pulmonary Circulation and Interstitial Space, pp. 327–338. University of Chicago, Chicago.
9. Schroter, R. C., and Sudlow, M. F. (1969). Flow patterns in models of human bronchial airways. Respir. Physiol. 9:371.
10. Heath, D., and Edwards, J. E. (1960). Configuration of elastic tissue of pulmonary trunk in idiopathic pulmonary hypertension. Circulation 21:59.
11. Rowe, R. D., and James, L. S. (1957). The normal pulmonary arterial pressure during the first year of life. J. Pediatr. 51:1.

12. Reid, L. (1968). Structural and functional reappraisal of the pulmonary artery system. *In* Scientific Basis of Medicine Annual Reviews, pp. 289–307.
13. Hislop, A., and Reid, L. (1973). Pulmonary arterial development during childhood: branching pattern and structure. Thorax 28:129.
14. Hislop, A., and Reid, L. (1973). Fetal and childhood development of the intrapulmonary veins in man—branching pattern and structure. Thorax 28:313.
15. Smiley, R. H., Jaques, W. E., and Campbell, G. S. (1966). Pulmonary vascular changes in lung lobes with reversed pulmonary blood flow. Surgery 59:529.
16. Reid, L., and Meyrick, B. (1976). Disturbance of the blood/gas barrier in pulmonary hypertension—in disease and animal models. *In* C. Hatzfeld (ed.), Distribution des échanges gazeux pulmonaires. Colloques INSERM (Paris) Vol. 51, pp. 155–164.
17. Arias-Stella, J., and Saldana, M. (1963). The terminal portion of the pulmonary arterial tree in people native to high altitudes. Circulation 28:915.
18. Abraham, A. S., Kay, J. M., Cole, R. B., and Pincock, A. C. (1971). Haemodynamic and pathological study of the effect of chronic hypoxia and subsequent recovery of the heart and pulmonary vasculature in the rat. Cardiovasc. Res. 5:95.
19. Heath, D., Castillo, Y., Arias-Stella, J., and Harris, P. (1969). The small pulmonary arteries of the llama and other domestic animals native to high altitudes. Cardiovasc. Res. 3:75.
20. Fung, Y. C., and Sobin, S. S. (1969). Theory of sheet flow in lung alveoli. J. Appl. Physiol. 26:472.
21. Fung, Y. C. (1974). Fluid in the interstitial space of the pulmonary alveolar sheet. Microvasc. Res. 7:89.
22. Sobin, S. S., Tremer, H. M., and Fung, Y. C. (1970). Morphometric basis of the sheet-flow concept of the pulmonary alveolar microcirulation in the cat. Circ. Res. 26:397.
23. Banister, J., and Torrance, R. W. (1960). The effects of the tracheal pressure upon flow: pressure relations in the vascular bed of isolated lungs. Q. J. Exp. Physiol. 45:352.
24. Permutt, S., Bromberger-Barnea, B., and Bane, H. N. (1962). Alveolar pressure, pulmonary venous pressure and the vascular waterfall. Med. Thorac. 19:239.
25. West, J. B., Dollery, C. T., and Naimark, A. (1964). Distribution of blood flow in isolated lung; relation to vascular and alveolar pressures. J. Appl. Physiol. 19:713.
26. Hughes, J. M. B., Glazier, J. B., Maloney, J. E., and West, J. B. (1968). Effect of extra-alveolar vessels on distribution of blood flow in the dog lung. J. Appl. Physiol. 25:701.
27. Lloyd, T. C., and Wright, G. W. (1960). Pulmonary vascular resistance and vascular transmural gradient. J. Appl. Physiol. 15:241.
28. Bruderman, I., Somers, K., Hamilton, W. K., Tooley, W. H., and Butler, J. (1964). Effect of surface tension on circulation in the excised lungs of dogs. J. Appl. Physiol. 19:707.
29. Pain, M. C. F., and West, J. B. (1966). Effect of the volume history of the isolated lung on distribution of blood flow. J. Appl. Physiol. 21:1545.

178 Hughes

30. Daly, B. D. T., Parks, G. E., Edmonds, C. E., Hibbs, C. W., and Norman, J. C. (1975). Dynamic alveolar mechanics as studied by videomicroscopy. Respir. Physiol. 24:217.
31. Glazier, J. B., Hughes, J. M. B., Maloney, J. E., and West, J. B. (1969). Measurements of capillary dimensions and blood volume in rapidly frozen lungs. J. Appl. Physiol. 26:65.
32. Rosenzweig, D. Y., Hughes, J. M. B., and Glazier, J. B. (1970). Effects of changes in transpulmonary and vascular pressures on pulmonary blood volume in the isolated dog lung. J. Appl. Physiol. 28:553.
33. Hoppin, F. G., Jr., Lee, G. C., and Dawson, S. V. (1975). Properties of lung parenchyma in distortion. J. Appl. Physiol. 39:742.
34. Roos, A., Thomas, L. J., Nagel, E. L., and Prommas, D. C. (1961). Pulmonary vascular resistance as determined by lung inflation and vascular pressures. J. Appl. Physiol. 16:77.
35. Sobin, S. S., Fung, Y. C., Tremer, H. M., and Rosenquist, T. H. (1972). Elasticity of the pulmonary alveolar microvascular sheet in the cat. Circ. Res. 30:440.
36. Baez, S., Lamport, H., and Baez, A. (1960). Pressure effects in living microscopic vessels. In A. L. Copley and G. Stainsky (eds.), Flow Properties of Blood, pp. 122–135. Pergamon Press, London.
37. Warrell, D. A., Evans, J. W., Clarke, R. O., Kingaby, G. P., and West, J. B. (1972). Pattern of filling in the pulmonary capillary bed. J. Appl. Physiol. 32:346.
38. Permutt, S., Caldini, P., Maseri, A., Palmer, W. H., Sasamori, T., and Zierler, K. (1969). Recruitment versus distensibility in the pulmonary vascular bed. In A. P. Fishman and H. Hecht (eds.), The Pulmonary Circulation and Interstitial Space, pp. 375–387. University of Chicago Press, Chicago.
39. West, J. B., Schneider, A. M., and Mitchell, M. M. (1975). Recruitment in networks of pulmonary capillaries. J. Appl. Physiol. 39:976.
40. Hales, S. (1731). Vegetable Staticks, p. 241. London.
41. Lee, G. de J., and Dubois (1955). Pulmonary capillary blood flow in man. J. Clin. Invest. 34:1380.
42. Wearn, J. T., Ernstene, A. C., Bromer, A. W., Barr, J. S., German, W. J., and Zschiesche, L. J. (1934). The normal behaviour of the pulmonary blood vessels with observations on the intermittence of the flow of blood in the arterioles and capillaries. Am. J. Physiol. 109:236.
43. Bevegard, S., Holmgren, A., and Jonsson, B. (1960). The effect of body position on the circulation at rest and during exercise, with special reference to the influence on the stroke volume. Acta Physiol. Scand. 49:279.
44. Maloney, J. E., Bergel, D. H., Glazier, J. B., Hughes, J. M. B., and West, J. B. (1968). Transmission of pulsatile pressure and flow through the isolated lung. Circ. Res. 23:11.
45. Macklin, C. C. (1946). Evidence of increase in the capacity of the pulmonary arteries and veins of dogs, cats and rabbits during inflation of the freshly excised lung. Rev. Can. Biol. 5:199.
46. Howell, J. B. L., Permutt, S., Proctor, D. F., and Riley, R. L. (1961). Effect of inflation of the lung on different parts of pulmonary vascular bed. J. Appl. Physiol. 16:71.
47. Marchand, P. (1951). The anatomy and applied anatomy of the mediastinal fascia. Thorax 6:359.

48. Tocker, A. M., and Langston, H. T. (1952). The perivascular space of the pulmonary vessels: an anatomic demonstration. J. Thorac. Surg. 23:539.

49. Permutt, S. (1965). Effect of interstitial pressure of the lung on pulmonary circulation. Med. Thorac. 22:118.

50. Hughes, J. M. B., Jones, Hazel A., Wilson, A. G., Grant, B. J. B., and Pride, N. B. (1974). Stability of intrapulmonary bronchial dimensions during expiratory flow in excised lungs. J. Appl. Physiol. 37:684.

51. Mead, J., Takishima, T., and Leith, D. (1970). Stress distribution in lungs: a model of pulmonary elasticity. J. Appl. Physiol. 28:596.

52. Benjamin, J. J., Murtagh, P. S., Proctor, D. F., Menkes, H. A., and Permutt, S. (1974). Pulmonary vascular interdependence in excised dog lobes. J. Appl. Physiol. 37:887.

53. Hughes, J. M. B., Glazier, J. B., Maloney, J. E., and West, J. B. (1968). Effect of lung volume on the distribution of pulmonary blood flow in man. Respir. Physiol. 4:58.

54. West, J. B., and Dollery, C. T. (1960). Distribution of blood flow and ventilation-perfusion ratio in the lung, measured with radioactive CO_2. J. Appl. Physiol. 15:405.

55. Glazier, J. B., Hughes, J. M. B., Maloney, J. E., and West, J. B. (1967). Vertical gradient of alveolar size in lungs of dogs frozen intact. J. Appl. Physiol. 23:694.

56. Milic-Emili, J., Henderson, J. A. M., Dolovich, M. B., Trop, D., and Kaneko, K. (1966). Regional distribution of inspired gas in the lung. J. Appl. Physiol. 21:749.

57. Krueger, J. J., Bain, T., and Patterson, J. L. (1961). Elevation gradient of intrathoracic pressure. J. Appl. Physiol. 16:465.

58. Anthonisen, N. R., and Milic-Emili, J. (1966). Distribution of pulmonary perfusion in erect man. J. Appl. Physiol. 21:760.

59. Euler, U. S. von, and Liljestrand, G. (1946). Observations on the pulmonary arterial blood pressure in the cat. Acta Physiol. Scand. 12:301.

60. Rahn, H., and Bahnson, H. T. (1953). Effect of unilateral hypoxia on gas exchange and calculated pulmonary blood flow in each lung. J. Appl. Physiol. 6:105.

61. Hertz, C. W. (1956). Unterfuchungen über den Einfluss der alveolaren Gasdrucke auf die intrapulmonale. Durchblutungsverteilung beim Menschen. Klin. Wochenschr. 34:472.

62. Himmelstein, A., Harris, P., Fritts, H. W., and Cournand, A. (1958). Effect of severe unilateral hypoxia on the partition of pulmonary blood flow in man. J. Thorac. Surg. 36:369.

63. Defares, J. G., Lundin, G., Arborelius, M., Stromblad, R., and Svanberg, L. (1960). Effect of "unilateral hypoxia" on pulmonary blood flow distribution in normal subjects. J. Appl. Physiol. 15:169.

64. Arborelius, M., Jr. (1966). Kr^{85} in the study of pulmonary circulation and ventilation during unilateral hypoxia. Scand. J. Respir. Dis. 62:105.

65. Arborelius, M., Jr. (1966). Respiratory gases and pulmonary blood flow: a bronchospirometric study. Ph.D. thesis, University of Lund. Falkmens Bokhandel, Malmo.

66. Barer, G. R., Howard, P., and Shaw, J. W. (1970). Stimulus-response curves for the pulmonary vascular bed to hypoxia and hypercapnia. J. Physiol. (Lond.) 211:139.

67. Grant, B. J. B., Jones, H. A., Davies, E. E., and Hughes, J. M. B. (1976).

Local regulation of pulmonary blood flow and ventilation-perfusion ratios in the coati mundi. J. Appl. Physiol. 40:216.

68. Ross, J. M., Fairchild, H. M., Weldy, J., and Guyton, A. C. (1962). Autoregulation of blood flow by oxygen lack. Am. J. Physiol. 202:21.

69. Hebb, C. (1969). Motor innervation of the pulmonary blood vessels of mammals. *In* A. P. Fishman and H. Hecht (eds.), The Pulmonary Circulation and Interstitial Space, pp. 195–222. University of Chicago Press, Chicago.

70. Daly, I. de B., and Hebb, C. (1966). Pulmonary and Bronchial Vascular Systems. Arnold, London.

71. Colebatch, H. J. H., Dawes, G. S., Goodwin, J. W., and Nadeau, R. A. (1965). The nervous control of the circulation in the foetal and newly expanded lungs of the lamb. J. Physiol. (Lond.) 178:544.

72. Barer, G. R., and McCurrie, J. R. (1969). Pulmonary vasomotor responses in the cat; the effects and interrelationships of drugs, hypoxia and hypertension. Q. J. Exp. Physiol. 54:156.

73. Porcelli, R. J., and Bergofsky, E. H. (1973). Adrenergic receptors in pulmonary vasoconstrictor responses to gaseous and humoral agents. J. Appl. Physiol. 34:483.

74. Howard, P., Barer, G. R., Thompson, B., Warren, P. M., Abbott, C. J., and Mungall, I. P. F. (1975). Factors causing and reversing vasoconstriction in unventilated lung. Respir. Physiol. 24:325.

75. Kazemi, H., Bruecke, P. E., and Parsons, E. F. (1972). Role of the autonomic nervous system in the hypoxic response of the pulmonary vascular bed. Respir. Physiol. 15:245.

76. Reeves, J. T., and Leathers, J. E. (1964). Hypoxic pulmonary hypertension of the calf with denervation of the lungs. J. Appl. Physiol. 19:976.

77. Malik, A. B., and Kidd, B. S. L. (1973). Adrenergic blockade and the pulmonary vascular response to hypoxia. Respir. Physiol. 19:96.

78. Silove, E. D., and Grover, R. F. (1968). Effects of alpha-adrenergic blockade and tissue catecholamine depletion on pulmonary vascular response to hypoxia. J. Clin. Invest. 47:274.

79. Duke, H. N., and Killick, E. M. (1952). Pulmonary vasomotor responses of isolated perfused cat lungs to anoxia. J. Physiol. (Lond.) 117:303.

80. Lloyd, T. C., Jr. (1970). Responses to hypoxia of pulmonary arterial strips in nonaqueous baths. J. Appl. Physiol. 28:566.

81. Nilsen, K. H., and Hauge, A. (1968). Effects of temperature changes on the pressor response to acute alveolar hypoxia in isolated rat lungs. Acta Physiol. Scand. 73:111.

82. Haas, F., and Bergofsky, E. H. (1972). Role of the mast cell in the pulmonary pressor response to hypoxia. J. Clin. Invest. 51:3154.

83. Dawson, C. A., Delano, F. A., Hamilton, L. H., and Stekiel, W. J. (1974). Histamine releasers and hypoxic vasoconstriction in isolated cat lungs. J. Appl. Physiol. 37:670.

84. Hauge, A. (1968). Role of histamine in hypoxic pulmonary hypertension in the rat: blockade or potentiation of endogenous amines, kinins and ATP, Circ. Res. 22:371.

85. Kay, J. M., Waymire, J. C., and Grover, R. F. (1974). Lung mast cell hyperplasia and pulmonary histamine-forming capacity in hypoxic rats. Am. J. Physiol. 226:178.

86. Mungall, I. P. F. (1976). Hypoxia and lung mast cells: influence of disodium cromoglycate. Thorax 31:94.

87. Silove, E. D., and Simcha, A. J. (1973). Histamine-induced pulmonary

vasodilatation in the calf: relationship to hypoxia. J. Appl. Physiol. 35:830.

88. Reeves, J. T., and Grover, R. F. (1974). Blockade of acute hypoxic pulmonary hypertension by endotoxin. J. Appl. Physiol. 36:328.

89. Vaage, J., Bjertnaes, L., and Hauge, A. (1975). The pulmonary vasoconstriction response to hypoxia: effects of inhibitors of prostaglandin synthesis. Acta Physiol. Scand. 95:95.

90. Sors, H., Even, P., Ruff, F., Duroux, P., and Dray, F. (1975). Radioimmunologic measurement of plasma prostaglandins and their 13-dehydro-15-keto derivates upstream and downstream from the lung during hypoxic pulmonary artery constriction in man. Eur. J. Clin. Invest., 5:72 (Abstr.).

91. Berkov, S. (1974). Hypoxic vasoconstriction in the rat: the necessary role of angiotensin II. Circ. Res. 35:256.

92. Fanburg, B. L., and Glazier, J. B. (1973). Conversion of angiotensin 1 to angiotensin 2 in the isolated perfused dog lung. J. Appl. Physiol. 35:325.

93. Hyman, A., Heymann, M., Levin, D., and Rudolph, A. (1975). Angiotensin is not the mediator of hypoxia-induced pulmonary vasoconstriction in fetal lambs. Circulation (Suppl. 2) 52:132 (Abst.).

94. McMurtry, I. F., Hiser, W. W., Reeves, J. T., and Grover, R. F. (1975). Disassociation of hypoxia- and antiotensin II-induced pulmonary vasoconstriction by saralastin. Fed. Proc. 34:438 (Abst.).

95. Lauweryns, J. M., and Goddeeris, P. (1975). Neuroepithelial bodies in the human child and adult lung. Am. Rev. Respir. Dis. 111:469.

96. Lauweryns, J. M., and Cokelaere, M. (1973). Hypoxia-sensitive neuroepithelial bodies: intrapulmonary secretory neuroreceptors, modulated by the CNS. Z. Zellforsch. 145:521.

97. Moosavi, H., Smith, P., and Heath, D. (1973). The Feyrter cell in hypoxia. Thorax 28:729.

98. Pearse, A. G. E. (1969). The cytochemistry and ultrastructure of polypeptide hormone producing cells of the APUD series and the embryologic, physiologic and pathologic implications of the concept. J. Histochem. Cytochem. 17:303.

99. Edwards, C., Heath, D., Harris, P., Castillo, Y., Gruger, H., and Arias-Stella, J. (1971). The carotid body in animals at high altitude. J. Pathol. 104:231.

100. Lancet. (1973). High-altitude chemodectoma. 1:1493.

101. Sykes, M. K., Davies, M. K., Chakrabarti, M. K., and Loh, L. (1973). The effects of halothane, trichloroethylene and ether on the hypoxic pressor response and pulmonary vascular resistance in the isolated, perfused cat lung. Br. J. Anaesth. 45:655.

102. Bjertnaes, L. J., Hauge, A., Nakken, K. F., and Bredesen, J. E. (1976). Hypoxic pulmonary vasoconstriction: inhibition due to anesthesia. Acta Physiol. Scand. 96:283.

103. Bredersen, J., Bjertnaes, L., and Hauge, A. (1975). Effects of anesthetics on the pulmonary vasoconstrictor response to acute alveolar hypoxia. Microvasc. Res. 10:236 (Abst.).

104. Daoud, K. S., Reeves, J. T., and Schoefer, J. W. (1972). Failure of hypoxic pulmonary vasoconstriction in patients with liver cirrhosis. J. Clin. Invest. 51:1076.

105. Filler, J., Smith, A. A. Stone, S., and Dancis. J. (1965). Respiratory control in familial dysautonomia. J. Paediatr. 66:509.

106. Hauge, A. (1969). Hypoxia and pulmonary vascular resistance: the relative

effects of pulmonary arterial and alveolar P_{O_2}. Acta Physiol. Scand. 76:121.

107. Hughes, J. M. B. (1975). Efficiency of gas exchange in the lung. Bull. Physiopathol. Respir. 11:921.

108. Weibel, E. R. (1969). The ultrastructure of the alveolar capillary membrane or barrier. *In* A. P. Fishman and H. Hecht (eds.), The Pulmonary Circulation and Interstitial Space, pp. 9–25. University of Chicago Press, Chicago.

109. Schneeberger-Keeley, E. E., and Karnovsky, M. J. (1968). The ultrastructural basis of alveolar capillary membrane permeability to peroxidase used as a tracer. J. Cell Biol. 37:781.

110. Schneeberger, E. E. (1976). Ultrastructural basis for alveolar-capillary permeability to protein. *In* R. Porter and M. O'Connor (eds.), Lung Liquids, Ciba Foundation Symposium 38, pp. 3–21. American Elsevier, Excerpta Medica, and North Holland, Amsterdam.

111. Blake, L. H., and Staub, N. C. (1972). Modeling of steady state pulmonary transvascular fluid and protein exchange in unanesthetized sheep. Physiologist 5:88 (Abstr.).

112. Boyd, R. D. H., Hill, J. R., Humphreys, P. W., Hormand, I. C. S., Reynolds, E. O. R., and Strang, L. B. (1969). Permeability of lung capillaries to macromolecules in foetal and newborn lambs and sheep. J. Physiol. (Lond.) 201:567.

113. Normand, I. C. S., Olver, R. E., Reynolds, E. O. R., Strang, L. B., and Welch, K. (1971). Permeability of lung capillaries and alveoli to nonelectrolytes in the foetal lamb. J. Physiol. (Lond.) 219:303.

114. Olver, R. E., and Strang, L. B. (1974). Ion fluxes across the pulmonary epithelium and secretion of lung liquid in the foetal lamb. J. Physiol. (Lond.) 241:327.

115. Fishman, A. P., and Pietra, C. G. (1976). Permeability of pulmonary vascular endothelium. *In* R. Porter and M. O'Connor (eds.), Lung Liquids, Ciba Foundation Symposium 38, pp. 29–38. American Elsevier, Excerpta Medica, and North Holland, Amsterdam.

116. Shirley, H. H., Wolfram, C. G., Wasserman, K., and Mayerson, H. S. (1957). Capillary permeability to macromolecules: stretched pore phenomenon. Am. J. Physiol. 190:189.

117. Strang, L. B. (1975). Foetal and newborn lung. *In* J. G. Widdicombe (ed.), MTP International Review of Science, Physiology Series I, Vol. 2, Respiratory Physiology, pp. 32–65. University Park Press, Baltimore.

118. Strang, L. B. (1976). The permeability of lung capillary and alveolar walls as determinants of liquid movements in the lung. *In* R. Porter and M. O'Connor (eds.), Lung Liquids, Ciba Foundation Symposium 38, pp. 49–58. American Elsevier, Excerpta Medica, and North Holland, Amsterdam.

119. Starling, E. H. (1896). Absorption of fluids from the connective tissue spaces. J. Physiol. (Lond.) 19:312.

120. Staub, N. C., Nagano, H., and Pearce, M. L. (1967). Pulmonary edema in dogs, especially the sequence of fluid accumulation in lungs. J. Appl. Physiol. 22:227.

121. Humphreys, P. W., Normand, I. C. S., Reynolds, E. O. R., and Strang, L. B. (1967). Pulmonary lymph flow and the uptake of liquid from the lungs of the lamb at the start of breathing. J. Physiol. (Lond.) 193:1.

122. Lauweryns, J. M., and Boussauw, L. (1969). The ultrastructure of pul-

monary lymphatic capillaries of newborn rabbits and of human infants. Lymphology 2:108.

123. Lauweryns, J. M., and Boussauw, L. (1973). The ultrastructure of lymphatic valves in the adult rabbit lung. Z. Zellforsch. 143:149.

124. Lauweryns, J. M., Baert, J., and Loecker, W. de (1975). Intracytoplasmic filaments in pulmonary lymphatic endothelial cells. Cell Tiss. Res. 163:111.

125. Guyton, A. C., and Lindsey, A. W. (1959). Effect of elevated left atrial pressure and decreased plasma protein concentration on the development of pulmonary oedema. Circ. Res. 7:649.

126. Iliff, L. D. (1971). Extra-alveolar vessels and edema development in excised dog lungs. Circl. Res. 28:524.

127. Chinard, F. P., and Enns, T. (1954). Transcapillary pulmonary exchange of water in the dog. Am. J. Physiol. 178:197.

128. Fazio, F., Clark, J. C., Buckingham, P. D., Rhodes, C. G., Hudson, F. R., Jones, H. A., Jones, T., and Hughes, J. M. B. (1975). An external counting method for regional measurements of extravascular lung water. Prog. Respir. Res. 9:249.

129. Fazio, F., Jones, T., MacArthur, C. G. C., Rhodes, C. G., Steiner, R. E. S., and Hughes, J. M. B. (1976). Measurement of regional pulmonary oedema in man using radioactive water (H_2 ^{15}O). Br. J. Radiol. 49:393.

130. Giuntini, C. (1971). Theoretical considerations on the measure of pulmonary blood volume and extravascular lung water in man. Bull. Physiopathol. Respir. 7:1125.

131. Goresky, C. A., Cronin, R. F. P., and Wangel, B. E. (1969). Indicator dilution measurements of extravascular water in the lungs. J. Clin. Invest. 48:487.

132. Goresky, C. A., Warnica, J. W., Burgess, J. H., and Nadeau, B. E. (1975). Effect of exercise on dilution estimates of extravascular lung water and on the carbon monoxide diffusing capacity in normal adults. Circ. Res. 37:379.

133. Naimark, A., Kirk, B. W., and Chernecki, W. (1971). Regional water volume, blood volume and perfusion in the lung. In C. Giuntini (ed.), Central Haemodynamics and Gas Exchange, pp. 144–160. Minerva Medica, Torino.

134. Muir, A. L., Hall, D. L., Despas, A., and Hogg, J. C. (1972). Distribution of blood flow in the lungs in acute pulmonary edema in dogs. J. Appl. Physiol. 33:763.

135. Levine, O. R., and Mellins, R. B. (1972). Effect of gravity on interstitial pressure of the lung in intact dogs. J. Appl. Physiol. 33:357.

136. Jones, T., Jones, H. A., Rhodes, C. G., Buckinham, P. D., and Hughes, J. M. B. (1976). Distribution of extravascular fluid volumes in isolated perfused lungs measured with H_2 ^{15}O. J. Clin. Invest. 57:706.

International Review of Physiology
Respiratory Physiology II, Volume 14
Edited by John G. Widdicombe
Copyright 1977   University Park Press   Baltimore

6
Control of
the Breathing Pattern

G. W. BRADLEY

Midhurst Medical Research Institute, Midhurst, Sussex, England

TIDAL VOLUME AND RESPIRATORY RATE   187
  "Hey Plot"   187
  Effect of Temperature   187
  Influence of Mechanical Loads   188
  Influence of Vagus Nerves   188

TIDAL VOLUME AND INSPIRATORY
  AND EXPIRATORY DURATIONS   188
  V_T and T_I in Steady State Conditions   188
  V_T and T_I with Volume Inflations Under
    Isocapnic Conditions in Anesthetized Animals   189
  Changes in T_E with Volume Inflations Under
    Isocapnic Conditions in Anesthetized Animals   190
  Effect of Carbon Dioxide   191
  Effect of Temperature   191
  V_T, T_I, and T_E in Man   193
  Effect of Anesthesia   194
  Effect of Sudden Changes in Chemoreceptor Drive   195
  Effect of Alternating Chemoreceptor Stimulation   195

MECHANISMS BY WHICH
  BREATHING PATTERN IS ALTERED   196
  Influence of Pneumotaxic Center   196
  "Pulmonary" Receptors   197
  Intercostal Nerve Afferents   199
  Temperature   199
  Exercise   200
  Cortical Influences   200

MODEL OF INSPIRATORY OFF-SWITCH   201
    Qualitative Description   201
    Mathematical Considerations   203
    Model Predictions and Observed Data   204
    Neurophysiological Basis   205
        A Pool   205
        B Pool   205
        C Pool   206

MODEL OF EXPIRATORY OFF-SWITCH   206

SOME PROBLEMS WITH THESE MODELS   208
    Apneusis   208
    Pneumotaxic Center   208
    Adaptive Phenomena   209
    Complexity of Discharge Patterns Within Brain Stem   209

The main aim of breathing is to provide appropriate ventilation to enable the lungs to transfer suitable amounts of oxygen and carbon dioxide in varying physiological situations. The fact that this is achieved, at least approximately, in a way that minimizes the work done (1), or force applied (2), against the mechanical structures of the respiratory system demonstrates the efficiency of the controlling mechanisms. Cunningham (3) has recently reviewed the literature on the regulation of respiration mainly from the standpoint of changes in total ventilation ($\dot{V}_E$). This review deals with the way the breathing pattern, i.e., the combination of tidal volume (V_T), inspiratory duration (T_I), and expiratory duration (T_E), is changed in a variety of circumstances, and also the means by which this regulation of breathing is achieved.

An examination of the neural mechanisms producing the respiratory rhythm in the brain stem aids in the appreciation of the breathing pattern. There are several reviews on this topic (4–6), but recent work has led to the formulation of a new model of the rhythm generator, and it is from this approach that current concepts of the generation of a respiratory rhythm are discussed in this chapter. The neurophysiological evidence supporting or opposing this model is examined. Other models have been presented previously in the literature (7–15) and are not fully discussed here. Each model has its proponents, and it is true to say that the neurophysiology of these central mechanisms is still far from fully understood.

TIDAL VOLUME AND RESPIRATORY RATE

"Hey Plot"

The pattern of breathing can be expressed graphically by plotting the relationship between V_T and $\dot{V}_E$. This approach was first introduced by Milic-Emili and Cajani (16) but was popularized by Hey et al. (17). Figure 1 shows a diagrammatic representation of the relationship between these two variables when ventilation is increased in humans; similar results have been obtained with anesthetized animals (18). The points obtained can usually be fitted reasonably by two linear curves which meet at a V_T of approximately half-vital capacity. Above this intercept, further increases in $\dot{V}_E$ are produced predominantly by increases in respiratory rate (f), and V_T changes little. Although a continuous curvilinear fit to the data might be more appropriate (18, 19), the use of linear approximations has the advantage of producing simple parameters which can be compared under different experimental conditions.

Contrary to the belief of older physiologists that hypercapnia primarily affected V_T whereas hypoxia changed respiratory rate (20), Hey et al. (17) demonstrated, by collecting data on normal subjects from a number of papers, that many different types of ventilatory stimuli increase ventilation in essentially similar ways. The relation between $\dot{V}_E$ and V_T is thus similar whether ventilation is increased by hypercapnia, hypoxia, metabolic acidemia, change in posture, exercise, or norepinephrine (17).

Effect of Temperature

One factor which does consistently change the Hey relation is a change in body temperature (17). An increase in body temperature, insufficient to exceed the panting threshold, causes a shift of the curve so that at any given level of ventilation the V_T is smaller and f is greater. This is true of conscious human

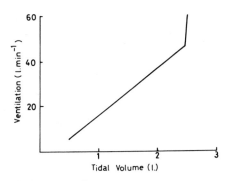

Figure 1. The relationship between $\dot{V}_E$ and V_T (the "Hey plot") with values representative of normal human subjects.

subjects (17, 21) and anesthetized animals (18). A fall in body temperature has the reverse effect.

Influence of Mechanical Loads

The mechanical forces against which the respiratory muscles have to work can influence the Hey relation. Thus, the respiratory rate is faster at a given level of $\dot{V}_E$ when an external elastic load is imposed on breathing (19, 22, 23). However, an increase of air flow resistance produced by the addition of an external resistive load has less consistent effects. Gilbert et al. (19) found that this procedure produced relatively slow breathing, but others (24, 25) could not confirm this.

When an external mechanical load does change the pattern of breathing, it seems to do so in a way which optimizes breathing (19). Voluntary influences may be important in this response, because anesthesia can abolish the changes in respiratory rate produced by elastic loading (26, 27).

Influence of Vagus Nerves

Since the classical experiments of Scott (28), it has been widely accepted that after vagotomy the respiratory rate remains constant as ventilation increases with changes in blood gases. However, the effect of hypercapnia on the respiratory rate after vagotomy is by no means clear. Many workers (18, 29–34) have found results similar to those of Scott, but others (35–39) found that vagotomy does not completely abolish the changes in respiratory rate with hypercapnia, although the response may be reduced. The reason for this discrepancy is difficult to find and seems unrelated to the species of animal used or the state of anesthesia. Vagal block in conscious man markedly reduces the increase in respiratory rate with hypercapnia but appears not to abolish it completely(40).

Whether or not changes in respiratory rate with hypercapnia are completely abolished after vagotomy, it is clear that vagal information is essential in the production of a normal response. Vagotomy changes the slope of the Hey relation in cats (18), and the inflection point is abolished. However, the increase in respiratory rate with exercise (30, 34, 41) and hyperthermia (31, 38, 42) persists after vagotomy, suggesting that the increase in ventilation in these circumstances acts through a mechanism different from that for hypercapnia. The similar Hey relations obtained with hypercapnia and exercise is perhaps, therefore, surprising.

TIDAL VOLUME, AND INSPIRATORY AND EXPIRATORY DURATIONS

V_T and T_I in Steady State Conditions

Priban (43) reported that even apparently regular breathing showed a tendency to cycle over a period of three to four breaths; V_T and f were negatively correlated, ventilation remaining more or less constant. Newsom-Davis and Stagg

(44) recorded normal breathing in resting man and found that V_T and T_I showed a strong positive correlation; the slope of this relationship—the mean inspiratory flow rate—remained constant at rest but increased progressively with $P_{A_{CO_2}}$. V_T, T_E, and V_T, $1/f$ were also positively correlated, the latter relationship confirming Priban's (43) findings.

V_T and T_I with Volume Inflations Under Isocapnic Conditions in Anesthetized Animals

When normal inspiration is assisted by positive pressure, inspiration is terminated early, but the tidal volume achieved is larger (see Figure 2,A). Clark and Euler (45) obtained a whole range of V_T and T_I values by varying the rate of lung inflation or by pulse inflations superimposed on normal inspiration. Large volume inflations were required to terminate inspiration if given soon after the beginning of inspiration, whereas smaller volumes sufficed if given later. Thus, contrary to the relation found during spontaneous breathing in steady state conditions, V_T and T_I are negatively correlated, and the form of the relationship can be described by a hyperbola. This form represents a central threshold which has to be reached before inspiration is terminated, and this threshold is highest at the beginning of inspiration, falling in an approximately hyperbolic fashion as inspiration progresses. This threshold can also be detected by stimulation of the central end of the vagus nerve, in that longer trains of stimuli are required to inhibit inspiration if given soon after the beginning of inspiration than are required if given later (46). The termination of inspiration thus depends on two factors: the form of the central threshold, and the rate of rise of volume (and,

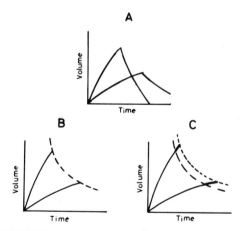

Figure 2. A, the relationship between volume and time from the beginning of an inspiration for a normal breath and for a breath assisted by positive pressure (larger breath). B, the *dashed line* is the volume threshold. Inspiration is terminated when the inspired volume reaches this threshold and, consequently, the volume threshold delineates the V_T/T_I relationship. C, fluctuations in the volume threshold with time produce a scatter in the V_T/T_I points along the direction of the inspired volume curve, i.e., along the thicker line between the two *dashed lines* which represent the extremes of the fluctuation.

therefore, inhibitory vagal information) during inspiration (Figure 2,B). It seems that, for vagal information, the termination of inspiration depends only on the information at the time the threshold curve is reached, because subthreshold volume inflations do not change T_I (45).

Small changes in the central threshold which might occur in steady state conditions will lead to variation in the time at which inspiration is cut off. When inspiration lasts longer, a larger V_T will be achieved, thereby producing the positive correlation between V_T and T_I which is found in these circumstances. Furthermore, the scatter in V_T and T_I points could depend on the angle at which the volume curve approaches the threshold curve. As will be apparent from Figure 2,C, a larger scatter of points might be expected at lower rates of $\dot{V}_E$, and this was demonstrated by Bradley et al. (42) in anesthetized animals.

When volume-related information from the lung is prevented from reaching the brain by vagotomy, T_I is no longer influenced by lung inflation (42). In these conditions, termination of inspiration depends primarily on brain stem mechanisms.

Changes in T_E with Volume Inflations Under Isocapnic Conditions in Anesthetized Animals

T_I and T_E are linearly related when ventilation is increased by hypercapnia (38, 45), although at slower rates of breathing produced by hypocapnia, T_E tends to be disproportionately large. Because of this linear relation, Clark and Euler (45) emphasized that, in normal conditions, T_E was determined by events terminating inspiration. However, T_E can be influenced when conditions are changed during expiration. Thus, Knox (47) found that volume inflations applied during expiration in anesthetized cats prolonged T_E. This can be seen with both pulse and step inflations, provided that they are given during the first 70% of expiration. Inflation in the last 30% of expiration is without effect on T_E, and this volume-insensitive time remains a constant fraction of T_E, even when the respiratory rate is changed by anesthesia or carbon dioxide. However, the magnitude of the response is depressed by anesthesia and increased by hypercapnia. Volume-related information from the lung is responsible for this reflex, because vagotomy abolishes the response.

Unlike the effects of lung volume on T_I, the response of T_E to changes in lung volume are not all-or-nothing in character. Volume pulses applied early during expiration will prolong T_E, showing that the mechanism exhibits integrative properties. Similarly, small step inflations applied early in expiration are more effective than similar steps applied later. Information received during expiration must be accumulated and used to influence the expiratory off-switch. However, larger step inflations may be more effective when given later on in expiration, suggesting that a further mechanism, related to the dynamic properties of a sudden change in lung volume, is also important.

Deflation produces the converse response (47) and, again, changes in volume toward the end of expiration (approximately the last 16%) are without effect.

Effect of Carbon Dioxide

The form of the V_T/T_I curve in anesthetized animals is similar whether it is delineated by volume inflation under isocapnic conditions or by increasing $\dot{V}_E$ with carbon dioxide (45). This suggests that carbon dioxide does not change the inspiratory threshold curve. This conclusion was confirmed quantitatively by Bradley et al. (42) with the use of various steady state levels of carbon dioxide and by comparing the curve obtained with that obtained by volume inflation.

Some shortening of T_I with hypercapnia may persist after vagotomy (38–40), despite the fact that the effect of artificial inflation of the chest is completely abolished. Anesthesia may be important in the response, because vagotomized decerebrate cats do not generally show a decrease in T_I with carbon dioxide but will do so if pentobarbitone is given (39). Because volume-related information is not important in the response, the effect of carbon dioxide must be operating through central mechanisms or peripheral chemoreceptors. The importance of anesthesia suggests that carbon dioxide influences the threshold curve by at least two different mechanisms which can be differentially suppressed by anesthesia. It should be noted, however, that Euler et al. (18) could find no change in T_I by increasing carbon dioxide after vagotomy in cats anesthetized with pentobarbitone.

In view of the possible effect of carbon dioxide in anesthetized vagotomized animals, it is surprising that carbon dioxide failed to influence the threshold curve in the intact animal by allowing smaller volumes to terminate inspiration with hypercapnia. The answer may be in the tendency for carbon dioxide to depress the pulmonary stretch receptor discharge (49, 50), thereby ensuring that larger tidal volumes are required to produce the same inhibitory potential. This peripheral depression could counteract the effect of carbon dioxide on the central nervous mechanisms.

In the intact animal, T_E decreases with hypercapnia despite the high lung volume at the beginning of expiration and the increased sensitivity of the vagal reflex (47), both of which will tend to prolong T_E. The length of the previous inspiration seems to influence T_E directly, as can be seen from the linear relation between T_I and T_E which persists after vagotomy (38). Furthermore, a high initial lung volume with hypercapnia will be followed by a quick fall due to increased expiratory activity and, in the intact animal, to a fall in laryngeal resistance (51). The effect of this operating through the inflation and deflation reflexes would be difficult to predict. Further studies focusing on expiratory duration would be of interest.

Effect of Temperature

Changes in body temperature have a marked effect on the inspiratory threshold curve. At a higher temperature than normal, smaller volumes will suffice to terminate inspiration at a particular T_I value, i.e., the V_T/T_I curve is shifted to the left (33, 38, 42) (see Figure 3). These changes have been analyzed quantita-

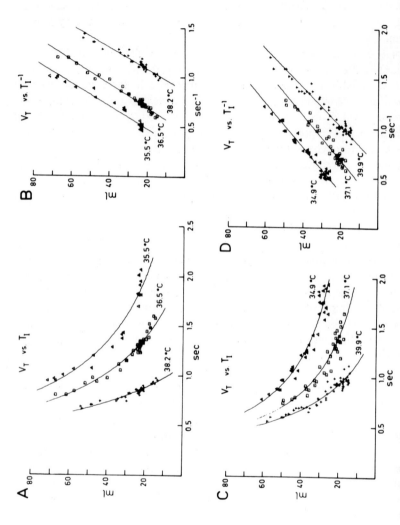

Figure 3. The influence of temperature on the volume threshold curve. A and C show the relationship between V_T and T_I at different temperatures in two different anesthetized cats. B and D show the equivalent relationship between V_T and the reciprocal of T_I. Reprinted with permission of Acta Physiol. Scand. 92:351 (1974).

tively by Bradley et al. (42) who showed that in the relationship

$$V_T = C\,T_I^{-1} + V_0 \qquad (1)$$

an increase in temperature affected the parameter V_0 rather than C, i.e., the effect of an increase in temperature can best be described as a shift of the whole V_T/T_I curve in a downward direction. Possible effects of temperature on functional residual capacity were excluded as a cause of this shift.

Even after vagotomy, T_I progressively shortens with an increase in body temperature (33, 38, 42). Grunstein et al. (33) concluded that this effect on central brain stem mechanisms terminating inspiration could explain the shift in the V_T/T_I curve seen before vagotomy. Nevertheless, effects of temperature on pulmonary stretch receptor discharge (49) should be considered as a possible contributory factor in the response.

T_E is reduced by an increase in temperature even though the reflex effect of volume inflation during expiration is more sensitive (52). As with hypercapnia, there are other possible influences on expiration, such as a reduced V_T and T_I, which could account for this apparent paradox.

V_T, T_I, and T_E in Man

Clark and Euler (45) found differences in the V_T/T_I relation between conscious man and anesthetized cats (Figure 4). As ventilation increases in man, T_I is initially constant as volume gets larger (range 1), but when a certain threshold is exceeded (which varies from person to person), T_I starts decreasing. This phase (range 2) is very similar to the relationship found in anesthetized cats. With very large tidal volumes, a third phase (range 3) is observed in which T_I once again lengthens. This is sometimes seen in anesthetized animals with large volume inflations (42). Range 1 was interpreted as a region in which inspiration was terminated by bulbo-pontine mechanisms. The differences between man and other animals might, therefore, only be quantitative, with the bulbopontine

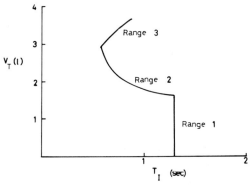

Figure 4. A diagrammatic representation of the relationship between V_T and T_I found in conscious man.

"pacemaker" set at a relatively faster rate in man, thereby encroaching on the volume threshold curve in a region over which breathing normally operates at rest.

In some cases, range 2 was short and for practical purposes T_I was constant with changing V_T. This might explain the results of other workers who have found a constant T_I with varying V_T in the majority of subjects during hypercapnia, hypoxia, and exercise (53, 54). Kay et al. (55) found a consistent decrease in T_I with exercise and hypercapnia, but the changes were small. In contrast to this, decreases in T_E with hypercapnia and exercise are more consistent and larger (53–55). Changes in T_E provide the largest contribution to the rise in respiratory rate which is seen with hypercapnia, hypoxia, and exercise in man.

The observation by Clark and Euler (45) that T_I is often prolonged at the higher levels of V_T (range 3) is surprising in view of the inflection point in the Hey relation above which further increases in V_E are achieved mainly or solely by decreasing the duration of the breath. Because T_I and T_E are approximately linearly related, it is not possible to invoke a markedly reduced T_E to explain this discrepancy. Range 3 is probably related to large augmented breaths or "sighs" which humans and other animals take from time to time. As Clark and Euler (45) pointed out, this inspiratory augmentation is variable and often too limited in extent to be described accurately.

Most workers have failed to find either a range 3 or the opposite when ventilation is increased in normal subjects, but this may be because ventilation was not increased sufficiently. On the other hand, Garrard and Lane (56) obtained results consistent with the Hey relation in that V_T reached a maximum above which changes in ventilation were due to reduction in breath duration. Similar results were obtained by Gardner (57); although V_T did not reach a maximum, he found a break point in the V_T/T_I and V_T/T_E curves above which shortening of T_I and T_E, rather than increases in V_T, predominated.

Grunstein et al (33) found that, when ventilation was increased by hypercapnia in anesthetized cats, a maximum V_T might be reached, although T_I and total breath duration might decrease further. This also would be consistent with the Hey relation. However, Bradley et al. (42) found that in anesthetized cats artificial inflation of the lung with large volumes often caused a prolongation of T_I, producing a range 3 in the V_T/T_I curve. In this case, the different sort of stimulus might have influenced the result, artificial lung inflation possibly stimulating irritant receptors more than an equivalent increase in lung volume due to hypercapnia.

Effect of Anesthesia

The results in man have all been obtained in conscious subjects, which might explain the different responses obtained between man and other animals. It is of interest that the V_T/T_I curve in conscious cats (58) is similar to that for man, in that T_I only shortens at high levels of ventilation. However, this relationship differs from a range 1 in humans in that T_I often shows some lengthening with mild hypercapnic stimulation. Pentobarbitone changes the response to that described previously for anesthetized animals. Certainly, pentobarbitone can influence respiratory reflexes (59–62) and it alters the V_T/T_I curve when given to decerebrate animals (39). A study of the V_T/T_I curve in anesthetized humans would be of interest.

Effect of Sudden Changes in Chemoreceptor Drive

When the chemoreceptor drive is suddenly altered, V_T changes before the respiratory rate responds (63, 64). Similarly T_I lags behind changes in V_T when carbon dioxide concentration is suddenly increased or decreased, producing a hysteresis in the V_T/T_I plot (38, 39, 65) around the steady state V_T/T_I curve (Figure 5). A hysteresis is sometimes seen in the T_I/T_E relation (38).

Cutting the carotid sinus nerves does not abolish the V_T/T_I hysteresis (39) which cannot, therefore, result from the central and peripheral chemoreceptors having different reflex effects. The response is not due to transient changes in functional residual capacity and can occur after vagotomy (39). It appears to be due to the properties of the central mechanism governing breathing.

Effect of Alternating Chemoreceptor Stimulation

Breath-by-breath values of ventilation can be made to alternate if alveolar P_{CO_2} is changed in alternate breaths in man, provided that a steady hypoxia is also present (66). This effect is enhanced by exercise (67) and is due to accentuation of oscillations in the gas concentration in blood travelling from the lung to the peripheral chemoreceptors. Smoothing of these oscillations by inserting a mixing chamber in the supply to the peripheral chemoreceptors abolishes the alternations in V_T seen in anesthetized cats under similar experimental conditions (68).

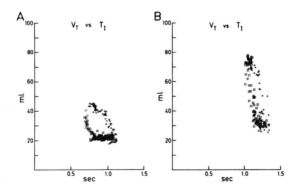

Figure 5. V_T/T_I relationship in response to a sudden increase in the concentration of inhaled carbon dioxide, from a cat anesthetized with pentobarbitone. *A*, before bilateral vagotomy and *B*, after bilateral vagotomy. *Crosses* show the transient response to a rapid increase in $F_{A_{CO_2}}$ from 3.5 to 7.0% and *squares* show the response to a fall in $F_{A_{CO_2}}$ back to 3.6%. Reprinted with permission of Acta Physiol. Scand. 92:341 (1974).

The response to an increase in afferent peripheral chemoreceptor activity of short duration, whether induced by electrical stimulation of the carotid sinus nerve (69, 70) or by changes in blood gas tensions (70, 71), depends precisely on the time during the respiratory cycle the stimulus is given. T_I and T_E may be shortened or lengthened, and the response obtained will, therefore, depend upon the time relation between the oscillating signal at the peripheral chemoreceptors and the phase of the breathing cycle. This in turn depends upon the circulation time between the pulmonary capillaries and the peripheral chemoreceptors, which is likely to differ between individuals and to change slightly from time to time in any one individual. It is not surprising, therefore, that several patterns of responses can be discerned when V_T, T_I, and T_E are measured as alternate breaths of carbon dioxide are given (67). Nevertheless, certain general statements can be made. T_I seems relatively stable, although T_E frequently shows marked oscillations. Inspiratory volume and mean inspiratory flow rate alternate frequently and substantially, but expiratory volume and flow are generally more stable. Consequently, functional residual capacity alternates because of the differences between inspiratory and expiratory volumes.

MECHANISMS BY WHICH BREATHING PATTERN IS ALTERED

There have been several recent reviews describing the properties of peripheral chemoreceptors (72–74) and central chemosensitive areas (75) and, therefore, it is not proposed to discuss these important mechanisms in this review. Respiratory reflexes from the heart and systemic circulation (76) are probably of secondary importance compared with the other reflexes described here and will not be considered further.

Influence of Pneumotaxic Center

Section of the brain stem in the mid-pontine region produces slow, deep breathing (30, 56, 77, 78), although this tends to revert to normal with time (78). The important area that is excluded by this section has been located in the dorsolateral part of the upper pons in the region of the nucleus parabrachialis medialis (79, 80) and is equivalent to what Lumsden (7) called the pneumotaxic center. When destruction of this area is combined with vagotomy, apneustic breathing results (8, 9, 81–83). This is characterized by marked prolongation of the inspiratory phase of the respiratory cycle, which can last for several minutes. Clearly this area is important in the termination of inspiration.

Further information about the function of the pneumotaxic center was obtained by looking at the V_T, T_I, and T_E response to hypercapnia after lesions had been placed in these structures (58). Destruction of the centers results in larger V_T, T_I, and T_E values, but the V_T/T_I and $V_T/(1/f)$ curves are of a shape similar to those found in the intact animal, merely being shifted to the right. Larger volume inflations are, therefore, needed to terminate inspiration at a particular T_I value, which suggests that the normal function of the pneumotaxic center is to reduce the threshold which has to be exceeded by an inhibitory signal before inspiration is curtailed. The recent results of Euler et al. (84) are in substantial agreement with these findings, but Tang (30) found that hypercapnia had little effect on the depth of breathing when the pneumotaxic centers had been destroyed.

Inspiration can be terminated early by stimulation of the nucleus parabrachialis medialis (85), larger shocks being required early on in inspiration. Although this nucleus obviously influences the central threshold governing the termination of inspiration, it seems that the fall in the central threshold as inspiration progresses does not reside in this nucleus. The excitatory influence of the nucleus parabrachialis medialis has been elegantly demonstrated by Euler et al. (84). The strength of stimulus (applied to one nucleus) required to terminate inspiration was determined before and after destruction of the remaining nucleus. This produced a parallel shift in the stimulus strength versus T_I relation, such that larger stimulus strengths were required after destruction of the other nucleus.

Other workers have obtained more complicated responses to stimulation in the pneumotaxic region. Cohen (86) found two different centers: an inspiratory facilitatory and an expiratory facilitatory. Stimulation of either center during inspiration shortened T_I, but the rate of rise of phrenic activity was greater than normal when the inspiratory facilitatory center was stimulated and less than normal when the expiratory facilitatory center was stimulated. Effects on T_E could also be obtained by stimulating these centers, the inspiratory facilitatory center shortening T_E and the expiratory facilitatory center prolonging T_E. Bertrand and Hugelin (80) also obtained different responses, depending upon which part of the nucleus parabrachialis medialis was stimulated. This area may, therefore, have a function more complex than has previously been supposed.

"Pulmonary" Receptors

It is now believed that there are only four types of receptor which are to be found in the tracheobronchial tree and lung parenchyma: pulmonary stretch receptors, cough receptors, irritant receptors, and J receptors (87). All of these can influence the breathing pattern, but pulmonary stretch receptors are the most likely to convey volume-related information. It is generally accepted that they inhibit inspiration (87), although this view does not go unchallenged (88). Irritant receptors may be responsible for the occasional deep breaths seen in spontaneously breathing animals (probably related to range 3 in the V_T/T_I relation), but more usually they cause hyperpnea. They are activated by inhalation of irritant gases and smoke, as well as by a number of pathological conditions (87). Stimulation of J receptors produces apnoea followed by rapid breathing, but it seems that they are not active in normal conditions (87).

Receptors from the larynx and pharynx can influence the breathing pattern (87), but in the majority of animal experiments these areas are bypassed by tracheostomy.

Differences in response to hypercapnia seen between man and other animals may be due to different reflex responses to pulmonary stretch receptor activation. Although the responses of these receptors to changes in lung volume are similar in man and other animals (89), the inflation reflex is generally weaker in man (90) and probably not operative until tidal volumes of 400–800 ml are reached (91). Thus, vagal block in conscious, normal man does not change the breathing pattern at rest (92) but reduces the respiratory rate during hypercapnia (92) when the tidal volumes are larger. This could explain the finding of a range 1 in the V_T/T_I relation in man when the tidal volume is insufficient to inhibit inspiration reflexes. However, it should be noted that the strength of the inflation reflex is usually tested by determining the length of apnea produced by lung inflation. This prolongation of expiration (attributed to pulmonary stretch receptor discharge) is due to delay in the operation of the expiratory off-switch, which may have a different threshold from the action of pulmonary stretch receptors in activating the inspiratory off-switch.

The action of pulmonary stretch receptors during inspiration may depend upon the phasic nature of the discharge. Bartoli et al (93) showed that maintained lung inflation in dogs had minor and inconsistent effects on T_I when blood gases were held constant by cardiac bypass. On the other hand, the effects of inflation on T_E were clear cut and consistent with the results of Knox (47) described above. Paralysis with gallamine produced prolongation of T_I, which was attributed to the removal of phasic pulmonary stretch receptor discharge. Some tonic influence on T_I was present, however, because vagotomy in the paralyzed state led to further prolongation of T_I. This tonic influence appears to be independent of volume. The failure to influence T_I by maintained lung inflation is difficult to reconcile with results obtained in animals without cardiac bypass. In cats, dogs, and rabbits, D'Angelo and Agostini (94) found that T_I was reduced and T_E prolonged when the end expiratory pressure was held above functional residual capacity. Similarly, maintained lung inflation in paralyzed dogs produces apnea followed by short phrenic bursts (short T_I) and long expirations (95).

If the tonic discharge is important, changes in functional residual capacity must be considered when the V_T/T_I curves in different circumstances are compared. The threshold curve defines the amount of inhibitory activity required to terminate inspiration at a given time during inspiration. The V_T/T_I curve is only a reflection of this threshold curve, and the relation between the two will depend on the connection between V_T and vagal inhibitory activity. This activity may change if the breath is taken from a different functional residual capacity, because the absolute peak inspiratory volume and, therefore, the peak inhibitory activity, will be different even with the same V_T. A similar argument applies to effects of temperature and hypercapnia on pulmonary stretch receptor discharge (49).

Intercostal Nerve Afferents

Reflexes from receptors within the intercostal muscles can influence the regulation of breathing. Remmers (96) has shown that intercostal muscle spindles stimulated by chest compression (presumably in the external intercostal muscles) can reduce phrenic activity and slow the respiratory rate. The slowing of respiratory rate is due to a prolongation of T_E, T_I being shorter than control. Interestingly, this shortening of T_I was more easily provoked if the compression were applied during the later parts of inspiration, perhaps reflecting the change in central threshold. Electrical stimulation of the external intercostal nerve can also shorten T_I and prolong T_E (97).

Apparently results contradictory to these were obtained by Decima and Euler (98), who demonstrated an excitation of phrenic activity produced by an increased discharge of muscle spindle afferents from either the external or internal intercostal muscles of the lower thoracic segments. In fact, it seems that the inhibitory influence on the phrenic nerve is produced by stimulation of muscle spindles in midthoracic segments, whereas the excitatory influence is only produced from the lower thoracic segments (99). The latter reflex is purely spinal, whereas the inhibitory influence passes via pathways in the ventrolateral part of the spinal cord (100, 101) to the brain stem.

Whether these reflexes are important in physiological conditions is questionable. Bradley et al. (42) could find no change in T_I with lung inflation after vagotomy, although occlusion of the trachea at end expiration (61) or application of smaller elastic loads (102) may shorten inspiration through the reflex described by Remmers. Gautier (48) found that dorsal rhizotomy in anesthetized rabbits produced a fall in V_T and an increase in f. The fall in V_T is to be expected when the feedback to the intercostal muscles is disrupted, but the rise in f may be due to disruption of the reflex inhibition from intercostal muscle spindles in the midthoracic region. It should be noted that response to passive inflation through this reflex should cause lengthening of T_I and shortening of T_E, which is the reverse of the response obtained from pulmonary stretch receptors.

Temperature

A rise in temperature increases the respiratory rate through stimulation of peripheral thermosensitive receptors (76), thermosensitive areas in the hypothalamus (4), and even thermosensitive areas in the spinal cord and medulla (103). Changes in breathing can be seen before the panting threshold is reached, and the responses to changes in temperature reviewed here have been limited to this range. When the panting threshold is reached, the reflex response to hypercapnia is altered (18).

Exercise

The respiratory response to exercise is complex and far from fully understood. The topic has been reviewed by Dejours (104), and, more recently, by Cunningham (3). In summary, it can be said that there are at least two components in the response to exercise, a fast and a slow one. The fast component may partly be due to a coordinated response initiated by the diencephalon, in which limb movements and the respiratory and cardiovascular systems are involved (105). Undoubtedly, mechanical stimulation resulting from muscle activity can also produce an increase in ventilation reflexes, although there is dispute as to which receptors are involved (106–110). The motor pathways mediating this reflex may partly be routed through the sympathetic system, which shows increased activity, with consequent increase in peripheral chemoreceptor activity, when the hind limbs of anesthetized cats are subjected to passive movement (111). Several factors could be responsible for the slow component of the increase in ventilation, and these are reviewed elsewhere (104).

In view of the complex nature of the response to exercise it is surprising that the changes in breathing pattern with exercise and alteration of blood gas tensions are so similar. However, no one has made a quantitative comparison of the V_T, T_I, and T_E responses in the two conditions. The major difference is the undisputed increase in respiratory rate which is seen with exercise even after vagotomy.

Cortical Influences

The basic breathing pattern and vagal reflexes are similar in both decerebrate and anesthetized animals. The mechanisms responsible for generation of the respiratory rhythm and the central connections for the respiratory reflexes must, therefore, lie within the brain stem. Nevertheless, higher centers can change the breathing pattern (4), and this mechanism could be responsible for some of the differences noted between conscious and anesthetized animals.

Aminoff and Sears (112) have shown that stimulation of the trunk area in the sensorimotor cortex can excite expiration and inhibit inspiration at the spinal level. Pathways serving this function are different from the pathways conveying the rhythmical breathing input. In this context, it is of interest that in some patients who have had a high cervical cordotomy, spontaneous breathing is impaired (with danger of respiratory failure during sleep) while voluntary control is normal (113). The converse situation can also occur with loss of voluntary control of breathing (114).

The importance of higher centers on the control of breathing was apparent in recovery experiments in cats in which bilateral lesions were made in the nucleus parabrachialis medialis (78). Although such lesions produced a temporary slowing of breathing, this recovered over a period of 1–3 months. On reanesthetizing the animals and cutting the vagus nerves, a state of apneusis was obtained but eupneic breathing was restored when the animals awoke. Further evidence illustrating the power of higher centers over respiratory reflexes is shown by the abolition of the apneic response to vagal stimulation in conscious cats if a noise or flash of light is given at the same time (115).

MODEL OF INSPIRATORY OFF-SWITCH

Bradley et al. (116) have proposed a model of the inspiratory off-switch, with the intention of collating data that were available at the time in the hope that questions raised might lead to profitable investigation in the future. Of necessity, the model is rather speculative and may well prove to be oversimplified. Herczynski and Karczewski (117) have recently proposed a model of breathing which, at first sight, seems different from that of Bradley et al. (116). However, there are many points of similarity and it is mainly the approach which differs. Essential differences in the models are mentioned below. Other models of the rhythm generator are reviewed elsewhere (4–6). They do not lend themselves to a quantitative analysis in the way that the models of Bradley et al. (116) and Herczynski and Karczewski (117) do, but are based mainly on the results of neurophysiological investigation of the brain stem.

Qualitative Description

The basic structure of the model is shown in Figure 6. The A pool consists of neurons with a slowly increasing inspiratory activity (i) which can be influenced by chemoreceptor stimulation and, possibly, by temperature. This activity projects to the spinal motoneurons (seen in the shape of the phrenic activity) and to a further group of neurons within the brain stem—the B pool. Within the B pool, i interacts with the vagal volume signal (v) in an additive fashion, producing an output (g) which is passed on to the C pool. In the absence of vagal information, i and g have the same form.

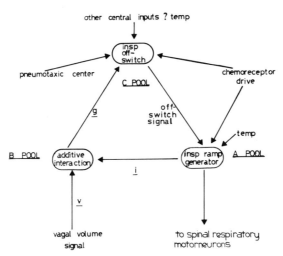

Figure 6. Model structure of the inspiratory off-switch mechanism. For description see text.

The C pool is assumed to have a threshold (c) which has to be reached by the g activity before the inspiratory off-switch is activated. Thus

$$g = c \qquad (2)$$

is the basic inspiratory off-switch equation. The threshold of the C pool may be influenced by chemoreceptor drive, temperature, and the nucleus parabrachialis medialis. It is assumed constant with time, although Herczynski and Karczewski (117) considered a central threshold falling during inspiration. This difference, however, is more apparent than real, because the latter authors consider the threshold after interaction with the vagal activity. After vagotomy, the threshold against time is constant.

In order to provide for the possibility of T_I remaining relatively constant with changing chemoreceptor drive after vagotomy, and because central inspiratory activity rises with increases in chemoreceptor activity, it is necessary to postulate that the threshold c also rises in these circumstances. This is illustrated in Figure 7 with two different levels of chemoreceptor activity. The relative influence of this chemoreceptor activity on the g activity and the threshold c will determine whether or not T_I is constant. It is possible that anesthetics disrupt the balance (39), producing mismatch.

The presence of vagal activity increases the rate of rise of g and the threshold is reached earlier (Figure 8,A). The larger the contribution from the vagus, the earlier will c be reached. The two *arrowed lines* in Figure 8, A and B, show the amount of vagal activity which would be required to terminate inspiration at that particular inspiratory duration. Clearly, Figure 8,B is a mirror image of the g activity and could be converted into a V_T/T_I plot if the relation between volume and vagal activity were known. It should be noted that this model assumes that only the vagal activity at the time the off-switch operates is important (see Clark and Euler (45)), whereas Herczynski and Karczewski (117) assume integration of vagal information.

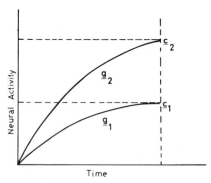

Figure 7. Inspiration is terminated when the rise in inhibitory input to the C pool (g) reaches the threshold (c). This is shown for two levels of chemoreceptor drive which, in this case, produces equivalent changes in the rate of rise of g and in the threshold c.

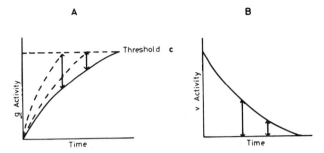

Figure 8. *A*, the *solid line* shows the increase in *g* without the addition of vagal information. The *dashed lines* show the influence of vagal information on the *g* activity at two different rates of lung inflation. The greater the rate of inflation, the earlier inspiration is terminated. The *arrows* show the amount of vagal activity required to terminate inspiration at that time. *B*, a plot of the vagal activity required to terminate inspiration at different times after the beginning of inspiration. The *arrows* are equivalent to those in *A*.

A rise in body temperature could cause a fall in the threshold *c* or an increase in the rate of rise of *g*, because either of these would increase the respiratory rate. This is considered in more detail later.

Mathematical Considerations

Making a number of assumptions, Bradley et al. (116) produced a formula which describes the function of their model. Some of these assumptions have been described above in the qualitative analysis of the model, but to these can be added the following:

1. The mathematical form of the *i* activity,

$$i(t) = i_{\text{sat}} \cdot \frac{t}{t + t_a} \tag{3}$$

where i_{sat} is asymptote, t is time, and t_a controls the rate of rise of activity.
2. *i* and *c* have drive-dependent as well as drive-independent parts. The drive-dependent parts of *i* and *c* are $f_1(x)$ and $f_2(x)$, respectively, where (x) represents the chemical drive. The drive-dependent part of *i* is modified by a transmission factor, α, at the B pool, becoming $\alpha f_1 x$ before reaching the C pool. Mismatch, $d(x)$, is defined as the difference between these drive-dependent functions as they interact at the C pool, i.e.,

$$d(x) = \alpha f_1(x) - f_2(x) \tag{4}$$

Using the basic switch equation, $g = c$, and assuming that *i* and *v* interact in a simple additive fashion, the following formula can be derived:

$$\beta v_t = u - d(x) - \alpha i_{\text{sat}} \cdot \frac{T_I}{T_I + t_a} \tag{5}$$

where α and β are transmission factors at the B pool and u defines the dependence of the threshold c on factors other than chemoreceptor drive; v_t is vagal activity present at the termination of inspiration. If there is no mismatch the formula simplifies.

Assuming values for all the parameters included and using the relation between lung volume (V) and vagal activity (v)

$$v = k \, (V - V_z)^{0.5} \qquad (6)$$

it is possible to derive a V_T/T_I plot which can be compared with experimental results. The effects of changing the values of different parameters can then be studied.

Model Predictions and Observed Data

The decrease in T_I sometimes seen with hypercapnia after vagotomy could be due to a failure of the threshold c and activity g to increase by equivalent amounts. It seemed surprising, however, that such mismatch did not manifest itself in a shift of the V_T/T_I curve with the vagus nerve intact. By choosing appropriate values of parameters, Bradley et al. (116) were able to show that a mismatch can be obtained which could be easily seen after vagotomy but which would be small, and possibly lost in the "noise," before vagotomy. The effect of carbon dioxide on pulmonary stretch receptor discharge could also contribute to a minimization of the shift with the vagus nerves intact.

Temperature changes produce marked shifts in the V_T/T_I curve and, according to the above model, this could be due to changing the threshold c or the rate of rise of the i activity (by changing i_{sat}). If temperature affects only the threshold, then the model shows that the v/T_I plot is shifted vertically; but when converted to a V_T/T_I curve, both the shape and the horizontal asymptote change. This is at variance with experimental results (42), although the effect on shape may have been too small to detect.

A rise in i_{sat} with temperature, on the other hand, increases the rate of rise of the i activity without markedly affecting its peak value (the chemoreceptor drive-dependent component being dominant). This agrees with the effect of temperature on the phrenic activity (reflecting the A pool activity) seen in apneustic conditions (84) and, furthermore, the model predictions of such a parameter change fit the experimental findings of Bradley et al (42) quite closely. It seems most likely, therefore, that temperature exerts its effect on the A pool activity, rather than on the threshold of the C pool.

The transient response to step changes in $P_{A_{CO_2}}$ applied to the model can be made to produce hysteresis effects, if the response of the two central mechanisms sensitive to changes in carbon dioxide are postulated to have different time constants. However, the model predicts a greater hysteresis effect when the vagus nerves are cut, which was not observed experimentally. This disagreement with experimental results could be explained if one assumed that the carbon dioxide sensitivity of the pulmonary stretch receptors is of importance and that this third time constant is somewhat faster than those of central origin.

Neurophysiological Basis

A Pool There are many neurons within the brain stem which show activity in time with respiration, but the functional equivalent of the A pool neurons must lie below the midpons, because section in this region does not destroy the rhythm-generating mechanism. There are two areas caudal to this level where discharge patterns similar to those expected from A pool neurons are found: the lateral part of the medulla in the vicinity of the nucleus retroambigualis and near the nucleus of the solitary tract. The neurons of the nucleus retroambigualis are predominantly either inspiratory or expiratory and provide the descending input to the segmental motoneurons (118, 119). They could be equivalent to the A pool neurons, but it is difficult to exclude the possibility that the rhythm generator mechanism lies elsewhere and that these neurons represent a relay station. The close similarity between the individual discharge patterns of these neurons and the total phrenic discharge, even with minor fluctuations in the inspiratory pattern, suggests that these neurons are not primarily involved in the generation of the respiratory rhythm (120). Also, no projection of these cells to neurons which are thought to be equivalent to the B pool neurons has been found (119), although this would be expected according to the above model.

Merrill (119) is of the opinion that the primary rhythm generator resides outside the nucleus retroambigualis, although interconnections between cells of this region could be responsible for switching from inspiration to expiration. Certainly, there are neurons near the nucleus of the tractus solitarius which could fulfil the function of the A pool neurons. These neurons have a discharge pattern similar to that of the phrenic nerve and are inhibited by lung inflation (R_α neurons of Baumgarten and Kanzow (10); similar neurons have been found by other workers (121, 122)). They project to the spinal cord (123), but whether they project to the cells of the nucleus retroambigualis is unknown.

B Pool Other respiratory neurons near the nucleus of the tractus solitarius show persistent activity, even when the phrenic discharge has been inhibited by lung inflation, provided that the inflation is maintained (10, 121, 122) (R_β neurons). They therefore appear to be closely related to pulmonary stretch receptors, and the nucleus of the tractus solitarius is known to be the dorsal nucleus for the vagus nerve (124). However, even when the animal was paralyzed and the ventilator stopped, an inspiratory discharge persisted in these neurons. Central inspiratory activity (*i* activity), as well as vagal afferent activity, must therefore project to them, making them ideal candidates for the B pool neurons.

The tractus solitarius complex is clearly an important area in the regulation of the breathing pattern, although the recent work of Koepchen et al. (125) has cast doubt on its central role in the rhythm-generating mechanism. These authors showed that bilateral destruction of these areas did not abolish breathing, although the respiratory frequency was markedly reduced. If the B pool is situated near the nucleus of the tractus solitarius, then total destruction of this area on both sides should completely destroy the rhythm generator according to the model of Bradley et al. (116), particularly if the A pool also resides near that structure. It is possible that the important areas were not completely destroyed in the experiments of Koepchen et al. (125), or, alternatively, several potential rhythm-generating mechanisms may exist for breathing, rather like the different pacemaker systems controlling the heart beat. If the latter is true, then destruction of even a central component may not abolish breathing, although the breathing pattern that remains may bear little relation to normal breathing.

Other workers (see Wyss (126)) have also shown that destruction of parts of the nucleus of the tractus solitarius can change the breathing pattern without destroying respiratory rhythm. There is evidence in rabbits that the rostral and caudal parts of the nucleus have different roles to play in reflexes elicited by stimulation of the vagus nerves. Thus, the expiratory response to high frequency vagal stimulation is abolished by destruction of the rostral part of the nucleus, whereas the inspiratory response to low frequency stimulation is abolished by destruction of the caudal part (126).

C Pool   The discharge of C pool neurons is thought to begin at the termination of inspiration and then to decline throughout expiration (116). Neurons with peak activity at the beginning of expiration have been recorded by several workers (13, 14, 127, 128), although the activity often ceases well before the end of expiration. Some of these neurons may be efferent to the larynx, but others may be involved in the termination of inspiration. It has been suggested that phase-spanning neurons with activity during late inspiration and early expiration are involved in the inspiratory off-switch (79, 80). Although these neurons show late inspiratory activity, this does not necessarily exclude them from being C pool neurons. They may have the same function as the neurons with activity limited to early expiration. Many of these phase-spanning neurons are found in the pneumotaxic center (79, 80), but because midpontine section does not abolish the basic rhythm generator, these cells could not be the C pool neurons. However, similar neurons have been found in the medulla, although there is no discrete area in which they predominate.

MODEL OF EXPIRATORY OFF-SWITCH

Increasingly more attention is now being paid to the termination of expiration. It is, perhaps, surprising that T_I has commanded so much attention when, at least in conscious humans, changes in respiratory rate are predominately due to changes in T_E. As further information becomes available, it may be possible to postulate an expiratory off-switch along lines similar to the inspiratory model. Such a switch is implicit in the model of Herczynski and Karczewski (117), but this model has not so far been extended to include the influence of temperature and chemoreceptor drive.

Knox (47) postulated that the inhibitory activity terminating inspiration continues to act in a slowly decaying manner during expiration until a lower threshold is reached, whereupon the next inspiration begins. In the model of Bradley et al. (116), it is suggested that the activity of the C pool serves this inhibitory function and that volume inflation during expiration can prolong expiration by increasing activity within this pool, so delaying the point at which the lower threshold is reached.

One problem with this simple model is that vagotomy prolongs T_E, although it prevents volume-related information from the lungs, with its tendency to lengthen T_E, from reaching the brain. An opposing and more powerful influence on T_E appears to be the length of the previous inspiration. Vagotomy would, therefore, lengthen T_E primarily by lengthening T_I. This could be due to a larger peak inhibitory activity in the C pool at the beginning of expiration, taking longer to decay to its lower threshold value. Why the peak inhibitory activity in the C pool should be higher with larger T_I remains unexplained.

Bartoli et al. (93) found that, in conditions of cardiopulmonary bypass in paralyzed dogs, vagotomy had no consistent effect on T_E. They postulated that in such conditions the pulmonary stretch receptor activity at end expiration had little influence on T_E. An increase in the activity, however, lengthened T_E and a decrease, produced by deflation, shortened T_E. Both these findings would be consistent with pulmonary stretch receptor activity lengthening T_E, inflation increasing this activity and deflation decreasing it. However, it is hard to see why the activity at a normal end-expiratory volume in conditions of bypass failed to have any influence on T_E.

Changes in chemoreceptor drive can influence the termination of expiration in several ways:

1. The sensitivity of pulmonary stretch receptors is reduced by hypercapnia and a preceding large lung inflation (129).
2. With an increased chemoreceptor drive, the initially high pulmonary stretch receptor activity at end inspiration (due to a large tidal volume) will fall rapidly as a consequence of increased expiratory activity and relaxation of the larynx (51). Furthermore, the end-expiratory lung volume is likely to be reduced due to increased expiratory activity.
3. The shorter T_I obtained as chemoreceptor drive is increased can directly influence the length of the following expiration. Thus, if inspiration is cut short by electrical stimulation of a vagus nerve during inspiration, in an animal with both vagus nerves cut, T_E is also reduced (46).
4. There is evidence that the threshold for termination of expiration is changed by alteration in chemoreceptor drive. Prolonged expiration produced by lung inflation is less when the chemoreceptor drive is increased by hypercapnia or hypoxia (130).

Clearly, the events leading to the termination of expiration are at least as complex as those involved in the termination of inspiration and need further analysis.

SOME PROBLEMS WITH THESE MODELS

Apneusis

The apneustic breathing which is produced by midpontine section is abolished by a further section at the pontomedullary junction. This led Lumsden (7) to suggest that an apneustic center, excitatory to inspiration, existed in the lower pons. The discovery of phase-spanning neurons in this region, discharging in late expiration and early inspiration, which could be excitatory to inspiration, lends some support to this idea (79). Furthermore, the findings of Pitts et al. (8) that electrical stimulation in this region produced inspiration were thought to be evidence in favor of this view. However, careful comparison of the anatomical position of Lumsden's apneustic center and Pitt's inspiratory center shows that the latter is somewhat caudal to the apneustic center and probably in the upper part of the medulla (6). It would seem to be equivalent to the nucleus reticularis gigantocellularis, which controls tonic, rather than phasic, inspiratory activity (131).

Current concepts of apneusis are at variance with the idea of an apneustic center. It is now thought that apneusis results when the inhibitory activity takes a long time to reach the central threshold, which is raised because of the removal of the pneumotaxic center influence. The fact that section at the pontomedullary junction abolishes apneusis suggests that an integral part of the rhythm-generating mechanism lies above this level. Most of the neurons in the lower pons are phase-spanning neurons, as mentioned above, and do not have a suitable discharge to be considered as A, B, or C pool neurons. They could have a role to play in the termination of expiration, but it is termination of inspiration which is changed when this part of the pons is cut away. Clearly, this is difficult to explain on the current concepts, as is also the recovery of rhythmical breathing, albeit sometimes gasping, by section at the pontomedullary junction. Perhaps damage produced by this section is quite extensive, and the breathing seen is unphysiological in the sense that the mechanisms responsible for the rhythm in these circumstances are entirely different from the mechanisms operating in the intact animal.

Pneumotaxic Center

According to the inspiratory off-switch model of Bradley et al. (116), rostral pontine structures exert a tonic influence on the C pool, thereby lowering the threshold which has to be exceeded before inspiration is terminated. If this is the sole function of the nucleus parabrachialis medialis, it seems strange that nearly all the neurons in this area are phasic. In recent years, this area has been extensively explored (80, 132), and the distribution of the different types of respiratory neurons found there has been mapped (132). It has been suggested that the pneumotaxic center functions as a respiratory oscillator (80), but, alternatively, the neurons of this center may be driven by the medullary oscillator. The suppression of activity within the nucleus parabrachialis medialis by pentobarbitone (133), without marked changes in normal breathing, suggests that the latter view is more likely. This view is also supported by the experiments of Cohen (134) and Hukuhara (133), who have shown that surgical interruption of the pathways between the medulla and pons abolishes the respiratory activity of the neurons within the pneumotaxic center, rather than that of medullary respiratory neurons. Whatever the outcome of this dispute, it would be surprising if the pneumotaxic center simply exerts a tonic influence on the medullary neurons.

Adaptive Phenomena

Any comprehensive model of the breathing pattern should explain the finding that the breathing pattern can alter while a stimulus is maintained, even in the absence of changes in blood gas tensions. Thus, prolonged lung inflation can initially completely inhibit phrenic nerve discharge, but, if maintained, the discharge eventually returns to near normal (95). Similarly, repetitive stretch of the Achilles tendon increases phrenic discharge, but the full reflex effect does not persist when the stimulus is maintained (41).

A different, but possibly related, phenomenon is the slow decline in ventilation which follows active hyperventilation produced by electrical stimulation of the carotid sinus nerve (135). This contrasts with the hypoventilation or apnea which follows passive hyperventilation. The same effect can be seen by recording the phrenic discharge of paralyzed animals when a stimulus is removed (136).

Such phenomena are thought to result from properties of the central respiratory mechanism (136), but our knowledge of these mechanisms is not yet sufficiently comprehensive to explain them.

Complexity of Discharge Patterns Within Brain Stem

The multiplicity of discharge patterns which have been described in the brain stem (13, 14, 78, 80, 133, 137) makes it likely that one would be able to find some neurons with discharge patterns to match almost any model. Furthermore, the range of discharge patterns seen is reduced by anesthesia and may change with time, perhaps showing a rhythmical discharge only intermittently; consequently, the true position may be more complicated than is normally apparent. Some of these neurons may have nothing to do with the generation of a respiratory rhythm, possibly functioning as interconnections between respiratory and other reflexes. Others may represent the motor supply to facial muscles, larynx, or other respiratory structures. It is also possible that some neurons with slightly different discharge patterns really belong to the same group, because it seems unlikely that even neurons belonging to one functioning group should discharge in precisely the same manner without showing some statistical scatter.

Nevertheless, the multiplicity of discharge patterns and their varying response to lung inflation (13, 138) and carbon dioxide (14) suggest that the current models are oversimplified. Even so, such models can be, and have been, useful as a stimulus and guide to further research.

ACKNOWLEDGMENTS

The author expresses his appreciation to Professor Curt von Euler for his stimulus and help over the last few years and to my colleagues Dr. M. I. M. Noble and Dr. Diane Trenchard for useful discussion.

REFERENCES

1. Otis, A. B., Fenn, W. O., and Rahn, H. (1950). Mechanics of breathing in man. J. Appl. Physiol. 2:592.
2. Mead, J. (1960). Control of respiratory frequency. J. Appl. Physiol. 15:325.
3. Cunningham, D. J. C. (1974). Integrative aspects of the regulation of breathing: a personal view. In J. G. Widdicombe (ed.), MTP International Review of Science, Physiology Series I, Vol. 2, Respiratory Physiology I, p. 303. University Park Press, Baltimore.
4. Wang, S. C., and Ngai, S. H. (1964). General organisation of central respiratory mechanisms. In W. O. Fenn and H. Rahn (eds.), Handbook of Physiology, Section #3: Respiration, Vol. 1, p. 487. American Physiology Society, Washington, D. C.
5. Karczewski, W. A. (1974). Organisation of the brain stem respiratory complex. In J. G. Widdicombe (ed.), MTP International Review of Science, Physiology Series I, Vol. 2, Respiratory Physiology I, p. 197. University Park Press, Baltimore.
6. Mitchell, R. A., and Berger, A. J. (1975). Neural regulation of respiration. Am. Rev. Respir. Dis. 111:206.
7. Lumsden, T. L. (1923). Observations on the respiratory centres in the cat. J. Physiol. (Lond.) 57:153.
8. Pitts, R. F., Magoun, H. W., and Ranson, S. W. (1939). Interrelations of the respiratory centers in the cat. Am. J. Physiol. 126:689.
9. Wang, S. C., Ngai, S. G., and Frumin, M. J. (1957). Organization of central respiratory mechanisms in the brain stem of the cat: genesis of normal respiratory rhythmicity. Am. J. Physiol. 190:333.
10. Baumgarten, R. von., and Kanzow, E. (1958). The interaction of two types of inspiratory neurons in the region of the tractus solitarius of the cat. Arch. Ital. Biol. 96:361.
11. Burns, B. D., and Salmoiraghi, G. C. (1960). Repetitive firing of respiratory neurones during their burst activity. J. Neurophysiol. 23:27.
12. Salmoiraghi, G. C., and Baumgarten, R. von. (1961). Intracellular potentials from respiratory neurones in brain-stem of cat and mechanism of rhythmic respiration. J. Neurophysiol. 24:203.
13. Nesland, R., and Plum, F. (1965). Subtypes of medullary respiratory neurones. Exp. Neurol. 12:337.
14. Cohen, M. I. (1968). Discharge patterns of brain-stem respiratory neurones in relation to carbon dioxide tension. J. Neurophysiol. 31:142.

15. Hugelin, A., and Bertrand, F. (1973). Organisation of the pneumotaxic oscillator in the cat. *In* W. A. Karczewski and J. G. Widdicombe (eds.), International Symposium on Neural Control of Breathing. Acta Neurobiol. Exp. 33:275.

16. Milic-Emili, G., and Cajani, F. (1957). La frequenza dei respiri in funzione della ventilazione polmonare durante il ristoro. Bull. Soc. It. Biol. Sper. 33:821.

17. Hey, E. N., Lloyd, B. B., Cunningham, D. J. C., Jukes, M. G. M., and Bolton, D. P. G. (1966). Effects of various respiratory stimuli on the depth and frequency of breathing in man. Respir. Physiol. 1:193.

18. Euler, C. von., Herrero, F., and Wexler, I. (1970). Control mechanisms determining rate and depth of respiratory movements. Respir. Physiol. 10:93.

19. Gilbert, R., Howland-Auchincloss, J., Baule, G., Peppi, D., and Long, D. (1971). Breathing pattern during CO_2 inhalation obtained from motion of the chest and abdomen. Respir. Physiol. 13:238.

20. Haldane, J. S., Meakins, J. C., and Priestley, J. G. (1919). The respiratory response to anoxaemia. J. Physiol. (Lond.) 52:420.

21. Vejby-Christensen, H., and Strange-Petersen, E. (1973). Effect of body temperature and hypoxia on the ventilatory CO_2 response in man. Respir. Physiol. 19:322.

22. Cotes, J. E., Johnson, G. R. Morgon, C., Williams, E. L., and Wood, M. M. (1970). Exercise tachypnoea during elastic loading of inspiration: relationship to other variables. J. Physiol. (Lond.) 207:86P.

23. Rebuck, A. S., Jones, N. L., and Pengelly, L. D. (1973). Tidal volume response to exercise in patients with stiff lungs and normal subjects with inspiratory elastic loading. Bull. Physiopathol. Respir. 9:1266.

24. Cotes, J. E., Johnson, G. R., and McDonald, A. (1970). Breathing frequency and tidal volume relationship to breathlessness. *In* Ruth Porter (ed.), Breathing: Hering-Breuer Centenary Symposium, p. 297. J. & A. Churchill, Lond.

25. Gee, J. B. L., Burton, G., Vassallo, C., and Gregg, J. (1968). Effects of external airway obstruction on work capacity and pulmonary gas exchange. Am. Rev. Respir. Dis. 98:1003.

26. Freedman, S., and Campbell, E. J. M. (1970). The ability of normal subjects to tolerate added inspiratory loads. Respir. Physiol. 10:213.

27. Margaria, C. E., Iscoe, S., Pengelly, L. D., Couture, J., Don, H., and Milic-Emili, J. (1973). Immediate ventilatory response to elastic loads and positive pressure in man. Respir. Physiol. 18:347.

28. Scott, F. H. (1908). On the relative parts played by nervous and chemical factors in the regulation of respiration. J. Physiol. (Lond.) 37:301.

29. Nesland, R. S., Plum, F., Nelson, J. R., and Siedler, H. D. (1966). The graded response to stimulation of medullary respiratory neurons. Exp. Neurol. 14:57.

30. Tang, P. C. (1967). Brain stem control of respiratory depth and rate in the cat. Respir. Physiol. 3:349.

31. Phillipson, E. A., Hickey, R. F., Bainton, C. R., and Nadel, J. A. (1970). Effect of vagal blockade on regulation of breathing in conscious dogs. J. Appl. Physiol. 29:475.

32. Rosenstein, R., McCarthy, L. E., and Borison, H. L. (1973). Rate versus depth of breathing independent of alveolar oxygen in decerebrate cats. Respir. Physiol. 19:80.

33. Grunstein, M. M., Younes, M., and Milic-Emili, J. (1973). Control of tidal volume and respiratory frequency in anaesthetized cats. J. Appl. Physiol. 35:463.
34. Lahiri, S., Mei, S. S., and Kao, F. F. (1975). Vagal modulation of respiratory control during exercise. Respir. Physiol. 23:133.
35. Hammouda, M., and Wilson, W. H. (1932). The vagus influences giving rise to the phenomena accompanying expansion and collapse of the lungs. J. Physiol. (Lond.) 74:81.
36. Rice, H. V. (1938). Respiratory vagal reflexes and carbon dioxide. Am. J. Physiol. 124:535.
37. Bouverot, P. (1973). Vagal afferent fibres from the lung and regulation of breathing in awake dogs. Respir. Physiol. 17:325.
38. Widdicombe, J. G., and Winning, A. (1974). Effects of hypoxia, hypercapnia and changes in body temperature on the pattern of breathing in cats. Respir. Physiol. 21:203.
39. Bradley, G. W., Euler, C. von., Marttila, I., and Roos, B. (1974). Transient and steady state effects of CO_2 on mechanisms determining rate and depth of breathing. Acta Physiol. Scand. 92:341.
40. Guz, A., Noble, M. I. M., Widdicombe, J. G., Trenchard, D., and Muschin, W. W. (1966). The effect of bilateral block of vagus and glossopharyngeal nerves on the ventilatory response to CO_2 of conscious man. Respir. Physiol. 1:206.
41. Kindermann, W., and Pleschka, K. (1973). Phrenic nerve response to passive muscle stretch at different arterial CO_2 tensions. Respir. Physiol. 17:227.
42. Bradley, G. W., Euler, C. von, Marttila, I., and Roos, B. (1974). Steady state effects of CO_2 and temperature on the relationship between lung volume and inspiratory duration (Hering-Breuer threshold curve). Acta Physiol. Scand. 92:351.
43. Priban, I. P. (1963). An analysis of some short-term patterns of breathing in man. J. Physiol. (Lond.) 166:425.
44. Newsom-Davis, J., and Stagg, D. (1975). Interrelationships of the volume and time components of individual breaths in resting man. J. Physiol. (Lond.) 245:481.
45. Clark, F. J., and Euler, C. von. (1972). On the regulation of depth and rate of breathing. J. Physiol. (Lond.) 222:267.
46. Boyd, T. E., and Maaske, C. A. (1939). Vagal inhibition of inspiration and accompanying changes of respiratory rhythm. J. Neurophysiol. 2:533.
47. Knox, C. K. (1973). Characteristics of inflation and deflation reflexes during expiration in the cat. J. Neurophysiol. 36:284.
48. Gautier, H. (1973). Respiratory responses of the anaesthetized rabbit to vagotomy and thoracic dorsal rhizotomy. Respir. Physiol. 17:238.
49. Schoener, E. P., and Frankel, H. M. (1972). Effect of hyperthermia and P_{aCO_2} on the slowly adapting stretch receptor. Am. J. Physiol. 222:68.
50. Mustafa, M. E. K. Y., and Purves, M. J. (1972). The effect of CO_2 upon discharge from slowly adapting stretch receptors in the lungs of rabbits. Respir. Physiol. 16:197.
51. Bartlett, D., Remmers, J. E., and Gautier, H. (1973). Laryngeal regulation of respiratory airflow. Respir. Physiol. 18:194.
52. Euler, C. von, and Trippenbach, T., personal communication.
53. Cunningham, D. J. C., and Gardner, W. N. (1972). The relation between

tidal volume and inspiratory and expiratory times during steady state CO_2 inhalation in man. J. Physiol. (Lond.) 227:50P.

54. Jenett, S., Russell, T., and Warnock, K. A. (1974). The duration of inspiration during changing states of ventilation in man. J. Physiol. (Lond.) 238:54P.

55. Kay, J. D. S., Strange-Petersen, E., and Vejby-Christensen, H. (1975). Mean and breath by breath pattern of breathing in man during steady state exercise. J. Physiol. (Lond.) 251:657.

56. Garrard, C. S., and Lane, D. J., (1973). The regulation of respiratory pattern. Bull. Physiopathol. Respir. 9:1267.

57. Gardner, W. N. (1975). Analysis of breathing patterns in man. Bull. Physiopathol. Respir. 11:78P.

58. Gautier, H., and Bertrand, F. (1975). Respiratory effects of pneumotaxic center lesions and subsequent vagotomy in chronic cats. Respir. Physiol. 23:71.

59. May, A. J., and Widdicombe, J. G. (1954). Depression of the cough reflex by pentobarbitone and some opium derivatives. Br. J. Pharmacol. 9:335.

60. Robson, J. G., Houseley, M. A., and Solis-Quiroga, O. H. (1963). The mechanism of respiratory arrest with sodium pentobarbital and sodium thiopental. Ann. N. Y. Acad. Sci. 109:491.

61. Sant'Ambrogio, G., and Widdicombe, J. G. (1965). Respiratory reflexes acting on the diaphragm and inspiratory intercostal muscles of the rabbit. J. Physiol. (Lond.) 180:766.

62. Bouverot, P., Crance, J. P., and Dejours, P. (1970). Factors influencing the intensity of the Breuer-Hering inspiration-inhibiting reflex. Respir. Physiol. 8:376.

63. Pearson, S. B., and Cunningham, D. J. C. (1973). Some observations on the relation between ventilation, tidal volume and frequency in man in various steady and transient states. In W. A. Karczewski and J. G. Widdicombe (ed.), International Symposium on Neural Control of Breathing. Acta Neurobiol. Exp. 33:177.

64. Miller, J. P., Cunningham, D. J. C., Lloyd, B. B., and Young, J. M. (1974). The transient respiratory effects in man of sudden changes in alveolar CO_2 in hypoxia and in high oxygen. Respir. Physiol. 20:17.

65. Gardner, W. N. (1974). The pattern of breathing following step changes of alveolar P_{CO_2} in man. J. Physiol. (Lond.) 242:75P.

66. Marsh, R. H. K., Lyen, K. R., McPherson, G. A. D., Pearson, S. B., and Cunningham, D. J. C. (1973). Breath-by-breath effects of imposed alternate-breath oscillations of alveolar CO_2. Respir. Physiol. 18:80.

67. Cunningham, D. J. C., and Ward, S., personal communication.

68. Wolff, C. B. (1975). The effects of alternative breaths of CO_2 and air on carotid arterial pH and breath by breath tidal volume in the anaesthetized cat. J. Physiol. (Lond.) 244:63P.

69. Eldridge, F. L. (1972). The importance of timing on the respiratory effects of intermittent carotid sinus nerve stimulation. J. Physiol. (Lond.) 222:297.

70. Black, A. M. S., and Torrance, R. W. (1971). Respiratory oscillations in chemoreceptor discharge in the control of breathing. Respir. Physiol. 13:221.

71. Eldridge, F. L. (1972). The importance of timing on the respiratory effects of intermittent carotid body chemoreceptor stimulation. J. Physiol. (Lond.) 222:319.

72. Biscoe, T. J. (1971). Carotid body: structure and function. Physiol. Rev. 51:437.
73. Neil, E., and Howe, A. (1972). Arterial chemoreceptors. *In* E. Neil (ed.), Handbook of Sensory Physiology III/1, Enteroceptors, p. 47. Springer-Verlag, Berlin.
74. Torrance, R. W. (1974). Arterial chemoreceptors. *In* J. G. Widdicombe (ed.), MTP International Review of Science, Physiology Series I, Vol. 2, Respiratory Physiology I, p. 247. University Park Press, Baltimore.
75. Loeschcke, H. H. (1974). Central nervous chemoreceptors. *In* J. G. Widdicombe (ed.), MTP International Review of Science, Physiology Series I, Vol. 2, Respiratory Physiology I, p. 167. University Park Press, Baltimore.
76. Widdicombe, J. G. (1964). Respiratory reflexes. *In* W. O. Fenn and H. Rahn (eds.), Handbook of Physiology, Section 3: Respiration, Vol. 1, p. 585. American Physiology Society, Washington, D.C.
77. Ngai, S. H., and Wang, S. C. (1957). Organization of central respiratory mechanisms in the brain stem of the cat: localization by stimulation and destruction. Am. J. Physiol. 190:343.
78. St. John, W. M., Glasser, R. L., and King, R. A. (1972). Rhythmic respiration in awake vagotomized cats with chronic pneumotaxic area lesions. Respir. Physiol. 15:233.
79. Cohen, M. I., and Wang, S. C. (1959). Respiratory neuronal activity in pons of cat. J. Neurophysiol. 22:33.
80. Bertrand, F., and Hugelin, A. (1971). Respiratory synchronizing function of nucleus parabrachialis medialis: pneumotaxic mechanisms. J. Neurophysiol. 34:189.
81. Stella, G. (1938). On the mechanism of production and the physiological significance of "apneusis". J. Physiol. (Lond.) 93:10.
82. Breckenridge, C. G., and Hoff, H. E. (1950). Pontine and medullary regulation of respiration in the cat. Am. J. Physiol. 160:385.
83. Tang, P. C. (1953). Localization of the pneumotaxic center in the cat. Am. J. Physiol. 172:645.
84. Euler, C. von, Marttila, I., Remmers, J. E., and Trippenbach, T., personal communication.
85. Euler, C. von, and Trippenbach, T. (1975). Cyclic excitability changes of the inspiratory "off-switch" mechanism. Acta Physiol. Scand. 93:560.
86. Cohen, M. I. (1971). Switching of the respiratory phases and evoked phrenic responses produced by rostral pontine electrical stimulation. J. Physiol. (Lond.) 217:133.
87. Widdicombe, J. G. (1974). Reflex control of breathing. *In* J. G. Widdicombe (ed.), MTP International Review of Science, Physiology Series I, Vol. 2, Respiratory Physiology I, p. 273. University Park Press, Baltimore.
88. Fishman, N. H., Phillipson, E. A., and Nadel, J. A. (1973). Effect of differential vagal cold blockade on breathing pattern in conscious dogs. J. Appl. Physiol. 34:754.
89. Guz, A., and Trenchard, D. (1971). Pulmonary stretch receptor activity in man: a comparison with dog and cat. J. Physiol. (Lond.) 213:329.
90. Widdicombe, J. G. (1961). Respiratory reflexes in man and other mammalian species. Clin. Sci. 21:163.
91. Guz, A., Noble, M. I. M., Trenchard, D., Cochrane, H. L., and Makey, A.

R. (1964). Studies on the vagus nerves in man: their role in respiratory and circulatory control. Clin. Sci. 27:293.

92. Guz, A., Noble, M. I. M., Eisele, J. H., and Trenchard, D. (1970). The role of vagal inflation reflexes in man and other animals. *In* R. Porter (ed.), Breathing: Hering-Breuer Centenary Symposium, p. 17. Churchill, London.

93. Bartoli, A., Bystrzycka, E., Guz, A., Jain, S. K., Noble, M. I. M., and Trenchard, D. (1973). Studies of the pulmonary vagal control of central respiratory rhythm in the absence of breathing movements. J. Physiol. (Lond.) 230:449.

94. D'Angelo, E., and Agostoni, E. (1975). Tonic vagal influences on inspiratory duration. Respir. Physiol. 24:287.

95. Stanley, N. N., Altose, M. D., Cherniack, N. S., and Fishman, A. P. (1975). Changes in strength of lung inflation reflex during prolonged inflation. J. Appl. Physiol. 38:474.

96. Remmers, J. E. (1970). Inhibition of inspiratory activity by intercostal muscle afferents. Respir. Physiol. 10:358.

97. Remmers, J. E., and Marttila, I. (1975). Action of intercostal muscle afferents on the respiratory rhythm of anaesthetized cats. Respir. Physiol. 24:31.

98. Decima, E. E., and Euler, C. von. (1969). Excitability of phrenic motoneurones to afferent input from lower intercostal nerves in the spinal cat. Acta Physiol. Scand. 75:580.

99. Remmers, J. E. (1973). Extra-segmental reflexes derived from intercostal afferents: phrenic and laryngeal responses. J. Physiol. (Lond.) 233:45.

100. Krieger, A. J., Christensen, H. D., Sapru, H. N., and Wang, S. C. (1972). Changes in ventilatory patterns after ablation of various respiratory feedback mechanisms. J. Appl. Physiol. 33:431.

101. Remmers, J. E., and Tsiaras, W. G. (1973). Effect of lateral cervical cord lesions on the respiratory rhythm of anaesthetized decerebrate cats after vagotomy. J. Physiol. (Lond.) 233:63.

102. Bradley, G. W. (1972). The response of the respiratory system to elastic loading in cats. Respir. Physiol. 16:142.

103. Chai, C. Y., and Lin, M. T. (1973). Effects of thermal stimulation of medulla oblongata and spinal cord in decerebrate rabbits. J. Physiol. (Lond.) 234:409.

104. Dejours, P. (1964). Control of respiration in muscular exercise. *In* W. O. Fenn and H. Rahn (eds.), Handbook of Physiology, Section 3, Respiration, Vol. 1, p. 631. American Physiology Society, Washington, D.C.

105. Wilson, M. F., Clarke, N. P., Smith, O. A., and Rushmer, R. F. (1961). Interrelation between central and peripheral mechanisms regulating blood pressure. Circ. Res. 9:491.

106. Comroe, J. H., and Schmidt, C. F. (1943). Reflexes from the limbs as a factor in the hyperpnoea of muscular exercise. Am. J. Physiol. 138:536.

107. Bessou, P., Dejours, P., and Laporte, Y. (1959). Effets ventilatoires réflexes de la stimulation de fibres afférentes de grand diamètre d'origine musculaire chez le chat. Compt. Rend. Soc. Biol. 153:477.

108. Flandrois, R., Lacour, J. R. Islas-Maroquin, J., and Charlot, J. (1967). Limbs mechanoreceptors inducing the reflex hyperpnoea of exercise. Respir. Physiol. 2:335.

109. Hodgson, H. J. F., and Matthews, P. B. C. (1968). The ineffectiveness of

excitation of the primary endings of the muscle spindle by vibration as a respiratory stimulant in the decerebrate cat. J. Physiol. (Lond.) 194:555.

110. Gautier, H., Lacaisse, A., and Dejours, P. (1969). Ventilatory response to muscle spindle stimulation by succinylcholine in cats. Respir. Physiol. 7:383.

111. Biscoe, T. J., and Purves, M. J. (1967). Factors affecting the cat carotid chemoreceptor and cervical sympathetic activity with special reference to passive hind-limb movements. J. Physiol. (Lond.) 190:425.

112. Aminoff, M. J., and Sears, T. A. (1971). Spinal integration of segmental, cortical and breathing inputs to thoracic respiratory motoneurones. J. Physiol. (Lond.) 215:557.

113. Plum, F. (1970). Neurological integration of behavioural and metabolic control of breathing. In R. Porter (ed.), Breathing: Hering-Breuer Centenary Symposium, p. 159. Churchill, London.

114. Newsom-Davis, J. (1974). Control of the muscles of breathing. In J. G. Widdicombe (ed.), MTP International Review of Science, Physiology Series I, Vol. 2, Respiratory Physiology I, p. 221. University Park Press, Baltimore.

115. Frankstein, S. I. (1970). Neural control of respiration. In R. Porter (ed.), Breathing: Hering-Breuer Centenary Symposium, p. 53. Churchill, London.

116. Bradley, G. W., Euler, C. von, Marttila, I., and Roos, B. (1975). A model of the central and reflex inhibition of inspiration in the cat. Biol. Cybernetics 19:105.

117. Herczynski, R., and Karczewski, W. A. (1976). Neural control of breathing: a system analysis. Acta Physiol. Pol. 27:2.

118. Kirkwood, P. A., and Sears, T. A. (1973). Monosynaptic excitation of thoracic expiratory motoneurones from lateral respiratory neurones in the medulla of the cat. J. Physiol. (Lond.) 234:87P.

119. Merrill, E. G. (1974). Finding a respiratory function for the medullary respiratory neurons. In R. Bellairs and E. G. Gray (eds.), Essays on the Nervous System, p. 451. Clarendon Press, Oxford.

120. Mitchell, R. A., and Herbert, D. A. (1974). The effect of carbon dioxide on the membrane potential of medullary respiratory neurons. Brain Res. 75:345.

121. Euler, C. von, Hayward, J. N., Marttila, I., and Wyman, R. J. (1973). Respiratory neurones of the ventrolateral nucleus of the solitary tract of cat: vagal input, spinal connections and morphological identification. Brain Res. 61:1.

122. Bystrzycka, E., Nail, B. S., and Purves, M. J. (1975). Afferent neurones in the central pathway of the Hering-Breuer reflex. J. Physiol. (Lond.) 245:107P.

123. Euler, C. von, Hayward, J. N., Marttila, I., and Wyman, R. J. (1973). The spinal connections of the inspiratory neurones of the ventrolateral nucleus of the cat's tractus solitarius. Brain Res. 61:23.

124. Lam, R. L., and Tyler, H. R. (1952). Electrical responses evoked in visceral afferent nucleus of rabbit by vagal stimulation. J. Comp. Neurol. 97:21.

125. Koepchen, H. P., Lazar, H., and Borchert, J. (1974). On the role of nucleus infrasolitarius in the determination of respiratory periodicity. Proceedings of the XXVI Congress International Union of Physiological Sciences, p. 81. New Delhi.

126. Wyss, O. A. M. (1954). The mode of functioning of the respiratory centre. Helv. Physiol. Acta (Suppl. X)12:5.

127. Haber, E., Kohn, K. W., Ngai, S. H., Holaday, D. A., and Wang, S. C. (1957). Localization of spontaneous respiratory neuronal activities in the medulla oblongata of the cat: a new location of the expiratory centre. Am. J. Physiol. 190:350.
128. Waldren, I. (1970). Activity patterns in respiratory muscles and in respiratory neurones of the rostral medulla of cat. J. Physiol. (Lond.) 208:373.
129. Pórszás, J., Barankay, T., and Pórszász-Gibiszer, K. (1965). Tonic expiratory vagal afferent fibres from the pulmonary stretch receptors. Acta Physiol. Acad. Scientiarum Hungaricae 27:125.
130. Younes, M., Vaillancourt, P., and Milic-Emili, J. (1974). Interaction between chemical factors and duration of apnoea following lung inflation. J. Appl. Physiol. 36:190.
131. Anderson, P., and Sears, T. A. (1970). Medullary activation of intercostal fusimotor and alpha motoneurones. J. Physiol. (Lond.) 209:739.
132. Bertrand, F., Hugelin, A., and Vibert, J. F. (1974). A stereologic model of pneumotaxic oscillator based on spatial and temporal distribution of neuronal bursts. J. Neurophysiol. 37:91.
133. Hukuhara, T. (1973). Neuronal organization of the central respiratory mechanisms in the brain stem of the cat. Acta Neurobiol. Exp. 33:219.
134. Cohen, M. I. (1958). Intrinsic periodicity of the pontile pneumotaxic mechanism. Am. J. Physiol. 195:23.
135. Eldridge, F. L. (1973). Posthyperventilation breathing: different effects of active and passive hyperventilation. J. Appl. Physiol. 34:422.
136. Eldridge, F. L. (1974). Central neural respiratory stimulatory effect of active respiration. J. Appl. Physiol. 37:723.
137. Batsel, H. L. (1964). Localization of bulbar respiratory center by microelectrode sounding. Exp. Neurol. 9:410.
138. Cohen, M. I. (1969). Discharge patterns of brain-stem respiratory neurons during Hering-Breuer reflex evoked by lung inflation. J. Neurophysiol. 32:356.

International Review of Physiology
Respiratory Physiology II, Volume 14
Edited by John G. Widdicombe
Copyright 1977   University Park Press   Baltimore

7
Comparative Physiology of Respiration: Functional Analysis of Gas Exchange Organs in Vertebrates

J. PIIPER AND P. SCHEID

Max Planck-Institut für experimentelle Medizin, Göttingen, Germany

EXTERNAL GAS EXCHANGE: GENERAL PRINCIPLES   220
    Basic Overall Equations: Conductances   222
    Internal Transport Medium: Blood   223
    External Medium: Air Versus Water   223

VARIOUS GAS EXCHANGE ORGANS:
  ANATOMY AND MODELS   229
    Fish Gills   230
    Bird Lungs   230
    Alveolar Lungs   231
    Skin   231

MODELS: QUANTITATIVE ANALYSIS   231
    Relative Partial Pressure Difference   232
    Total Conductance   236
    Limitation Index   236

SKIN BREATHING: A SIMPLE MODEL FOR EVALUATION
  OF DIFFUSION AND PERFUSION LIMITATION   237

APPLICATION OF MODEL ANALYSIS   240

REAL SYSTEMS VERSUS MODELS   243
    Complications Due to Anatomical Arrangement   243
      Medium Dead Space   243

       Blood: Arrangement of Blood Vessels in Relation to Gas
          Exchange Organs   243
Inhomogeneities   245
       Functional Inhomogeneities of Parallel Units   245
       Temporal Variations in Conductances and in Partial
          Pressures   245
Additional Transfer Resistances   246
       Diffusion in Medium and Blood   246
       Kinetics of Chemical Reactions   247
Complications Arising from Blood Chemistry   247
       Dependence of β on P   247
       Bohr and Haldane Effects   247

The comparative physiology of respiration has been treated and reviewed by a number of authors in treatises of mammalian-oriented respiration physiology (1, 2), in handbooks and textbooks covering the entire comparative animal physiology (3–7), and in monographs dedicated to the comparative physiology of respiration (8–13). The reviews dealing with respiration in a single vertebrate class are noted below.

The scope of this chapter is restricted to qualitative description and quantitative analysis of the performance of the main types of gas exchange organs encountered in vertebrates. Use is made of simplified models whose gas exchange behavior is investigated in theory, and some selected sets of experimental data are analyzed on the basis of the models.

This study is not intended to be a review article quoting and summarizing world literature of the field. It is mainly an extension of the authors' previous work (14, 15), undertaken with the aim of presenting a general framework for understanding the external gas exchange in animals. A more comprehensive treatment of comparative physiology of gas exchange based on similar lines of approach has been recently presented by Dejours (13).

In this chapter, some general principles useful for analysis of external gas exchange are considered first; it will then be shown how simple models of gas exchange organs may be deduced from their complicated anatomical structure. General formulae for the model analysis are followed by their application to physiological measurements in a few selected species. At the end, restrictions and limitations of the approach are discussed.

EXTERNAL GAS EXCHANGE: GENERAL PRINCIPLES

In a generalized model of an external gas exchange organ of vertebrates (Figure 1), flowing internal medium, *blood*, comes into diffusional exchange contact

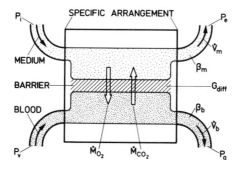

Figure 1. General model for analysis of external gas exchange.

with an outer *medium,* also streaming in most cases (exception: skin breathing). The transfer of O_2 and CO_2 between the medium and blood takes place through a separating tissue *barrier.* The different types of gas exchange system are characterized by the *specific arrangement* of the medium and blood flows resulting from the anatomical structure.

Generally the gas exchange organ consists of a large number of similar units in functionally parallel arrangement (e.g., secondary lamellae in fish gills, parabronchi in avian lungs, alveoli in mammalian lungs, a large number of blood capillary segments in all systems). In the models, all these structures can be represented by one single idealized unit which is functionally equivalent to the whole organ.

The following basic quantities (listed with typical units) are required for a quantitative analysis of gas exchange. (The concepts and terminology which are devised with particular consideration for requirements of comparative physiology of gas exchange (16) will be used throughout this article.)

1. *Transfer rate, $\dot{M}$,* amount of gas exchanged per unit of time, e.g., O_2 uptake and CO_2 output (mmol min^{-1}).
2. *Concentration, C,* of a gas species in medium or blood (mmol liter^{-1}).
3. *Partial pressure, P,* of a gas species (Torr = mm Hg).
4. *Capacitance coefficient,* β, defined as increment in concentration per increment in partial pressure, $\Delta C/\Delta P$ (mmol l^{-1} Torr^{-1}); if in liquids no chemical binding is involved, β is equal to physical *solubility coefficient,* α.
5. *Flow rate, $\dot{V}$,* of external medium and blood (ml min^{-1}).
6. *Diffusing capacity, D,* of tissue barrier (mmol min^{-1} Torr^{-1}).

Throughout this chapter, the following subscripts will be used:

m, medium;
b, blood;
g, gas;
i, inspired (= medium entering gas exchange organ);

e, expired (= medium leaving gas exchange organ);
v, venous (= blood entering gas exchange organ);
a, arterial (= blood leaving gas exchange organ).

In order to obtain the simplest possible solutions for gas exchange properties of the various models, the following *assumptions,* whose validity will be discussed later, are made.

1. The gas exchange system is in *steady state,* meaning constancy in time of all variables. In particular, ventilation and blood flow are assumed to be constant, i.e., nontidal and nonpulsatile.
2. The β_m and β_b values are *constant,* i.e., independent of the partial pressures in the partial pressure range occurring in the system.

Basic Overall Equations: Conductances

From Fick's principle (based on the conservation of mass), the following relationships are obtained for the convective transport by ventilation:

$$\dot{M} = \dot{V}_m \cdot (C_i - C_e) = \dot{V}_m \cdot \beta_m \cdot (P_i - P_e) \tag{1}$$

and for the convective transport by blood flow:

$$\dot{M} = \dot{V}_b \cdot (C_a - C_v) = \dot{V}_b \cdot \beta_b \cdot (P_a - P_v) \tag{2}$$

It is useful to define the conductance as the ratio of transfer rate to the underlying partial pressure difference, $\dot{M}/\Delta P$. Thus, the convective conductance by ventilation (= medium flow) is

$$G_{vent} = \dot{V}_m \cdot \beta_m \tag{3}$$

and by perfusion (= blood flow):

$$G_{perf} = \dot{V}_b \cdot \beta_b \tag{4}$$

Similarly, the overall transport equation for diffusive transport through the medium/blood barrier is

$$\dot{M} = G_{diff} \cdot (\bar{P}_m - \bar{P}_b) \tag{5}$$

where $\bar{P}_m$ and $\bar{P}_b$ designate spatial mean partial pressures on the medium side and on the blood side of the barrier, respectively. G_{diff} stands for the diffusive conductance and may be expressed according to Fick's law of diffusion as:

$$G_{diff} = D = \mathrm{D} \cdot \alpha \cdot \frac{A}{x} \tag{6}$$

in which D and α designate diffusion coefficient and solubility coefficient in the tissue barrier, separating medium, and blood, considered as a flat sheet of area, *A,* of uniform thickness, *x,* and with uniform properties. The product of diffusion coefficient and solubility coefficient, D · α, termed as Krogh's diffusion constant or permeation coefficient, is a measure of the specific diffusional permeability of a material. It is evident that G_{diff} can be obtained either from physiological measurements (equation 5) or from anatomical determinations in conjunction with physical properties (equation 6). It is one of the major objects of the model analysis of this chapter to show how G_{diff} may be obtained from physiological determinations.

Internal Transport Medium: Blood

The decisive property of blood with respect to conveyance of O_2 and CO_2 is the chemical binding of these gases. The amount of O_2 and CO_2 taken up or released by a unit blood volume per unit change of partial pressure, that is, the capacitance coefficient, β_b, is increased by a considerable factor over that of water or saline solution. It follows from the dissociation curves that β_b for both O_2 and CO_2 is variable. In fact, β_b constitutes the slope of the dissociation curves plotted as concentration (chemically bound + physically dissolved) against partial pressure.

The following factors influence $(\beta_b)_{O_2}$: chemical structure of hemoglobin; concentration of hemoglobin (concentration of red cells or hematocrit); temperature; pH and P_{CO_2} (Bohr effect); intraerythrocyte concentration of organic phosphates as "specific regulators," e.g., adenosine triphosphate (ATP), 2,3-diphosphoglycerate (2,3-DPG), and inositol pentaphosphate (IPP). The reversible association of O_2 to hemoglobin has been studied in great detail and the results have been reviewed in a number of articles (17–26).

The capacitance coefficient for CO_2, $(\beta_b)CO_2$, depends upon the buffering properties of blood, which in turn are influenced by the concentration and specific buffering properties of hemoglobin, plasma proteins, phosphates, hemoglobin oxygenation (Haldane effect), and temperature. The interdependence of O_2 and CO_2 (Bohr and Haldane effects) increases both $(\beta_b)_{CO_2}$ and $(\beta_b)_{O_2}$.

The dependence of $(\beta_b)CO_2$ and $(\beta_b)O_2$ upon the partial pressure ranges introduces difficulties into a quantitative analytical treatment of gas exchange (see below). For the overall transport (equation 2), it suffices to take the slope of the straight line crossing the dissociation curve at the arterial and venous values. For calculations aimed at analysis of medium-blood gas transfer, particular step-by-step techniques are used (Bohr integration).

Further problems leading to deviation of the real blood from idealized blood used for model calculations are finite reaction times in association and dissociation of O_2 and CO_2, diffusional resistance offered by blood, etc., which factors will be discussed below.

External Medium: Air Versus Water

The properties of primary importance in determining the carriage of O_2 and CO_2 by the external medium are the respective β values. For air or a gas phase it follows from the ideal gas law,

$$P \cdot V = M \cdot R \cdot T \tag{7}$$

(P, pressure or partial pressure; V, volume; M, amount of substance; R, gas constant; T, absolute temperature), that the capacitance coefficient

$$\beta = \frac{M}{V \cdot P} = \frac{1}{R \cdot T} \tag{8}$$

is equal for all gas species (insofar as the gas mixture can be considered "ideal").

For O_2 in water, the β value is in every respect equal to physical solubility, depending upon temperature and concentration of solutes (salinity).

For CO_2 in water containing bicarbonate (and/or other buffer substances), the buffering reactions must be taken into account which lead to an effective increase of β_{CO_2} caused by formation (or disintegration) of bicarbonate due to changes in P_{CO_2}. The underlying chemical reactions in sea water (28) involve formation of HCO_3^- in the presence of the bicarbonate/carbonate and boric acid/borate buffer systems:

$$CO_2 + CO_3^{2-} + H_2O \rightleftharpoons 2\,HCO_3^- \tag{9}$$

$$CO_2 + H_2BO_3^- + H_2O \rightleftharpoons HCO_3^- + H_3BO_3 \tag{10}$$

Due to bicarbonate formation with increasing P_{CO_2} (or bicarbonate disintegration with decreasing P_{CO_2}) the "effective CO_2 dissociation curve" of sea water has a higher slope than can be accounted for by the physical solubility alone.

Differences in β values between O_2 and CO_2 and between respective values in water and air (Table 1) lead to some important consequences (28–30):

1. Because β_{O_2} is much less for water than for air, water-breathing animals must ventilate much more than air breathers in order to achieve the same O_2 uptake (cf. equation 1) (31).

2. Because in water β_{CO_2} exceeds β_{O_2}, this high water ventilation forcibly means low $(P_e - P_i)_{CO_2}$ differences. For air, $\beta_{CO_2} = \beta_{O_2}$, and thus with air ventilation $(P_e - P_i)_{CO_2}$ is similar to $(P_i - P_e)_{O_2}$ (the ratio being equivalent to the metabolic respiratory quotient, RQ, in steady state).

These considerations may be used to predict blood and body P_{O_2} and P_{CO_2} values in various water and air breathers, provided the process that limits gas

Table 1. Comparison of physicochemical properties of respired gases in water and air

Property	Air/Water[a]		CO_2/O_2	
	CO_2	O_2	Air	Water
Capacitance coefficient, β	1.05	30	1.0	29
Diffusion coefficient, D	8,000	7,000	0.8	0.7
Krogh's diffusion constant, K	8,000	200,000	0.8	20

[a]Approximate values. For air, $K = D_g \cdot \beta_g$; for water, $K = D_w \cdot \alpha_w$.

exchange is known, i.e., convection of medium or diffusion through tissue barrier. If convection in water limits gas exchange, as is the case for fishes with gas exchange predominantly through gills, the much higher value of β_{CO_2} compared with β_{O_2} results in a much higher gas exchange conductance for CO_2 than for O_2, $(G_{vent})_{CO_2} \gg (G_{vent})_{O_2}$ (cf. equation 3) which leads to small P_{CO_2} values in body and blood. As shown in Figure 2, the highest possible P_{CO_2} values that may be attained when O_2 extraction from water is complete is only about 5 Torr. Arterial P_{CO_2} in water-breathing elasmobranchs and teleosts is usually about 2 Torr (see Table 2).

In skin-breathing animals, in which diffusion in tissue limits gas exchange, CO_2 release is favored over O_2 uptake because the diffusion constant of Krogh, D × α, is much higher for CO_2 than for O_2 (Table 1 and Figure 2) and, therefore, $(G_{diff})_{CO_2} \gg (G_{diff})_{O_2}$ (cf. equation 6). This is true for both air and water as media bordering upon the skin so long as these media do not limit gas exchange appreciably. Low blood P_{CO_2} values have indeed been found in the exclusively skin-breathing salamander, *Desmognathus fuscus*, in air (Table 2).

Thus, the important difference in respect of blood P_{CO_2} is not between water-breathing and air-breathing but rather between transport in water (or tissue) and transport in air as the process limiting gas exchange. In the lungs of mammals and birds, gas transfer is via a tissue barrier into gas spaces (alveoli, parabronchi), and in this transfer CO_2 is favored compared to O_2. However, the limiting process in these lungs is convection by ventilating gas and, therefore, G_{vent} is the decisive parameter for overall gas exchange. Because $\beta_{O_2} = \beta_{CO_2}$

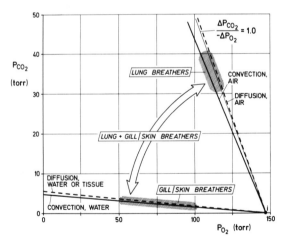

Figure 2. The CO_2-O_2 diagram for transport of respiratory gases by convection (of air or water) or diffusion (in air, water, or tissue), RQ being 0.9 (32). The identity line, $\Delta P_{CO_2} : \Delta P_{O_2} = 1.0$, is attained for convective transport in air at RQ = 1.0. Ranges for partial pressures of CO_2 and O_2 observed in arterialized blood of air breathers and water breathers are indicated by *shaded areas*. Dual (bimodal/trimodal) breathers are located in the intermediate range indicated by the *double arrow*.

Table 2. Arterial P_{CO_2} and relative extrapulmonary (branchial and/or cutaneous) CO_2 output in various animals exhibiting pure aerial, pure aquatic, or dual gas exchange

	Species	Arterial P_{CO_2} (Torr)	Extrapulmonary $\dot{M}_{CO_2}$ (%)	Gas exchange organs
Aerial	Man	40	0	lungs
	Electrophorus electricus (33, 34)	30	80	buccal cavity (air), skin (water)
	Protopterus aethiopicus (35)	25	70	lungs, gills
	Rana catesbeiana (36)	13		lungs, skin (air)
	Rana clamitans (52)		80	lungs, skin (air)
Dual	*Amphiuma tridactylum* (37, 38)	11	80	skin (water), lungs
	Necturus maculosus (39)	4.4	99	skin (water), gills, lungs
	Neoceratodus forsteri (40)	3.6	100	gills, lungs
	Desmognathus fuscus (41)	5.2	100	skin (air)
Aquatic	*Scyliorhinus stellaris* (42)	1.9	100	gills

[a]Cutaneous $\dot{M}_{CO_2}$.

for gas, $(G_{vent})_{CO_2} = (G_{vent})_{O_2}$, and thus both O_2 and CO_2 face resistances to gas exchange that are of the same order of magnitude. Thus, for a given O_2 partial pressure gradient between body and environment, much larger body P_{CO_2} values are encountered in lung-breathers (see Table 2, Figure 2). Similar considerations hold for gas exchange in bird eggs (33), in which diffusion in air is limiting, because diffusion coefficients for O_2 and CO_2 in air are similar.

Most amphibians and many fishes and reptiles display dual (bimodal) gas exchange, i.e., simultaneously with air (in lungs and/or skin) and water (in gills and/or skin). In many amphibians with gills persisting in the adult stage, even trimodal gas exchange is encountered. If gas exchange is predominantly via gills and skin (no matter whether air or water borders upon the skin), conditions for CO_2 exchange are more favorable than those for O_2 uptake, and low body and blood P_{CO_2} results.

If gas exchange takes place simultaneously via lungs and via extrapulmonary organs, O_2 and CO_2 are unequally allotted to these alleys, the RQ being lower (than mean metabolic RQ) for the lungs and higher for the extrapulmonary pathways (Table 3). This is a direct consequence of physics of gases (Table 1): the $CO_2:O_2$ ratio for the capacitance coefficient β is much higher for water (and tissue) than for air, transfer of CO_2 is favored in skin and gills, and transfer of O_2 is favored in lungs.

The lines in the O_2-CO_2 diagram (Figure 2) for dual breathers are intermediate between the lines for water and tissue and those for air, the exact value for body P_{CO_2} depending upon the significance of pulmonary versus extrapulmonary gas exchange and also on O_2 extraction. For example, unlike *Amphiuma tridactylum*, arterial P_{CO_2} is relatively high in *Electrophorus electricus* (Table 2), although extrapulmonary CO_2 exchange is estimated to be about equally high in both. However, the arterial P_{O_2} is much lower in *E. electricus*, indicating that overall gas exchange conductance is lower in this animal, and thus blood and body P_{O_2} and P_{CO_2} fall on parts of the lines in the CO_2-O_2 diagram that are more to the left.

Some interesting consequences arise from the fact that fish gills are not only organs for external respiration, i.e., exchange of O_2 and CO_2, but also the site of ion exchange with water (43). Of particular interest is the participation of gills in the regulation of acid-base balance.

In carnivorous elasmobranch fishes, as in mammals, the ureotelic catabolism of proteins results in an acidotic tendency as H^+ ions are produced, essentially as an end product of the oxidation of sulfur-containing amino acids (cysteine, cystin, and methionine) (44), and probably to a great part excreted in expiratory water, urine flow being very small. Because H^+ would displace the reaction equilibrium

$$H^+ + HCO_3^- \rightarrow CO_2 + H_2O \qquad (11)$$

to the right, an increased expired-inspired P_{CO_2} difference would result for the same inspired-expired CO_2 content difference. This means that the effective

Table 3. Partition of O_2 uptake ($\dot{M}_{O_2}$) and CO_2 output ($\dot{M}_{CO_2}$) between lungs and extrapulmonary gas exchange organs (gills and/or skin) in amphibians at 25°C, $RQ = \dot{M}_{CO_2}/\dot{M}_{O_2}$.

		Extrapulmonary		RQ		Extrapulmonary exchange: medium and organ
		$\dot{M}_{O_2}$ (%)	$\dot{M}_{CO_2}$ (%)	Extrapulmonary	Pulmonary	
Urodela	Necturus maculosus (47)	96	99	0.85	0.19	water; gills and skin
	Cryptobranchus alleganiensis (48)	92	98	0.86	0.22	water; skin
	Siren lacertina (49)	50	78	1.43	0.40	water; gills and skin
	Amphiuma means (50)	44	77	1.55	0.36	water; skin
	Ambystoma maculatum (51)	46	87	1.13	0.17	air; skin
	Taricha granulosa (51)	32	75	2.03	0.30	air; skin
Anura	Rana clamitans (52)	36	79	2.57	0.27	air; skin
	Bufo terrestris (53)	31	75	2.46	0.37	air; skin

slope of the CO_2 dissociation curve of respired water, β_{CO_2}, would be decreased. In a steady state, however, the effect should be minor even with a high protein diet (45).

In teleost fishes, the protein catabolism is ammonotelic, meaning a physiological metabolic alkalosis, because the ammonia, NH_3, is a base. It probably is secreted as NH_4HCO_3, according to the following reactions:

$$NH_3 + H_2O \rightarrow NH_4^+ + OH^- \tag{12}$$

$$OH^- + CO_2 \rightarrow HCO_3^- \tag{13}$$

The "metabolic" increase of HCO_3^- relative to P_{CO_2} in expired water leads to an increase in effective β_{CO_2}, which has been found experimentally (46). In the steady state, however, the magnitude of the effect should also be rather limited due to the fact that much more CO_2 is produced than NH_3, even if all energy is derived from protein catabolism.

For the ideal models (see below), β is the only significant property of the medium with respect to gas transfer. In real gas exchange organs, however, a number of other properties are important.

1. Diffusion properties, characterized by the diffusion coefficient, D, or Krogh's diffusion constant, K (= D · α), determine the development of partial pressure gradients inside the medium (interlamellar water in fish gills; surrounding air or water in skin breathing; "stratification" in mammalian lungs; see below).

2. Viscosity, η, is a major property determining the mechanical resistance to respiratory medium flow, both with air and water breathing.

3. Density, ρ, determines the inertia of the medium and is, therefore, of importance in the respiratory flow whose rate varies with time, e.g., the respiratory cycle.

These factors all tend to make water breathing more costly, i.e., requiring more energy per volume of medium respired, than air breathing, because K is much smaller (cf. Table 1) and ρ and η much higher in water than in air (water to air ratio for ρ is 815 and for η 63).

VARIOUS GAS EXCHANGE ORGANS: ANATOMY AND MODELS

Gas exchange organs in vertebrates display a considerable amount of variation and represent adaptations to varied requirements. Basically, four general types of gas exchange organs can be distinguished, each of these corresponding to a different physical model.

1. Gills of fish—countercurrent system (model I).
2. Parabronchial lungs of birds—crosscurrent system (model II).
3. Alveolar lungs of mammals (reptiles and amphibians)—ventilated pool system (model III).
4. Skin, particularly of amphibians—infinite pool system (model IV).

Fish Gills

The fish gill apparatus (54–57) comprises gill arches carrying a double row of gill filaments which carry the secondary lamellae (Figure 3). The secondary lamellae form a fine sieve for respiratory water flow. Venous blood is driven by the heart through the ventral aorta and afferent branchial arteries to the lacunae (capillaries) of the secondary lamellae, where arterialization takes place. The arterialized blood is collected by the efferent branchial arteries into the arterial system. It follows from the anatomical arrangement, particularly in teleosts, that water flow past, and blood flow in, the secondary lamellae must be countercurrent. Due to the presence of the branchial system in elasmobranchs, difficulties for the free interlamellar space outflow were predicted. However, the clear demonstration of an outflow channel by Kempton (58) has made the presence of countercurrent flow in elasmobranch gills highly probable.

Bird Lungs

The avian respiratory system (59–64) is based on a design which is very different from that of mammals (Figure 4). The respiratory system consists of two functionally different parts: a) air sacs, which change their volume during the respiratory cycle, but in which practically no gas exchange takes place (65), and b) lungs, consisting of a set of parallel parabronchi connecting with (secondary) bronchi at both ends, where gas exchange takes place.

The parabronchial lung is practically volume-constant and is ventilated, in flow-through manner, during both inspiration and expiration, the air flow direction being mostly unidirectional. Gas exchange takes place in the periparabronchial tissue layer which mainly consists of interwoven air capillary and blood capillary networks. The arrangement of the circulatory system with respect to complete separation of right (venous) and left (arterial) heart and thereby of venous and arterialized blood is the same as in mammals.

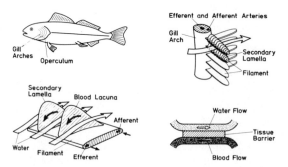

Figure 3. Schematic diagram of the gill apparatus in teleosts to show the relationship between the anatomical structure and the simplified model used for analysis of gas exchange.

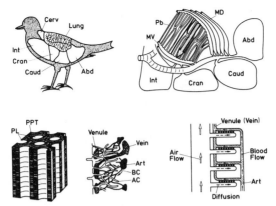

Figure 4. Schematic diagram showing the air sac-lung apparatus in a bird and how a model for gas exchange is deduced from the arrangement of air capillaries (AC) and blood capillaries (BC) in the periparabronchial tissue (PPT). Four paired air sacs usually occur in birds—the cervical (Cerv), cranial (Cran), and caudal thoracic (Caud) and abdominal (Abd) air sacs, and the unpaired interclavicular (Int). MV and MD, mediodorsal and medioventral secondary bronchi; Pb, parabronchus; PL, parabronchial lumen; Art, arteriole.

Alveolar Lungs

In the mammalian lung, the airways form a highly branching (23–30 generations in human lungs) closed dead-end system (66). Gas exchange takes place between the terminal airways (alveoli) and the blood capillary network. In contrast to the avian respiratory tract, the terminal airways are the site both for tidal volume change and gas exchange.

Skin

Skin breathing (67) is important in all amphibians, being the exclusive site of gas exchange in salamanders, in which lungs are reduced or absent and gills are not developed (as in the family Plethodontidae and in a few species of other families). Gas exchange takes place between the cutaneous, subepidermal, capillary network and the ambient air or water.

MODELS: QUANTITATIVE ANALYSIS

In Figure 5, the simplified models are depicted that will be used for quantitative analysis (14, 15) in the four gas exchange systems described above. It is evident that the only difference between these systems is in the specific arrangement of medium and blood flow (cf. Figure 1). In the models of Figure 5, many details have been omitted to allow a general, simplified analysis. Some implications of this neglect will be discussed later.

If the conductances G_{vent}, G_{perf}, and G_{diff} are known for a given model, its overall gas transfer performance can be computed. For example, the partial

232   Piiper and Scheid

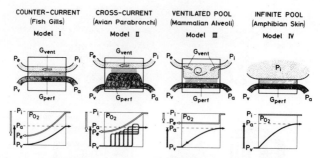

Figure 5. Schema of the typical specific arrangement of medium-to-blood contact in the four models used. *Bottom,* typical curves showing partial pressure changes for O_2 in medium and blood along the exchange area.

pressures in the effluent medium and blood, P_e and P_a, and the transfer rate $\dot{M}$ can be calculated for any given set of values of the partial pressures in inflowing medium and blood, P_i and P_v. Often the value of $\dot{M}$, representing the metabolic requirement, is fixed. In this case, the values P_e, P_a, and P_v can be computed for given P_i and conductance values. On the other hand, the conductance values can be calculated on the basis of experimentally determined P_i, P_e, P_a, P_v, and $\dot{M}$.

Relative Partial Pressure Differences

The gas exchange performance of the four systems are described here by equations relating partial pressure differences in medium and blood to the various conductances. For standardization, any partial pressure difference is related to the maximum possible difference, i.e., to $(P_i - P_v)$. Thus, three relative partial pressure differences, Δp, may be defined as follows:

$$\frac{P_i - P_e}{P_i - P_v} = \Delta p_{\text{vent}} \tag{14}$$

$$\frac{P_e - P_a}{P_i - P_v} = \Delta p_{\text{tr}} \tag{15}$$

$$\frac{P_a - P_v}{P_i - P_v} = \Delta p_{\text{perf}} \tag{16}$$

It is evident from equations 14–16 that only two values of Δp are needed to describe a given model because all three add up to unity.

The Δp values have the meaning of relative resistances attributable to the process indicated in the subscript. This is easily realized for Δp_{vent} and Δp_{perf}, which approach zero as the ventilation or the perfusion, respectively, are increased to infinity. On the other hand, if ventilation is the only limiting process in gas transfer, Δp_{vent} approaches unity. The same applies to Δp_{perf}.

The exact meaning of the quantity Δp_{tr} (transfer Δp) is more complex. For the "ideal lung" (ventilated pool model), it is identical with the relative diffusion resistance, varying in theory between 0 and 1. The same applies for skin breathing. In the countercurrent and crosscurrent models, however, Δp_{tr} can assume negative values, as can be seen from the *overlapping arrows* in Figure 5. Therefore, in general, it should not be considered as a value for the relative diffusion resistance in gas transfer. Instead, it may be viewed as a composite quantity determined a) by diffusion resistance and b) by the inherent properties of the model. Accordingly, Δp_{tr} can be split into two components, Δp_o, representing the model-specific transfer conditions (i.e., $\Delta p_{tr} = \Delta p_o$ for $G_{diff} \to \infty$), and Δp_{diff}, the diffusion limitation part:

$$\Delta p_{tr} = \Delta p_o + \Delta p_{diff} \tag{17}$$

The Δp values for the four models may be expressed as functions of two conductance ratios, e.g., $G_{vent}:G_{perf}$ and $G_{diff}:G_{perf}$ (Table 4). In Figure 6, Δp_{vent}, Δp_{perf}, and Δp_{tr} are plotted as functions of $G_{vent}:G_{perf}$ for all models (except infinite pool where $G_{vent}:G_{perf}$ is infinite) and for three selected $G_{diff}:G_{perf}$ values:∞, 1, and 0.2 (which cover the estimated physiological range; see below). There are marked differences between the models in respect of Δp_{vent}, Δp_{perf}, and Δp_{tr}. These differences are most pronounced with $G_{vent}:G_{perf}$ values not far from unity and with high G_{diff} (or $G_{diff}:G_{perf}$)

Table 4. Relative partial pressure differences, Δp, for four models

	Countercurrent	Crosscurrent	Ventilated pool	Infinite pool
Δp_{vent}	$\dfrac{1 - e^{-Z\,a}}{X - e^{-Z}}$	$1 - e^{-Z'}$	$\dfrac{1 - e^{-Y}}{X + 1 - e^{-Y}}$	0
Δp_{perf}	$\dfrac{X(1 - e^{-Z})}{X - e^{-Z}}$	$X(1 - e^{-Z'})$	$\dfrac{X(1 - e^{-Y})}{X + 1 - e^{-Y}}$	$1 - e^{-Y}$
Δp_{tr}	$\dfrac{X \cdot e^{-Z} - 1}{X - e^{-Z}}$	$e^{-Z'} - X(1 - e^{-Z'})$	$\dfrac{X \cdot e^{-Y}}{X + 1 - e^{-Y}}$	e^{-Y}
Δp_o	$-X^b; -\dfrac{1}{X}c$	$-X + (1 + X)e^{-1/X}$	0	0
Δp_{diff}	$\dfrac{X^2 - 1^b}{X - e^{-Z}}$;	$(X + 1)(e^{-Z'} - e^{-1/X})$	$\dfrac{X \cdot e^{-Y}}{X + 1 - e^{-Y}}$	e^{-Y}
	$\dfrac{e^{-Z}(X^2 - 1)^c}{X(X - e^{-Z})}$			

$^a X = \dfrac{G_{vent}}{G_{perf}}$; $Z = Y(1 - \dfrac{1}{X})$; $Z' = \dfrac{1 - e^{-Y}}{X}$; $Y = \dfrac{G_{diff}}{G_{perf}}$.

$^b X \leqslant 1.$

$^c X \geqslant 1.$

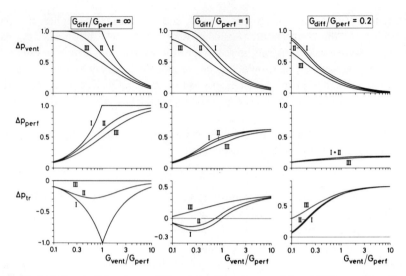

Figure 6. ·Relative partial pressure differences of the three models exhibiting medium flow. I, countercurrent model; II, crosscurrent model; III, ventilated pool model.

values. With decreasing G_{diff}, the differences between the models blur and become hardly perceptible between the countercurrent and crosscurrent models for $G_{diff} : G_{perf} = 0.2$.

Of particular interest is the overlapping of medium partial pressure range, from P_i to P_e, with that of the blood, from P_a to P_v, which occurs only in the countercurrent and crosscurrent models and reveals their high efficiency. This aspect is illustrated in Figure 7, particularly at $G_{diff} = \infty$. The highest, "ideal" efficiency is reached at $G_{vent} : G_{perf} = 1$ by the countercurrent model. Here arterial blood fully equilibrates with inspired water, and expired medium equilibrates with venous blood. With the crosscurrent system, there is still some overlap (i.e., Δp_{tr} is negative), but with the uniform pool model only an equality of partial pressure in gas and blood can be reached by equilibration (the same holds for the infinite pool model).

The effect of changes in $G_{vent} : G_{perf}$ is also displayed in Figure 7. With deviations of $G_{vent} : G_{perf}$ from unity, there can no longer be a complete equilibration for both water and blood in the countercurrent model. Starting from $G_{vent} : G_{perf} = 1$, increasing blood flow or decreasing ventilation (i.e., $G_{vent} : G_{perf} < 1$) causes arterial blood to no longer reach equilibration with inflowing medium. On the other hand, reducing blood flow or increasing ventilation (i.e., $G_{vent} : G_{perf} > 1$) leads to nonattainment of equilibration between expired medium and inflowing blood. With crosscurrent, the maximum overlap is less than in the countercurrent system and varies relatively less with variations of $G_{vent} : G_{perf}$.

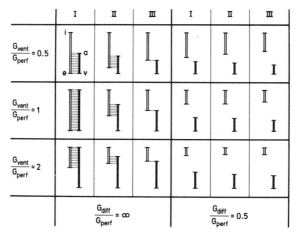

Figure 7. Ranges of partial pressures in medium and blood for some values of the conductance ratios in models I, II, III, (see Figure 6.)

For any given $G_{vent}:G_{perf}$ and $G_{diff}:G_{perf}$ ratio, the length of the bars for either medium or blood is a measure of the total gas transfer rate, $\dot{M}$, which may serve to compare the gas exchange efficacies of the models. The sequence of decreasing efficiency

$$countercurrent > crosscurrent > ventilated\ pool$$

is particularly well visible for $G_{vent}:G_{perf} = 1$.

To the right in Figure 7, the situation for relatively strong diffusion limitation ($G_{diff}:G_{perf} = 0.5$) is shown. For all models, the efficiency is much reduced compared with $G_{diff}:G_{perf} = \infty$, and the differences between the models become blurred.

It is evident from this analysis that it is the ratio of conductances that determines the gas exchange behavior. Of particular interest is the ratio $G_{vent}:G_{perf}$, which, according to equations 3 and 4, is

$$G_{vent}:G_{perf} = (\beta_m \cdot \dot{V}_m):(\beta_b \cdot \dot{V}_b)$$

(18)

In general, it is thus not sufficient to consider the ventilation to perfusion ratio, $\dot{V}_m:\dot{V}_b$, as is usually done for alveolar gas exchange, but rather the ratio of capacitance coefficients has to be taken into account. This is particularly true when $\beta_m:\beta_b$ differs significantly from unity, as is the case for CO_2 in lungs and for both O_2 and CO_2 in water breathers. The importance of the ratio $(\beta_m \cdot V_m):(\beta_b \cdot \dot{V}_b)$ has been first pointed out by Hughes and Shelton (57) in connection with gas exchange in fish gills.

The foregoing analysis is not only valid for respiratory gases, but also for inert gas transfer in the models. Here some simplifications arise from the fact that β means physical solubility of the gas in water, tissue, and blood. Particularly for tissue and blood, solubility values are generally close to identical. In this case, the $G_{diff}:G_{perf}$ ratio becomes independent of solubility, depending upon the diffusion coefficient of the inert gas only.

Total Conductance

On the basis of the general definition of conductance, a total conductance, G_{tot}, can be defined as transfer rate per (total) partial pressure difference between inspired medium and inflowing blood,

$$G_{tot} = \frac{\dot{M}}{P_i - P_{\bar{v}}} \tag{19}$$

The total conductance is a function of the "individual" conductances G_{vent}, G_{perf}, and G_{diff}. It is easily recognized that G_{tot} must be smaller than the smallest individual G value. One may also consider the reciprocal parameter, the resistance $R = 1/G$. The total resistance is higher than any individual resistance.

The following relationships result from the definitions of G_{tot}, G_{vent}, and G_{perf}:

$$G_{tot} = G_{vent} \cdot \Delta p_{vent} \tag{20}$$

$$G_{tot} = G_{perf} \cdot \Delta p_{perf} \tag{21}$$

Using these relationships together with Table 4, the G_{tot} values can be calculated as functions of G_{vent}, G_{perf}, and G_{diff}. In Figure 8, G_{tot} is calculated for the countercurrent, crosscurrent, and ventilated pool models.

The transfer rate $\dot{M}$ is proportional to G_{tot} for any given total partial pressure difference, $P_i - P_v \cdot G_{tot}$ constitutes a relative measure for the gas transfer efficiency of any particular system. The sequence of the models in terms of efficiency is again best seen in Figure 8 for $G_{diff} = \infty$. Under these conditions, G_{tot} of the countercurrent system equals G_{perf} if $G_{vent}:G_{perf} \geqslant 1$, and equals G_{vent} if $G_{vent}:G_{perf} \leqslant 1$. The decreasing differences between the models with decreasing G_{diff} are well documented.

Limitation Index

Another way of expressing the relative role of a component factor in limiting the total transfer rate is to calculate to what extent the process under study reduces the total transfer rate or the total conductance. Thus, the limitation index, L_x, of a process x (ventilation, perfusion, or diffusion) may be defined as

$$L_x = 1 - \frac{\dot{M} \text{ (limited by x)}}{\dot{M} \text{ (not limited by x)}} \tag{22}$$

$$L_x = 1 - \frac{G_{tot} \text{ (limited by x)}}{G_{tot} \text{ (not limited by x)}} \tag{23}$$

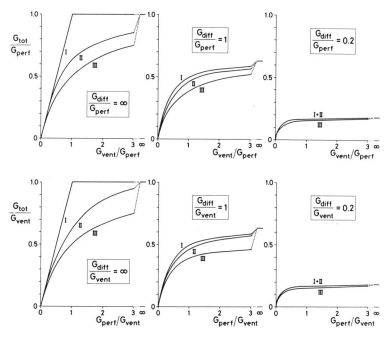

Figure 8. Total conductance, relative to perfusive (*upper panel*) or ventilatory conductance (*lower panel*), for selected values of diffusive conductance in models I, II, III (see Figure 6).

Thus, the following limitation indices can be defined:

$$\text{Ventilation limitation index, } L_{\text{vent}} = 1 - \frac{G_{\text{tot}} \text{ (actual)}}{G_{\text{tot}}(G_{\text{vent}} = \infty)} \qquad (24)$$

$$\text{Perfusion limitation index, } L_{\text{perf}} = 1 - \frac{G_{\text{tot}} \text{ (actual)}}{G_{\text{tot}}(G_{\text{perf}} = \infty)} \qquad (25)$$

$$\text{Diffusion limitation index, } L_{\text{diff}} = 1 - \frac{G_{\text{tot}} \text{ (actual)}}{G_{\text{tot}} (G_{\text{diff}} = \infty)} \qquad (26)$$

For example, $L_{\text{diff}} = 0.60$ means that the total conductance is reduced by 60% from the "ideal" value, i.e., the value in absence of any diffusion limitation (which is in this case 1.0:0.4 = 2.5 times the actual value). Expressions for the three limitation indices in the four models are presented in Table 5.

SKIN BREATHING: A SIMPLE MODEL
FOR EVALUATION OF DIFFUSION AND PERFUSION LIMITATION

Model IV, for skin breathing, is a degenerate model and represents a particular extreme case of the models I, II, and III. If G_{vent} is increased to infinity (e.g.,

Table 5. Limitation indices, L, for four models

	Model I (countercurrent)	Model II (crosscurrent)	Model III (ventilated pool)	Model IV (infinite pool)
L_{vent}	$\dfrac{e^{-Z}(X-1)+e^{-Y}(e^{-Z}-X)^a}{(X-e^{-Z})(1-e^{-Y})}$	$\dfrac{1-e^{-Y}-X(1-e^{-Z'})}{1-e^{-Y}}$	$\dfrac{1-e^{-Y}}{X+1-e^{-Y}}$	0
L_{perf}	$\dfrac{X-1+e^{-Y}/X\,(e^{-Z}-X)}{(X-e^{-Z})(1-e^{-Y}/X)}$	$\dfrac{e^{-Z'}-e^{-Y/X}}{1-e^{-Y/X}}$	$\dfrac{X/Y(Y-1+e^{-Y})}{X+1-e^{-Y}}$	$\dfrac{Y-1+e^{-Y}}{Y}$
L_{diff}	$\dfrac{X-e^{-Z}-A(1-e^{-Z})^b}{X-e^{-Z}}$	$\dfrac{e^{-Z'}-e^{-1/X}}{1-e^{-1/X}}$	$\dfrac{X\cdot e^{-Y}}{X+1-e^{-Y}}$	e^{-Y}

$^a X = \dfrac{G_{\text{vent}}}{G_{\text{perf}}}; Y = \dfrac{G_{\text{diff}}}{G_{\text{perf}}}; Z = Y(1-\tfrac{1}{X}); Z' = \dfrac{1-e^{-Y}}{X}$

$^b X \leqslant 1{:}A = 1; X > 1{:}A = X.$

by very high ventilation), Δp_{vent} and L_{vent} become zero in models I–III, and in this condition all these models are functionally identical with model IV. Therefore, although in a skin-breathing animal there is no ventilation in the sense of ventilatory flow produced by respiratory movements, the state is functionally equivalent to infinite ventilation. It also becomes evident that the various systems described differ only in respect of the relative arrangement of medium and blood flows.

Model IV represents the simplest system combining perfusion and diffusion limitation and, therefore, deserves particular attention. It is eminently suited for study of alveolar-capillary transfer in mammalian lungs, but can also be applied to examination of gas transfer in an infinitesimal segment of a parabronchial unit in avian lungs.

In Figure 9, the perfusion and diffusion limitation indices, L_{perf} and L_{diff}, are plotted as functions of the diffusion: perfusion conductance ratio, G_{diff}: G_{perf}. Some G_{diff}:G_{perf} ratio values for dog lungs and salamander skin, calculated on the basis of experimental data, are indicated. It can be seen that in lungs the alveolar-capillary transfer of N_2 is almost exclusively flow-limited. Even a gas with a diffusion coefficient in an alveolar-capillary barrier that is 20 times less than that of nitrogen (corresponding to a molecular weight of more than 10,000) is expected to be unlimited by diffusion in alveolar-capillary transfer. For this consideration, the solubility of inert gases is immaterial because it is about equal in the alveolar-capillary membrane and in blood: both G_{perf} and G_{diff} are proportional to solubility.

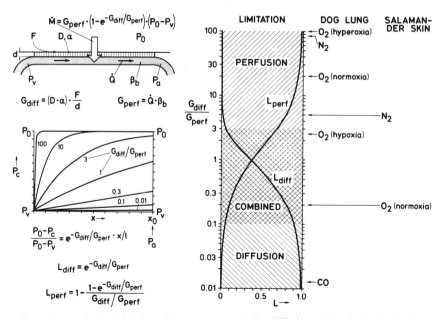

Figure 9. Analysis of skin breathing as an example for diffusion and perfusion limitation.

But the picture changes when the solubility or capacitance coefficient in blood alone is increased, as is the case for O_2, CO_2, and CO. For exchange of O_2 and CO, the chemical bonding with hemoglobin produces a very marked increase in β_b, thereby increasing G_{perf} and decreasing $G_{diff}:G_{perf}$ as compared with the ratio for inert gases. The extremely high affinity of hemoglobin for CO is responsible for a very high β_b and a very low $G_{diff}:G_{perf}$ ratio, meaning pure diffusion limitation. For O_2, β_b depends on the level of P_{O_2}. Thus, in alveolar lungs, alveolo-capillary O_2 uptake is mainly perfusion-limited in normoxia, exclusively perfusion-limited in hyperoxia, and markedly diffusion-limited in hypoxia (Figure 9). In salamander skin, with its much thicker diffusion barrier, $G_{diff}:G_{perf}$ ratios for a given gas are much lower than in alveolar lungs. Thus, the transfer of inert gases is limited both by perfusion and diffusion, and O_2 and CO_2 are prevalently diffusion-limited.

APPLICATION OF MODEL ANALYSIS

The model analysis developed in the preceding sections will be applied to experimental data obtained on a representative species of each of the four types of gas exchange organs. The following examples are chosen for comparative analysis:

1. Larger spotted dogfish (*Scyliorhinus stellaris*), an elasmobranch fish, for the countercurrent model of fish gills (68).
2. Domestic hen (*Gallus domesticus*) for the crosscurrent model of avian para-bronchial lungs (69).
3. Dog (*Canis familiaris*) for the mammalian alveolar lung functionally analyzed on the basis of the ventilated pool model (70).
4. Common dusky salamander (*Desmognathus fuscus,* Plethodontidae), a lung-less and gill-less salamander, for skin breathing studied on the basis of the infinite pool model (41).

In order to demonstrate the characteristic behavior of the gas exchange organs, values measured in hypoxia (or hypoxia combined with hypercapnia) are used in some cases. There are two main reasons for this choice, the first being reduction of "inhomogeneity effects" (see below). Secondly, in hypoxia both G_{perf} and G_{vent} are increased, whereas G_{diff} is virtually unaffected. Hence, diffusion becomes the limiting process, G_{diff} being measurable with reasonable precision.

In Table 6 are presented the experimentally obtained values for O_2 uptake, CO_2 output, and partial pressures of CO_2 and O_2 at the four sites (inspired, expired, venous, and arterial) and the corresponding values of Δp. For the dog, ideal alveolar P_{O_2} and P_{CO_2} were used for P_e. In the hen, both initial para-bronchial, P_i, and end parabronchial partial pressures, P_e, are not easily obtained from inspired and expired values measured at the trachea. The values used in Table 6 are based on estimations from experimental data. For fish or sala-

Table 6. Experimental values used for analysis

	Model I Countercurrent (fish gills)[a]		Model II Crosscurrent (parabronchial lungs)[b]		Model III Ventilated pool (alveolar lungs)[c]		Model IV Infinite pool (skin)[d]	
	CO_2	O_2	CO_2	O_2	CO_2	O_2	CO_2	O_2
$\dot{M}$ (mmol/min)	0.062	0.065	0.85	1.09	6.07	6.70	0.16	0.19
P_i (Torr)	0.7	149	22.6	90.4	0.2	81	0.2	152
P_e (Torr)	1.25	57	45.4	63.3	39.1	38.7	5.2	61
P_a (Torr)	2.0	49	38.8	69.3	39.1	36.9	6.2	40
P_v (Torr)	2.6	10	46.8	37.6	46	22.9	0	0
Δp_{vent}	0.29	0.66	0.94	0.51	0.85	0.73	0.17	0.19
Δp_{perf}	0.31	0.28	0.33	0.60	0.15	0.24	0.83	0.81
Δp_{tr}	0.40	0.06	−0.27	−0.11	(0)	0.03		

[a]From the dogfish (2.2 kg body weight) in normoxia.
[b]From the chicken (1.6 kg body weight) in hypoxia and hypercapnia.
[c]From the dog (25 kg body weight) in hypoxia.
[d]From the salamander (6.1 g body weight) in normoxia.

mander, these problems do not arise. For the dog, arterial P_{O_2} was corrected further for venous admixture.

In Table 6, the much smaller range of P_{CO_2} values (from P_i to P_v) in the dogfish and the skin-breathing salamander in contrast to the bird and the mammal is well documented, the reason being the prevalent ventilation limitation in air-ventilating animals (see above). The P_{eO_2} values and the blood P_{O_2} in the dogfish are much lower than the normoxic values in mammals (alveolar P_{O_2} ≈ 100 Torr) and in birds, due to the fact that the ventilation is not high enough to compensate for the much reduced $(\beta_m)_{O_2}$ in water compared with air (see above).

Only in the case of the bird is the "relative transfer resistance," Δp_{tr}, negative. In fish, the values are positive, although on the basis of the countercurrent model they could be negative and, in fact, it was frequently observed that $(\Delta p_{tr})_{O_2}$ was negative (P_{O_2} in arterial blood is higher than in expired water). The observation of large variations in $(\Delta p_{tr})_{O_2}$ from positive to negative values, occurring in an individual fish, makes it likely that varying functional inhomogeneities play a role.

The quantities conductance, G, and limitation index, L, calculated from the values of Table 6, are compiled in Table 7. The following observations can be made:

1. In general, the diffusion resistance for CO_2 in lungs (hen and dog) is small, G_{diff} not being distinguishable from infinity with enough accuracy. Therefore, for dog and hen, G_{diff} is assumed to be infinity.

2. Remarkably, for fish gills and salamander skin the $G_{diff}:G_{perf}$ ratio is about equal for O_2 and CO_2. If, however, absolute values of G_{diff} are calculated, marked differences between CO_2 and O_2 are revealed, as expected from differences in solubility: for fish gills, $(G_{diff})_{CO_2}:(G_{diff})_{O_2} \approx 40$; for salamander

Table 7. Summary of values for conductance (in mmol min^{-1} $Torr^{-1}$) and limitation index calculated from Table 6

	Model I Dogfish gills		Model II Hen lung		Model III Dog lung		Model IV Salamander skin	
	CO_2	O_2	CO_2	O_2	CO_2	O_2	CO_2	O_2
G_{vent}	0.11	0.001	0.040	0.040	0.16	0.16	∞	∞
G_{perf}	0.10	0.002	0.11	0.034	0.88	0.48	0.16	0.009
G_{diff}	0.05	0.001	(∞)	0.063	(∞)	2.64	0.05	0.002
$G_{vent}:G_{perf}$	1.09	0.42	0.35	1.17	0.18	0.33	∞	∞
$G_{diff}:G_{perf}$	0.45	0.51	(∞)	1.85	(∞)	3.0	0.30	0.22
L_{vent}	0.13	0.33	0.67	0.29	0.85	0.74	0	0
L_{perf}	0.15	0.09	0.06	0.35	0.15	0.18	0.14	0.10
L_{diff}	0.69	0.37	(0)	0.11	(0)	0.01	0.74	0.80

skin, $(G_{diff})_{CO_2} : (G_{diff})_{O_2} \approx 20$. As the $(G_{perf})_{CO_2} : (G_{perf})_{O_2}$ ratios show a similar behavior, about equal $G_{diff} : G_{perf}$ ratios for CO_2 and O_2 are obtained.

3. $(G_{diff})_{O_2}$ is more than one order of magnitude less in the dogfish and the salamander than in the hen and the dog. This difference is confirmed by morphometric data: smaller surface area and higher thickness of the medium-blood barrier in elasmobranch gill and salamander skin.

4. For all animals selected, the G_{perf} values are higher for CO_2 than for O_2, due to higher $(\beta_b)_{CO_2}$ than $(\beta_b)_{O_2}$. For fish blood, this difference is most marked, because O_2 capacity, and hence $(\beta_b)_{O_2}$, is low and blood P_{CO_2} values are low with consequently high $(\beta_b)_{CO_2}$. In hypoxia and for blood of high O_2 capacity (hen and dog), the difference is less marked.

5. G_{vent} for O_2 and CO_2 are identical for the air-breathing hen and dog but differ for the water-breathing fish due to the much higher capacitance coefficient in water for CO_2 than for O_2 (see above).

6. For air-breathing animals, the high L_{vent} for CO_2 as compared with O_2 (in normoxia the diffusion limitation is much more marked; see above) is in agreement with the well known fact that in mammals (and man) transient hyperventilation, or local hyperventilation in lungs with regional differences in ventilation-perfusion ratio, leads to high gas exchange ratio.

REAL SYSTEMS VERSUS MODELS

Differences in performance between the idealized, simple models and real gas exchange organs are due to anatomical and functional complications of the latter. The following section aims at giving a brief, qualitative overview of the various complications.

Complications Due to Anatomical Arrangement

The anatomical complexity of real gas exchange organs may render it difficult to directly sample the medium and blood entering and leaving the organ.

Medium Dead Space When mammals inspire, at first, dead space gas (which corresponds to the end-expired gas of the preceding breath) and then fresh gas enter the gas exchange area of the lung, where both gas species are mixed. This can be most easily and quite satisfactorily taken into account by considering an effective tidal volume of inspired gas equal to total tidal volume minus dead space volume. This approach may also be used in birds. One of the clear advantages of the gill system is the functional absence of dead space due to unidirectional water flow.

Blood: Arrangement of Blood Vessels in Relation to Gas Exchange Organs Of more fundamental importance is the fact that arterialized blood leaving the gas exchange organ may become substantially modified by admixture of venous-like blood before entering the systemic arterial system. The extent of this "venous admixture" is primarily dictated by the arrangement of the circulatory system in relation to gas transfer organs (gills, lungs, skin) and to metabo-

lizing organs ("body"), which is very schematically pictured for various vertebrate groups in Figure 10.

Only in "typical" (i.e., exclusively water-breathing) fishes, with the "simple
circulation," and in mammals and birds, with "double circulation" (complete
separation of arterial and venous blood in the heart), is there a single clearly
defined kind of arterial blood leaving the gas exchange organ and flowing to
metabolizing tissues. In amphibians and reptiles, there are complications due to
the presence of several gas exchanging sites and partial (or even complete)
mixing of arterialized blood with venous blood. This, in connection with
periodic or low breathing rates and regulatory changes in distribution of blood
flow occurring during a respiratory cycle, makes a quantitative analysis of gas
exchange difficult. These and related topics have been treated in several recent
reviews (67, 71–74). Only a few remarks will be made here in connection with
Figure 10.

1. Skin breathing occurs in all vertebrate classes, particularly when the ratio of
surface area to body mass is high. For example, water turtles (75) and sea snakes
(76) have gas exchange with water when submerged, and bats have been shown
to exhibit considerable cutaneous CO_2 exchange (77). In primitive amphibians,
such as the heavily armored Stegocephalia, on the other hand, skin breathing
may have been unimportant (78).

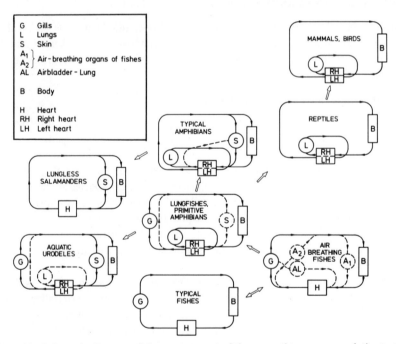

Figure 10. Schematic diagram of the arrangement of the gas exchange organs relative to the
circulatory system in the main vertebrate groups.

2. The degree of functional separation of venous and arterialized, pulmonary venous blood in lungfishes, amphibians, and reptiles is rather varied. In recent salamanders, the separation seems to be secondarily reduced, up to complete absence, in connection with the preponderance of skin breathing.

3. Because skin capillaries are generally arranged in parallel to systemic capillaries, the afferent skin blood is the same as arterial blood. Thus, in salamanders, the blood perfusing the cutaneous capillaries is mixed cardiac blood distributed to the skin by the arterial system. In frogs, less arterialized blood is conveyed to the skin by a branch to the pulmonary artery, but the arterialized blood from skin is returned to the heart along with the venous return from the body.

4. In the bony fishes (Osteichthyes), the "typical fish" condition seems to be secondary, because apparently all early osteichthyes had lung-like structures that subsequently were developed into the swim bladder in most bony fishes (78). The aquatic giant salamander *Cryptobranchus,* whose lung seems to be mainly hydrostatic (48), provides an interesting case of parallel evolution.

5. There is a great diversity of air-breathing organs and their circulatory arrangement in air-breathing fishes (79).

6. The development of the tetrapod pulmonary circulation and divided heart not only allowed separation of venous and arterialized blood, but also permitted development of low pulmonary capillary pressure simultaneously with high systemic arterial pressure.

7. Convergent parallel evolution from the reptilian state has resulted in a functionally very similar central circulation in mammals and birds.

8. The embryonic stages, which have not been considered in this chapter, show further complexity (e.g., fetal-maternal gas exchange system in placental mammals).

Inhomogeneities

Functional Inhomogeneities of Parallel Units   For analysis of steady state gas exchange, differences between parallel units in either $G_{vent}:G_{perf}$ or $G_{diff}:G_{perf}$, or in both, are of importance. For alveolar lungs such regional inhomogeneities exist, and their influence on gas exchange has been assessed in theory (80–82). In general, regional inhomogeneities lead to a reduction in gas exchange efficacy.

Functional inhomogeneities of parallel units are likely to occur in other types of vertebrate gas exchange systems as well, although they have not been worked out in similar detail as for mammals. Burger and Scheid (unpublished observations) found only a small venous admixture in birds, amounting to a few percent of cardiac output, and also a relatively small air shunt (equivalent to alveolar dead space ventilation). In fish, there is evidence for a functional blood shunt in the base of the secondary lamellae (83).

Temporal Variations in Conductances and in Partial Pressures   For model analysis, conductance values have been assumed to be constant in time. Although blood flow past the gas exchanging surface is pulsatile due to the cyclic action of the vertebrate heart, its effects on gas exchange appear to be small in alveolar lungs (84). Ventilation in mammals and birds is tidal, and, hence, ventilatory gas flow is not constant. For mammals the expiratory phase is functionally equivalent to a breathholding period with ensuing changes in alveolar and arterial P_{O_2} and P_{CO_2} (85–87). In birds, the effects of non-constant, tidal ventilation would be expected to be much more severe than in mammals, due to the smallness of the parabronchial gas volume. However, the functional breath-holding time encountered in mammals is virtually removed in birds by the parabronchial airflow during both inspiration and expiration with the "rectification" resulting from unidirectional gas flow (64). Unpublished experiments in this laboratory suggest that ventilation of parabronchi in ducks with a sinusoidal flow pattern instead of constant flow does not markedly impair gas exchange. Despite the cyclic action of the water-promoting buccal and opercular pumps, gill ventilation is almost continuous as suggested from record-ings of the differential pressure across the gill sieve (56). Effects on gas exchange are thus expected to be less pronounced than with the to-and-fro mode of mammalian ventilation.

Additional Transfer Resistances

Diffusion in Medium and Blood For model analysis, the resistances to gas transfer have been concentrated into three discrete components: the convective resistance of medium and blood, $1/G_{vent}$ and $1/G_{perf}$, and the diffusive resis-tance, $1/G_{diff}$. Strictly, the analysis holds only for the case in which diffusion is confined to the membrane separating blood and gas or, in addition, to a stagnant layer adhering to it. Diffusive resistances within the medium or blood lead to considerable complications of the model analysis.

In mammals, finite diffusivity of O_2 and CO_2 within the alveolar gas phase leads to concentration gradients between alveolar tidal air and alveolo-capillary membrane. Whether, and under which conditions, this "stratified inhomogeneity (= stratification)" (88) limits alveolar O_2 and CO_2 exchange is not definitely settled (89).

In avian lungs, gas is convectively transported through the parabronchial lumen but has to diffuse through the vestibula, infundibula, and particularly through the air capillaries in order to reach the blood-gas interface. This pathway must be overcome by diffusion. Theoretical analysis suggests that the diffusive resistance within the air capillaries is small compared with the overall diffusive resistance (90, 91), and unpublished experimental data from this laboratory support this result.

Diffusion resistance in water ventilating fish gills is expected to be much more severe than stratified resistances in either mammals or birds, because the diffusivity of gases in water is several orders of magnitude smaller than in gas (see Table 1). The effects of diffusion limitation in water passing between the secondary lamellae have been estimated by model calculations which suggest that the resistance imposed by interlamellar water is between 25 and 50% of the total diffusion resistance in teleosts (92) and in elasmobranchs (93) or even higher (94).

Diffusion inside the blood is expected to be of lesser significance for all classes of vertebrates, because the diffusion distances offered by the secondary lamellar lacunae and lung blood capillaries are small and convective mixing due to motion and deformation of red cells is likely to occur both in plasma and inside the red cells.

Kinetics of Chemical Reactions It has been assumed in the foregoing analysis that the various chemical reactions involved in O_2 and CO_2 exchange in gill lacunae or in lung capillaries are in steady state. This assumption implies that the reaction times involved are small compared with the contact time of blood at the gas exchange surface. Reaction kinetics of O_2 with hemoglobin, in solution and in erythrocytes, has been studied in much detail (20, 95), but a definite statement on their limiting role in vivo is not yet possible. For CO_2 liberation, the rate-limiting reaction appears to be the dehydration of H_2CO_3, which is substantially speeded by carbonic anhydrase present in the red cells (95). According to our present knowledge, chemical reaction rates and cell plasma exchange processes are not expected to be importantly exchange-limiting in mammalian lungs (84, 96, 97). At the lower body temperatures of poikilotherms, chemical reactions involved in both O_2 and CO_2 transport may become rate-limiting, although quantitative data are currently not available.

Complications Arising from Blood Chemistry

Dependence of β on P The blood dissociation curves for both O_2 and CO_2 are curved, their slopes, β_b, depending upon the partial pressures. There are essentially two ways in which problems arising from nonlinear dissociation curves in analysis of gas exchange can be handled. The first is to use approximation methods that account for the shape of the dissociation curve, such as the graphical Bohr integration for alveolar lungs (98), a modification of which has been applied to fish gills (99). The second method, used in this chapter, is to analyze data obtained in hypoxia and hypercapnia where the dissociation curves are virtually straight. Particular attention must be paid in birds because, due to the crosscurrent system, blood P_{O_2} and P_{CO_2} values potentially span the total range from P_i to P_v and may thus far exceed the range from P_a to P_v; hence, hypoxia must be deep enough to ensure restriction to a sufficiently linear part of the O_2 dissociation curve.

Bohr and Haldane Effects Due to the link between O_2 and CO_2 binding of blood provided by the Bohr and Haldane effects, $(\beta_b)_{O_2}$ depends not only on P_{O_2} but also on P_{CO_2}, and conversely $(\beta_b)_{CO_2}$ depends not only on P_{CO_2} but also on P_{O_2}. It has been suggested on model calculations that neglect of the Bohr and Haldane effects does not invalidate the quantitative analysis of alveolar gas exchange attempted here (100), and the same may be true for analysis of the gill system. Peculiar problems arise in the crosscurrent system, which appears to specifically magnify the influences provided by the Bohr-Haldane effect (101).

Thus, P_{CO_2} in end-parabronchial gas, P_e, may exceed not only the arterial P_{CO_2} but also the mixed venous P_{CO_2} during steady state gas exchange, which behavior seems impossible for any other system. In general, the Bohr and Haldane effects, which lead to an increase in effective slopes of the O_2 and CO_2 dissociation curves, enhance the efficiency of all gas exchange systems.

Note added in proof: Reference number 102 appeared while this article was in press. A few articles from this book had been available to us in manuscript form, but the volume contains many more papers that are of direct relevance to the subject covered here.

REFERENCES

1. Bethe, A. (1925). Atmung: Allgemeines und Vergleichendes. *In* Handbuch der normalen und pathologischen Physiologie, Vol. 2, pp. 1–36. Springer, Berlin.
2. Irving, L. (1964). Comparative anatomy and physiology of gas transport mechanisms. *In* Handbook of Physiology, Section 3, Respiration, Vol. 1, pp. 177–212. Am. Physiol. Soc., Washington, D.C.
3. Buddenbrock, W. von. (1939). Atmung, Blut, Erfolgsorgane, Blutkreislauf. *In* Grundriß der vergleichenden Physiologie, Ed. 2, Vol. 2, pp. 569–1228. Borntraeger, Berlin.
4. Prosser, C. L. (1973). Oxygen: respiration and metabolism. *In* C. L. Prosser (ed.), Comparative Animal Physiology, pp. 165–211. W. B. Saunders, Philadelphia.
5. Prosser, C. L. (1973). Respiratory functions of blood. *In* C. L. Prosser (ed.), Comparative Animal Physiology, pp. 317–361. W. B. Saunders, Philadelphia.
6. Schmidt-Nielsen, K. (1975). Adaptation and environment. *In* Animal Physiology. University Press, Cambridge.
7. Bert, P. (1870). Lecons sur la physiologie comparée de la respiration. Baillière, Paris.
8. Krogh, A. (1941). The Comparative Physiology of Respiratory Mechanisms. University of Pennsylvania Press, Philadelphia.
9. Hughes, G. M. (1963). Comparative Physiology of Vertebrate Respiration. Heinemann, London.
10. Negus, V. (1965). The Biology of Respiration. Livingstone, London.
11. Steen, J. B. (1971). Comparative Physiology of Respiratory Mechanisms. Academic Press, New York.
12. Jones, J. D. (1972). Comparative Physiology of Respiration. Edward Arnold, London.
13. Dejours, P. (1975). Principles of Comparative Respiratory Physiology. American-Elsevier, New York.
14. Piiper, J., and Scheid, P. (1972). Maximum gas transfer efficacy of models for fish gills, avian lungs and mammalian lungs. Respir. Physiol. 14:115.
15. Piiper, J., and Scheid, P. (1975). Gas transport efficacy of gills, lung and skin: theory and experimental data. Respir. Physiol. 23:209.
16. Piiper, J., Dejours, P., Haab, P., and Rahn, H. (1971). Concepts and basic quantities in gas exchange physiology. Respir. Physiol. 13:292.
17. Antonini, E. (1965). Interrelationship between structure and function in hemoglobin and myoglobin. Physiol. Rev. 45:123.

18. Antonini, E., and Brunori, M. (1971). Hemoglobin and Myoglobin in Their Reactions with Ligands. North Holland, London.
19. Bartels, H. (1964). Comparative physiology of oxygen transport in mammals. Lancet 19:599.
20. Bauer, C. (1974). On the respiratory function of hemoglobin. Rev. Physiol. Biochem. Pharmacol. 70:1.
21. Brenna, O., Luzzana, M., Pace, M., Perrella, M., Rossi, F., Rossi-Bernardi, L., and Roughton, F. J. W. (1972). The interaction between hemoglobin and its oxygen-linked ligands. In G. J. Brewer (ed.), Hemoglobin and Red Cell Structure and Function, p. 19. Plenum Press, New York.
22. Johansen, K., and Lenfant, C. (1972). A comparative approach to the adaptability of O_2-Hb affinity. In M. Rørth and P. Astrup (eds.), Oxygen Affinity of Hemoglobin and Red Cell Acid-Base Status, pp. 750–780. Munksgaard, Copenhagen.
23. Kreuzer, F., Roughton, F. J. W., Rossi-Bernardi, L., and Kernohan, J. C. (1972). Specific effect of CO_2 and bicarbonate on the affinity of hemoglobin for oxygen. In M. Rørth and P. Astrup (eds.), Oxygen Affinity of Hemoglobin and Red Cell Acid-Base Status, pp. 208–215. Munksgaard, Copenhagen.
24. Metcalfe, J., and Dhindsda, D. S. (1972). The physiological effects of displacements of the oxygen dissociation curve. In M. Rørth and P. Astrup (eds.), Oxygen Affinity of Hemoglobin and Red Cell Acid-Base Status, pp. 613–628. Munksgaard, Copenhagen.
25. Riggs, A. (1965). Functional properties of hemoglobins. Physiol. Rev. 45:619.
26. Roughton, F. J. W. (1964). Transport of oxygen and carbon dioxide. In Handbook of Physiology, Respiration, Vol. 1, pp. 767–825. Am. Physiol. Soc., Washington, D.C.
27. Harvey, H. W. (1957). The Chemistry and Fertility of Sea Waters. University Press, Cambridge.
28. Rahn, H. (1966). Aquatic gas exchange: theory. Respir. Physiol. 1:1.
29. Rahn, H. (1967). Gas transport from the external environment to the cell. In A. V. S. de Reuck and R. Porter (eds.), Development of the Lung. Ciba Foundation Symposium, pp. 3–23. J. and A. Churchill, London.
30. Dejours, P. Garey, W. F., and Rahn, H. (1970). Comparison of ventilatory and circulatory flow rates between animals in various physiological conditions. Respir. Physiol. 9:108.
31. Dejours, P. (1972). Comparison of gas transport by convection among animals. Respir. Physiol. 14:96.
32. Rahn, H., Wangensteen, O. D., and Farhi, L. E. (1971). Convection and diffusion gas exchange in air or water. Respir. Physiol. 12:1.
33. Garey, W. F., and Rahn, H. (1970). Normal arterial gas tensions and pH and the breathing frequency of the electric eel. Respir. Physiol. 9:141.
34. Farber, J., and Rahn, H. (1970). Gas exchange between air and water and the ventilation pattern in the electric eel. Respir. Physiol. 9:151.
35. Lenfant, C., and Johansen, K. (1968). Respiration in the African lung fish Protopterus aethiopicus. I. Respiratory properties of blood and normal pattern of breathing and gas exchange. J. Exp. Biol. 49:437.
36. Erasmus, B. de W., Howell, B. J., and Rahn, H. (1970/71). Ontogeny of acid-base balance in the bullfrog and chicken. Respir. Physiol. 11:46.
37. Toews, D. P., Shelton, G., and Randall, D. J. (1971). Gas tensions in the lungs and major blood vessels of the urodele amphibian, Amphiuma tridactylum. J. Exp. Biol. 55:47.

38. Guimond, R. W., and Hutchison, V. H. (1976). Gas exchange of the giant salamanders of North America. *In* G. M. Hughes (ed.), Respiration of Amphibious Vertebrates, pp. 313–338. Academic Press, Cambridge.
39. Lenfant, C., and Johansen, K. (1967). Respiratory adaptations in selected amphibians. Respir. Physiol. 2:247.
40. Lenfant, C., Johansen, K., and Grigg, G. C. (1966/67). Respiratory properties of blood and pattern of gas exchange in the lungfish *Neoceratodu forsteri* (Krefft). Respir. Physiol. 2:1.
41. Piiper, J., Gatz, R. N., and Crawford, E. C., Jr. (1976). Gas transport characteristics in an exclusively skin-breathing salamander, *Desmognathus fuscus* (Plethodontidae). *In* G. M. Hughes (ed.), Respiration in Amphibious Vertebrates, pp. 339–356. Academic Press, Cambridge.
42. Piiper, J., and Schumann, D. (1967). Efficiency of O_2 exchange in the gills (Plethodontidae). *In* G. M. Hughes (ed.), Respiration in Amphibious Vertebrates. Academic Press, Cambridge, in press.
42. Piiper, J., and Schumann, D. (1967). Efficiency of O_2 exchange in the gills of the dogfish, *Scyliorhinus stellaris*. Respir. Physiol. 2:135.
43. Motais, R., and Garcia-Romen, F. (1972). Transport mechanisms in the teleostean gill and amphibian skin. Ann. Rev. Physiol. 34:141.
44. Woodbury, J. W. (1965). Regulation of pH. *In* T. C. Ruch and H. D. Patton (eds.), Howell-Fulton: Physiology and Biophysics, Ed. 19, pp. 899–934. W. B. Saunders, Philadelphia.
45. Murdaugh, H. V., Jr., and Robin, E. D. (1967). Acid-base metabolism in the dogfish shark. *In* P. W. Gilbert, R. F. Mathewson, and D. P. Rall (eds.), Sharks, Skates and Rays, pp. 249–264. Johns Hopkins Press, Baltimore.
46. Dejours, P., Armand, J., and Verriest, G. (1968). Carbon dioxide dissociation curves of water and gas exchange of water breathers. Respir. Physiol. 5:23.
47. Guimond, R. W., and Hutchison, V. H. (1972). Pulmonary, branchial and cutaneous gas exchange in the mud puppy, *Necturus maculosus maculosus* (Rafinesque). Comp. Biochem. Physiol. 42*A*:367.
48. Guimond, R. W., and Hutchison, V. H. (1973). Aquatic respiration: an unusual strategy in the hellbender *Cryptobranchus alleganiensis alleganiensis* (Daudin). Science 182:1263.
49. Guimond, R. W., and Hutchison, V. H. (1973). Trimodal gas exchange in the large aquatic salamander, *Siren lacertina* (Linnaeus). Comp. Biochem. Physiol. 46*A*:249.
50. Guimond, R. W., and Hutchison, V. H. (1974). Aerial and aquatic respiration in the congo eel *Amphiuma means means* (Garden). Respir. Physiol. 20:147.
51. Whitford, W. G., and Hutchison, V. H. (1965). Gas exchange in salamanders. Physiol. Zool. 38:228.
52. Vinegar, A., and Hutchison, V. H. (1965). Pulmonary and cutaneous gas exchange in the green frog, *Rana clamitans*. Zoologica 50:47.
53. Hutchison, V. H., Whitford, W. G., and Kohl, M. (1966). Relation and body size and surface area to gas exchange in anurans. Physiol. Zoöl. 41:65.
54. Randall, D. J. (1970). Gas exchange in fish. *In* W. S. Hoar and D. J. Randall (eds.), Fish Physiology, Vol. IV, pp. 253–292. Academic Press, New York.
55. Johansen, K. (1971). Comparative physiology: gas exchange and circulation in fishes. Ann. Rev. Physiol. 33:569.

56. Hughes, G. M., and Morgan, M. (1973). The structure of fish gills in relation to their respiratory function. Biol. Rev. 48:419.
57. Hughes, G. M., and Shelton, G. (1962). Respiratory mechanisms and their nervous control in fish. Adv. Comp. Physiol. Biochem. 1:275.
58. Kempton, R. T. (1969). Morphological features of functional significance in the gills of the spiny dogfish *Squalus acanthias*. Biol. Bull. Mar. Biol. Lab., Woods Hole, 136:226.
59. King, A. S. (1966). Structural and functional aspects of the avian lungs and air sacs. Int. Rev. Gen. Exp. Zool. 2:171.
60. Duncker, H.-R. (1971). The lung air sac system of birds. Ergeb. Anat. Entwicklungsgesch. 45:1.
61. King, A. S., and Molony, V. (1971). The anatomy of respiration. *In* D. K. Bell and B. M. Freeman (eds.), Physiology and Biochemistry of the Domestic Fowl, Vol. I, pp. 93—169. Academic Press, London.
62. Lasiewski, R. C. (1972). Respiratory function in birds. *In* D. S. Farner and J. R. King (eds.), Avian Biology, Vol. II. pp. 287—342. Academic Press, New York.
63. Fedde, M. R. (1976). Respiration. *In* P. D. Sturkie (ed.), Avian Physiology, Ed. 3, pp. 122—145. Comstock, Ithaca, New York.
64. Piiper, J., and Scheid, P. (1973). Gas exchange in avian lungs: models and experimental evidence. *In* L. Bolis, K. Schmidt-Nielsen, and S. H. P. Maddrell (eds.), Comparative Physiology, pp. 161—185. North Holland, Amsterdam.
65. Magnussen, H., Willmer, H., and Scheid, P. (1976). Gas exchange in air sacs: contribution to respiratory gas exchange in ducks. Respir. Physiol. 26:
66. Thurlbeck, W. M., and Wang, N.-S. (1974). The structure of the lungs. *In* J. G. Widdicombe (ed.), MTP International Review of Science, Physiology Series I, vol. II, Respiratory Physiology I, pp. 1—30. University Park Press, Baltimore.
67. Foxon, G. E. H. (1964). Blood and Respiration. *In* J. A. Moore (ed.), Physiology of the Amphibia, pp. 151—209. Academic Press, New York.
68. Baumgarten-Schumann, D., and Piiper, J. (1968). Gas exchange in the gills of resting unanesthetized dogfish (*Scyliorhinus stellaris*). Respir. Physiol. 5:317.
69. Scheid, P., and Piiper, J. (1970). Analysis of gas exchange in the avian lung: theory and experiments in the domestic fowl. Respir. Physiol. 9:246.
70. Haab, P., Duc, G., Stuki, R., and Piiper, J. (1964). Les échanges gazeux en hypoxie et la capacité de diffusion pour l'oxygène chez le chien narcotisé. Helvet. Physiol. Acta 22:203.
71. Lenfant, C., Johansen, K., and Hanson, D. (1970). Bimodal gas exchange and ventilation-perfusion relationship in lower vertebrates. Fed. Proc. 29:1124.
72. Johansen, K., Lenfant, C., and Hanson, D. (1970). Phylogenetic development of pulmonary circulation. Fed. Proc. 29:1135.
73. White, F. N. (1970). Central vascular shunts and their control in reptiles. Fed. Proc. 29:1149.
74. Gans, C. (1970). Strategy and sequence in the evolution of the external gas exchanges of ectothermal vertebrates. Forma Functio 3:61.
75. Belkin, D. A. (1968). Aquatic respiration and underwater survival of two freshwater turtle species. Respir. Physiol. 4:1.

76. Graham, J. B. (1974). Aquatic respiration in the sea snake, *Pelamis platurus*. Respir. Physiol. 21:1.
77. Herreid, C. F., II, Bretz, W. L., and Schmidt-Nielsen, K. (1968). Cutaneous gas exchange in bats. Am. J. Physiol. 215:506.
78. Romer, A. S. (1972). Skin breathing—primary or secondary? Respir. Physiol. 14:183.
79. Johansen, K. (1970). Air breathing in fishes. *In* W. S. Hoar and D. J. Randall (eds.), Fish Physiology, Vol. IV, pp. 361–411. Academic Press, New York.
80. Rahn, H., and Farhi, L. E. (1964). Ventilation, perfusion and gas exchange—V_A/Q concept. *In* W. D. Fenn and H. Rahn (eds.), Handbook of Physiology, Section 3, Respiration, Vol. 1, pp. 735–766. American Physiological Society, Washington, D.C.
81. Piiper, J., and Sikand, R. S. (1966). Determination of D_{CO} by single breath method in inhomogeneous lungs: theory. Respir. Physiol. 1:75.
82. Wagner, P. D., Saltzman, H. A., and West, J. B. (1974). Measurement of continuous distributions of ventilation-perfusion ratios. J. Appl. Physiol. 36:588.
83. Steen, J. B., and Kruysse, A. (1964). The respiratory function of teleostean gills. Comp. Biochem. Physiol. 12:127.
84. Wagner, P. D., and West, J. B. (1972). Effects of diffusion impairment on O_2 and CO_2 time courses in pulmonary capillaries. J. Appl. Physiol. 33:62.
85. Otis, A. B. (1964). Quantitative relationships in steady-state gas exchange. *In* W. O. Fenn and H. Rahn (eds.), Handbook of Physiology, Section 3, Respiration, Vol. 1, pp. 681–698. American Physiological Society, Washington, D.C.
86. Hlastala, M. P. (1972). A model of fluctuating alveolar gas exchange during the respiratory cycle. Respir. Physiol. 15:214.
87. Lin, K. H., and Cumming, G. (1973). A model of time-varying gas exchange in the human lung during a respiratory cycle at rest. Respir. Physiol. 17:93.
88. Piiper, J., and Scheid, P. (1971). Respiration: alveolar gas exchange. Annu. Rev. Physiol. 33:131.
89. Sikand, R. S., Magnussen, H., Scheid, P., and Piiper, J. (1976). Convective and diffusive gas mixing in human lungs: experiments and model analysis. J. Appl. Physiol. 40:362.
90. Zeuthen, E. (1942). The ventilation of the respiratory tract in birds. Kgl. Danske Videnskab. Selskab Biol. Medd. 17:1.
91. Hazelhoff, E. H. (1943). Bouw en functie van de vogellong. Versl. gewone Vergad. Afd. Natuurk. Ned. Akad. Wet. 52:391. (English translation: (1951). Structure and function of the lung of birds. Poultry Sci. 30:3.)
92. Scheid, P., and Piiper, J. (1971). Theoretical analysis of respiratory gas equilibration in water passing through fish gills. Respir. Physiol. 13:305.
93. Scheid, P., and Piiper, J. (1976). Quantitative functional analysis of branchial gas transfer: theory and application to *Scyliorhinus stellaris* (Elasmobranchii). *In* G. M. Hughes (ed.), Respiration of Amphibious Vertebrates, pp. 17–38. Academic Press, London.
94. Hughes, G. M., and Hills, B. A. (1971). Oxygen tension distribution in water and blood at the secondary lamellae of the dogfish. J. Exp. Biol. 55:399.
95. Forster, R. E. (1964). Rate of gas uptake by red cells. *In* W. O. Fenn and

H. Rahn (eds.), Handbook of Physiology, Section 3, Respiration, Vol. 1, pp. 827–837. American Physiological Society, Washington, D.C.

96. Piiper, J. (1968). Rate of chloride-bicarbonate exchange between red cells and plasma. *In* CO_2: Chemical, Biochemical and Physiological Aspects, pp. 267–273. NASA Sp-188, Washington, D.C.

97. Forster, R. E. (1968). The rate of CO_2 equilibration between red cells and plasma. *In* CO_2: Chemical, Biochemical and Physiological Aspects, pp. 275–284. NASA SP-188, Washington, D.C.

98. Forster, R. E. (1964). Diffusion of gases. *In* W. O. Fenn and H. Rahn (eds.), Handbook of Physiology, Section 3, Respiration, Vol. 1, pp. 839–872. American Physiological Society, Washington, D.C.

99. Piiper, J., and Baumgarten-Schumann, D. (1968). Effectiveness of O_2 and CO_2 exchange in the gills of the dogfish (*Scyliorhinus stellaris*). Respir. Physiol. 5:338.

100. Hlastala, M. P. (1973). Significance of the Bohr and Haldane effects in the pulmonary capillary. Respir. Physiol. 17:81.

101. Meyer, M., Worth, H., and Scheid, P. (1976). Gas-blood CO_2 equilibration in parabronchial lungs of birds. J. Appl. Physiol. 41:302.

102. Hughes, G. M., ed. (1976). Respiration in Amphibious Vertebrates, Academic Press, London.

International Review of Physiology
Respiratory Physiology II, Volume 14
Edited by John G. Widdicombe
Copyright 1977   University Park Press   Baltimore

8
Control of Breathing in Diseases of the Respiratory System

F. PALEČEK

Institute of Pathophysiology, Faculty of Pediatrics, Charles University,
Praha, Czechoslovakia

BASIC FUNCTIONS OF BREATHING   257
    Coupling of Respiratory Functions   257
    Uncoupling of Central Motoneuron
        Output and Lung Movements   258

FEEDBACKS   258
    Methods of Studying Control Mechanisms in Respiratory Physiology   259
    Thoracoabdominal Feedback   259
    Pulmonary Feedback   260
    Chemical Feedback   261
        Tube Breathing   261
        Ventilatory Response to Carbon Dioxide   263
        Uncoupling of Minute and Alveolar Ventilation
        by Changes of Physiological Dead Space   265

BASIC PATHOPHYSIOLOGICAL MECHANISMS OF RESPIRATORY
INSUFFICIENCY WITH REGARD TO ARTERIAL P_{O_2} AND P_{CO_2}
    265
    Hypoxic Hypoxia Compared to
        Arterial Hypoxemia in Respiratory Insufficiency   266
    Carbon Dioxide Inhalation Compared to
        Arterial Hypercapnia in Respiratory Insufficiency   267

INCREASED FUNCTIONAL RESIDUAL CAPACITY   268
    Mechanics of Increased Functional Residual Capacity   268
    Control of Functional Residual Capacity   270
    Consequences   270
    Increased Functional Residual Capacity in
        Some Naturally Occurring and Modeled Lung Diseases   271

"NEW INPUTS"   271

FEEDBACK RELATIONSHIPS   272
   Thoracoabdominal and Pulmonary Feedback   272
     Resistance to Breathing   273
   Pulmonary and Chemical Feedback   274
     Hypoventilation Syndrome   275

CONCLUSIONS   277

From the vast amount of information available on the control of breathing, a short review of that which is relevant to the basic differences in the control of breathing between healthy and diseased organisms is presented. The diseases will be limited to those of the respiratory system. The physiological part is meant only to point out information that seems important for understanding the differences in disease and to define several terms to be used later. Of the recent reviews of closely related subjects, special attention should be paid to references 1–10.

Even in spacious handbooks on respiration, the information on the control of breathing in lung disease is relatively meager, compared with the wealth of information on the control of breathing in healthy lungs and on pulmonary function in disease. It seems that most workers in the field accept the attitude of a prominent respiratory physiologist: "Physiologists cannot expect the pathophysiologists to interpret measurements of the pathological until we have provided a quantitative framework of normality for reference" (11).

Therefore, among the objectives of this review is an attempt to discuss the following questions:

1. Is the control of breathing in lung disease different from that in health?
2. If so, what are the basic differences?
3. What are the trends of research?

Generally, there are two basic ways in which the control of breathing in disease may differ from that in health:

A. An impaired function of the effector may be found at the beginning of most disturbances, and the control system adjusts for the changed function. These instances have been thoroughly studied by clinicians; the conditions have been defined morphologically and functionally. Our concern is, how is the system adjusted when a part of it is failing?
B. Occasionally the respiratory system does not function properly, although the state of the effector does not seem to explain the whole condition. Then it may be inferred that there is a failure in the control system itself. As an example, chronic hypoventilation may be due to an inefficiency of the effector (12); but at other times, "hyposensitivity of the respiratory center"

or inefficiency of the chemoreceptor system is possible (13, 14). In such a case, the defect can be qualified as primarily that of the control system.

BASIC FUNCTIONS OF BREATHING

Breathing in man serves three basic functions:

1. Gas exchange—oxygen intake and carbon dioxide output—is the vital function. This function is maintained by the respiratory system in close coordination with the cardiovascular and blood systems.
2. Breathing is adjusted to other vegetative nonrespiratory functions of the body and is modified by them. Typical examples are body position, swallowing, vomiting, and reflexes from the airways, but there are also thermoregulation, circulation, etc.
3. Breathing subserves the functions of higher nervous activity when speaking, singing, and performing other voluntary actions that make use of the respiratory system (blowing musical instruments, etc.).

Obviously, the control systems of all three functional sets are interwoven, and their separation would be highly artificial (15). However, this review discusses primarily the control mechanisms from the point of the vital gas exchange function.

Coupling of Respiratory Functions

In physiological conditions, there is a tight mechanical coupling of chest and lung movements. Therefore, inadequate performance of the respiratory muscles will be sensed not only by the receptors of the chest wall, but also by pulmonary, especially stretch, receptors. Similarly, increased resistance of the lungs and airways (elastic and/or flow resistance) is sensed both by the lung receptors (as inadequate stretch) and by the receptors of the chest wall (as increased resistance to contraction).

Normally, increased contractions of the respiratory muscles are followed closely by increased volume changes of the chest cavity, including the lungs. A given degree of muscle work is linked to a defined degree of lung ventilation. With increased resistance to breathing, there is a discrepancy between the afferent inputs from the chest and pulmonary receptors: for a given amount of muscular work the chest and lung movements are less. The pertinent question is, can respiratory muscles sense the degree of work they are performing or the change of loading? "Loaded breathing" has been the subject of a recent symposium (16).

Similarly, just as there is a mechanical link between chest and lung movements, diffusion of oxygen and carbon dioxide links alveolar ventilation to lung perfusion. More or less complete uncoupling may occur in diffusion disturbances in the so-called "alveolar capillary block." Much more often, however, the regional quantitative mismatch of ventilation to perfusion is found. Ventilation-perfusion inequalities are actually regarded as the most common disorder of lung diseases (17). Local disturbances of surfactant production also seem to participate in various diseases of the lungs (18).

Uncoupling of Central Motoneuron Output and Lung Movements

Even in normal conditions, there is a difference between the central nervous and the peripheral patterns of breathing. The duration of inspiration monitored by respiratory motoneuron output is regularly longer than the corresponding chest movement or air flow (19). In complete muscular paralysis, the chest and lung movements typically are independent of the central motoneuron output, unless the ventilator is driven by modified phrenic potentials (20). In another situation, there may be no chest and lung movements at all, as in cardiopulmonary bypass.

It was shown in dogs (21) and in man (22) that ventilation may be adequate after partial curarization. It became insufficient, however, when the demands on ventilation were increased by added dead space, increased airway resistance, or a combination of both (21).

Another classic example of uncoupling is pneumothorax. In certain conditions, as in anesthetized dogs, pneumothorax may result in actual hyperventilation, as manifested by the decreasing values of arterial P_{CO_2} (23).

It seems justified that all situations of impaired transformation of the central breathing pattern into the corresponding lung movements be considered under this heading. The causes may lie in muscular diseases, chest deformities, increased lung stiffness, or lung resistance, etc.

FEEDBACKS

A negative feedback is regarded as a basic feature of any control system aiming at homeostasis (24). At the moment, three feedbacks can be identified in the respiratory control system: 1) the thoracoabdominal feedback, comprising afferentation from respiratory muscles and costovertebral joints; 2) the pulmonary feedback (or vagal and sympathetic feedback), including afferentation from pulmonary receptors; 3) the chemical feedback, including afferentation from peripheral and central chemoreceptors.

The thoracoabdominal feedback carries information about the action of respiratory muscles and of the movements of the thoracic cage. As the respiratory muscles serve simultaneously for breathing and for postural and other reflexes, only a part of the afferentation is relevant to breathing.

The pulmonary feedback corresponds functionally to minute ventilation. It carries information about lung volume and of the volume change with time.

With regard to the vital (gas exchange) function of breathing, the chemical feedback is most relevant. It carries information about the overall function of the respiratory system, i.e., of the adequacy of gas exchange. The corresponding respiratory functions are alveolar ventilation, gas diffusion, and regional ventilation-perfusion ratios.

The three feedback circuits provide complementary afferent inputs concerning the act of breathing. Under physiological conditions, all the inputs are in accord: the respiratory center output is realized in respiratory muscle contractions (thoracoabdominal feedback) which result in lung expansion (pulmonary feedback). The adequacy of the resulting gas exchange is monitored by the chemical feedback. In pathological conditions, however, the inputs from the three feedbacks may be different and the question of their relative importance becomes actual.

Methods of Studying Control Mechanisms in Respiratory Physiology

To open a feedback loop, the following approaches have been made: vagotomy, dorsal rhizotomy (25, 26), differential vagal blockade by cold (27–29) or direct current (30, 31), and complete vagal blockade by local anesthesia (32); section of spinal ascending paths (33, 34); attempts at selective destruction or blockade of the pulmonary stretch receptors by steam (35), dodecylnonaethylenoxiaether (36), oxyphenonium (37) and bupivacain (38, 39); recently, the blocking action of sulfur dioxide on the pulmonary stretch receptors (40); and functional blockade of the stretch receptors which is assumed to take place when reflex inhibition of breathing due to lung inflation is prevented by tracheal occlusion at the functional residual capacity (FRC) level (41).

Analyses of the discharge pattern in single vagal fibers (42) (see review 43), lung sympathetic fibers (44, 45), or afferent fibers from peripheral chemoreceptors (46–51) have provided a quantitative basis for the stimulus-discharge relationship.

Changing the chemical input in a defined way has become a classic method for studying the chemical feedback (52) (see reviews 1, 2).

Stimulation of lung receptors has been used (see review 43) or of vagal (see review 53) or carotid body afferents (54, 55).

Mathematical modeling of control processes of the respiratory system has developed as a separate discipline (24, 56–70).

Thoracoabdominal Feedback

Extensive reviews of the proprioceptive afferents in control of respiratory muscles, mainly at the spinal level, have been given by von Euler (71, 72) and Newsom Davis (73). The respiratory muscles also serve a postural function, and the role of their proprioceptive afferentation in the regulation of eupneic breathing in man has been questioned (74). However, indications of supraspinal projections of intercostal muscle afferents, mainly from the midthoracic region, have been further elaborated (75, 76). The intercostal-to-diaphragm inhibitory reflex is mediated by spinal tracts, located superficially in the lateral areas of the cervical spinal cord (34). The localization and function of these connections seem to be similar to those described by Krieger et al. (33). The effect of the midthoracic intercostal muscle afferents on respiratory rhythm has been analyzed (77).

In summary, two types of intercostal-to-phrenic reflexes have been established: a mainly facilitatory reflex originating from caudal thoracic structures and mediated by spinal structures (references in 72) and an inhibitory reflex, originating from midthoracic intercostal muscles and having a supraspinal projection (78). The latter reflex was manifested by external elastic loading in human subjects as an increase of the rate of breathing combined with decreased tidal volumes; in dogs an analogous effect was demonstrated, present also after vagotomy (75). In rabbits, a shortening of the expiratory phase as the result of lung volume increase became obvious only after vagotomy; with intrapulmonary pressure decrease the vagal and intercostal reflexes went in the same direction (76). The progressive increase of inspiratory efforts with elastic or resistive inspiratory loading depended on the increasing chemical drive (79, 80).

The abdominal expiratory muscles are under reflex control both at the spinal segmental level and by supraspinal afferents (81) and through a vagal reflex (82, 83). Their expiratory activity is uninfluenced by chemical drive in the absence of vagal feedback (84).

Pulmonary Feedback

The pulmonary feedback is mainly represented by pulmonary vagal afferents. The significance of pulmonary sympathetic centripetal fibers is not clear (44, 45).

The role of vagal control of breathing has been reassessed several times in recent years (53, 85). Because of detailed neurophysiological studies, knowledge about pulmonary receptors and their representation in vagal afferent fibers is continuously increasing (86). However, the results are far from complete enough to understand the whole functional significance of the pulmonary feedback.

Relatively most studied and therefore most obvious is the function of pulmonary stretch receptors. They have been identified morphologically (3, 87), and their topography has been determined by pharmacological (88) and mechanical (89–91) methods. It seems indisputable that the relevant information concerns lung volume, both static (equivalent to functional residual capacity, FRC) and dynamic (equivalent to tidal volume), and its changes both in magnitude and in speed (43, 92). The sensitivity of the system to FRC changes is extraordinary (93), although normally obscured by the phasic influences. The effect of vagal afferentation on tidal volume has been studied by "functional vagotomy," i.e., by tracheal occlusion at different lung volumes (94). The method indicated that the share of tonic vagal afferentation in regulating the pattern of breathing is true not only in the highly artificial conditions of extrapulmonary oxygenation (93), but also in intact, conscious dogs (95).

With maintained inflation, the amount of vagal inhibition of inspiration decreases (96). The decrease of inhibition has been ascribed to changes in blood gas composition (97, 98); excluding the blood gas changes, there are still two factors responsible—adaptation of the stretch receptors and changes in the central nervous complex (99).

The patterns of firing of stretch receptors are probably different in various species. The most common type in the dog, cat, and rabbit is the inflation-activated stretch receptor. In the rabbit, however, there is a significant proportion of deflation-activated stretch receptors (100). It is likely that the rat is, in this respect, similar to the rabbit (101).

Information on the subepithelial irritant receptors and alveolar type J receptors has been summarized (10, 86). In the dog, the irritant receptors have been localized (102); their functional properties, however, have been questioned (103).

The functional identification of airway receptors has been reviewed (104). The significance of the irritant, type J, and airway receptors in the control of breathing is not clear, although it seems likely that they are activated especially in pathological conditions.

Chemical Feedback

Chemical feedback has been frequently studied, and some excellent reviews are available (1, 2, 105–108). Therefore, many comments on its physiological role are omitted here.

Tube Breathing To check the hypothesis of the importance of carbon dioxide oscillations on the peripheral chemoreceptors, several unsuccessful (109, 110) and some successful (111–113) experiments have been performed (see review (1)). Among the successful approaches was the so-called "tube breathing." Tube breathing means breathing through an additional dead space of a fixed volume.

To discuss the control mechanisms involved in adjustment to tube breathing, it is convenient to use the respiratory hyperbola for graphical demonstration (Figure 1). (The respiratory hyperbola is identical with "ventilation lines" (114), "hyperbola" (110), "ventilatory hyperbola" (115), and "metabolic hyperbola" (2).) In Figure 1 the respiratory hyperbola is presented on the left (*A*) as a straight line, due to the logarithmic scale on both axes. On the right (*B*), it is redrawn as the typical hyperbola in conventional coordinates. (All control values are marked by symbols O.) The effective alveolar ventilation (*point A*) is determined by arterial P_{CO_2} (*point a*) and the point of intersection (*point B*) on the hyperbola. Minute ventilation (*E*) determines another point of intersection (*C*) on the hyperbola with the corresponding P_{CO_2} on the abscissa. The difference between *points A* and *B* on the ordinate corresponds to the physiological dead space ventilation. ("Physiological dead space" is used in the sense as defined by Bouhuys (116). However, terms such as "total dead space" (117) or "effective dead space" might be preferred.) All values immediately after switching to tube breathing are marked by symbols 1. Adding the extra dead space is shown on the ordinate ($+V_D$). Alveolar ventilation moves vertically and determines a new hyperbola, corresponding to the decreased carbon dioxide output (*thin line*). Minute ventilation moves horizontally toward the new hyperbola. All response values of the control system are marked by symbols 2. To

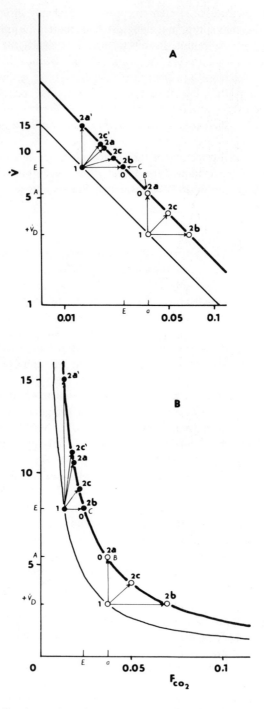

Figure 1. Respiratory hyperbola and tube breathing. For description see text.

provide carbon dioxide output corresponding to carbon dioxide production (assumed to be unchanged), ventilation has to move back toward the original hyperbola. This adjustment can follow one of three usual courses. Adjustment to position *2a* would be ideal, maintaining isocapnia–"isocapnic response." Position *2b* would provide the original carbon dioxide output without any ventilatory adjustment–"isoventilatory response." The typical response, *2c,* is mixed, aiming at somewhere between *2a* and *2b*. It is noteworthy that minute ventilation can assume several values to any of the alveolar ventilation responses, depending on the pattern of breathing, i.e., on the combination of tidal volume and frequency of breathing for a given value of minute ventilation. The mechanisms controlling the pattern of breathing have been thoroughly studied in recent years (118–121) (see reviews 1 and 10). Special attention has been paid to the control of expiration by laryngeal resistance (119, 122–126).

The isoventilatory response presumes no change in ventilation. In the mixed and isocapnic responses, subindices *a* and *c* mark the values of minute ventilation when its increase is achieved solely by an increase of tidal volume. The subindices *a'* and *c'* denote values when the increase is solely due to the increase of breathing frequency. The real values would lie somewhere in between (assuming that at least one of the variables is increasing).

The ventilatory response to tube breathing is caused by a combination of hypoxic and hypercapnic drives, which can, however, be fully compensated by increased ventilation. In healthy human subjects, the response to tube breathing air is typically such that the arterial P_{O_2} is unchanged from its control values (127). When desirable, the original hypoxic drive can be removed by breathing high oxygen mixtures through the tube.

Ventilatory Response to Carbon Dioxide The isocapnic ventilatory response to increased carbon dioxide load has been observed in healthy man and in animals during physical exercise (see review 128) or in drug-induced increases of metabolic carbon dioxide production (129, 130). Oxygen consumption, increased 2–3 times and induced by sciatic nerve stimulation in cats and dogs, was isocapnic before and after spinal cord transsection (131). Also in patients with increased resting oxygen consumption due to skeletal muscle mitochondrial disorder (Luft's syndrome), the ventilation is maintained isocapnically (arterial P_{CO_2} = 37.8 Torr) at a higher level (132). Attempts to mimic increased carbon dioxide production by intravenous injections of carbon dioxide-loaded blood resulted in an isocapnic (113, 133) or a mixed (134, 135) ventilatory response.

Tube breathing through a dead space of 1.4 liters by healthy adult males gave a mixed ventilatory response (an increase of 7.4 Torr end-expiratory P_{CO_2} after 10 min of tube breathing) in 10 subjects (111). In two other subjects, however, when arterial P_{CO_2} was also measured, the increase of ventilation during tube breathing was almost isocapnic. An isocapnic response with tube breathing (volume 200 ml) was also observed in 12 tracheotomized, unconscious patients with major brain injuries (136).

A mixed response with tube breathing (in adult healthy subjects, tube volume 1.4 liters) was obtained by Goode et al. (112). The exact increase of

P_{CO_2} during tube breathing was not given, as end-tidal P_{CO_2} was artificially adjusted; the authors estimate the difference from ventilation-carbon dioxide lines to have been about 5–9 Torr. Fenner et al. (127) added increasing volumes of dead space from 145 to 445 ml to children (age 4–12 years), which amounted to approximately one-third to 4-fold of the resting tidal volume. The ventilatory response was mixed, the increase of end-tidal P_{CO_2} being directly proportional to the volume of dead space added. Dead space was also added to six healthy human subjects at three levels of physical exercise to study their patterns of breathing; carbon dioxide response curves were not constructed, however (137).

It is well to remember that the end-tidal P_{CO_2} values need not be identical with arterial P_{CO_2}. One can imagine that if alveolar dead space is present and decreases during tube breathing, then end-tidal P_{CO_2} will go up although arterial P_{CO_2} may remain at the same level.

Interesting results on chronic tube breathing of conscious dogs have been obtained by Barnett et al. (138). The tube volume was 5 to over 30 ml/kg of body weight (50–500 ml) and was added to a tracheostomy tube. Control arterial P_{CO_2} values were obtained with 5 ml/kg or less added dead space (corresponding approximately to the normal dead space bypassed). Addition of 5–20 ml/kg led to an isocapnic increase of ventilation for a time period up to 48 hr. Larger added dead space volumes (20–30 ml/kg) increased arterial P_{CO_2} by about 7 Torr within 24 hr. However, even the smaller dead spaces (5–20 ml/kg) increased arterial P_{CO_2} to the same extent, when left over 48 hr. The authors do not exclude the possible influence of increased flow resistance due to mucus accumulation with the prolonged tube breathing.

It seems that carbon dioxide inhalation, even in small concentrations, leads in healthy subjects to a mixed rather than an isocapnic response. Dejours et al. (139) deduced theoretically that with low carbon dioxide concentrations in inhaled air the changes of alveolar P_{CO_2} and alveolar ventilation would hardly exceed the error of measurement. They observed in three out of four healthy subjects increases of end-tidal P_{CO_2} of 1.2, 1.0, and 2.0 Torr when breathing 1% carbon dioxide in air; in the fourth subject the value was not significantly different from the control. Similar results are evident in Lambertsen's experiments (140), in which inhalations of 2% carbon dioxide—in spite of individual variability—resulted in a clear increase of alveolar P_{CO_2} (about 3 Torr). Even more convincing may be the experiments of Schaefer (141), who exposed 21 healthy men to 1.5% carbon dioxide over a period of 42 days. There was a significant increase of alveolar P_{CO_2} over the whole period; it seems that a significant increase occurred on the first measurement (presumably on the first day of exposure), although the maximum (about 4 Torr elevation) was observed after approximately 3 weeks. The author also mentions a significant difference between alveolar and arterial P_{CO_2} during the exposure, meaning that arterial P_{CO_2} must have increased even more.

An isoventilatory response to carbon dioxide inhalation is seen in bilaterally acutely phrenecotomized rabbits (142). An isoventilatory increase of arterial

P_{CO_2} (4.7 Torr on the average) was also observed in four cats 20 min after a meal (143). Their ventilatory response curves to carbon dioxide inhalation had similar slopes, however, before and after the meal. The supraspinal effects of splanchnic A δ_2 fibers may be taken into consideration (144).

Uncoupling of Minute and Alveolar Ventilation by Changes of Physiological Dead Space   The most physiological test of the control of breathing would seem to be an increase of the physiological dead space, obtained by having the subject change his body position from supine to erect. There are ample data on the concomitant changes of lung volumes and ventilation-perfusion ratios in this maneuver (see reviews 145–147). It would be interesting to know the corresponding data on arterial blood gas tensions and ventilation. Among the eight subjects of Riley et al. (148), in every instance their minute ventilation was higher when standing than when lying down, as was their physiological dead space. Moreover, in spite of the varying carbon dioxide output with posture, arterial P_{CO_2} was lower when standing (see also 149). Thus, it appears that another input apart from the chemical feedback was at work. These were all healthy subjects with the exception of one with pulmonary stenosis. It was also shown in healthy subjects that the ventilatory response to carbon dioxide rebreathing is independent of body position (150).

On the other hand, changes in the physiological dead space may be one of the factors responsible for differences in the ventilatory response to carbon dioxide. The most common construction of a carbon dioxide response curve correlates arterial P_{CO_2} with minute ventilation. Changes in the physiological dead space will influence the slope of the carbon dioxide response curve, but are seldom measured. The changes in the physiological dead space during carbon dioxide rebreathing were observed in control rats (151). It can be assumed that with ventilation-perfusion inequalities such changes might be even more pronounced (152).

The regulatory mechanisms in lung diseases characterized by increased physiological dead space may be assumed to be similar to those in tube breathing (see Figure 1).

BASIC PATHOPHYSIOLOGICAL MECHANISMS OF RESPIRATORY INSUFFICIENCY WITH REGARD TO ARTERIAL P_{O_2} AND P_{CO_2}

As mentioned in the opening paragraphs, this review does not attempt to discuss functional disorders and their classification. However, a brief and highly schematic summary is given with regard to the function of the chemical feedback in lung disease.

There is a relatively uniform pattern of blood gas levels in a variety of lung diseases. The most advanced disturbance is characterized by arterial hypoxemia and hypercapnia. This situation is defined as respiratory failure or respiratory insufficiency. According to the speed of development, it may be acute or chronic, although an episode of acute respiratory failure superimposed on a chronic one is not uncommon. In a less advanced stage or better compensated situation, arterial hypoxemia alone may be seen. An indication of the qualitative changes is given in Table 1. For details see references 146 and 153.

Thus, all situations of respiratory insufficiency are characterized by arterial hypoxemia; some of them, in the more advanced stages, also exhibit hypercapnia.

To study respiratory insufficiency, it seems important to consider the possible differences inherent in some methods used to produce hypoxia and/or hypercapnia compared to the situations occurring in naturally existing respiratory insufficiency.

Hypoxic Hypoxia Compared to Arterial Hypoxemia in Respiratory Insufficiency

The inhalation of air at low ambient pressures or of mixtures with low oxygen content is commonly used to study the effects of hypoxic hypoxia on the organism. In respiratory insufficiency, arterial hypoxemia is the consequence of a disturbance of ventilation, diffusion, or ventilation-perfusion inequalities. Severe hypoxemia can also be seen in some congenital heart malformations.

With regard to arterial chemoreceptors, the hypoxic stimuli are identical when breathing air with a low partial pressure of oxygen and when the low arterial P_{O_2} is the result of pulmonary disease or right-to-left shunt in a heart disease. What are the theoretically possible differences with regard to the control of breathing between both types of hypoxia?

1. Air with low P_{O_2} could stimulate structures in the airways or lungs or sensitize them to other stimuli (e.g., carbon dioxide).
2. One mechanism, at least, has been described which is sensitive primarily to alveolar hypoxia: the constriction of pulmonary vessels. In lung disease, alveolar hypoxia is much less generalized than with low oxygen breathing. Also pul-

Table 1. Blood gas changes in some respiratory disturbances

Condition	Uncompensated		Compensated	
	$P_{aO_2}{}^a$	P_{aCO_2}	P_{aO_2}	P_{aCO_2}
Hypoventilation	↓	↑	N	N
Impaired diffusion	↓	N	N	↓
			↓	N
$\dot{V}/\dot{Q}$ inequalities	↓	N	N	↓
Regional increased $\dot{V}/\dot{Q}$	↓	↑	↓	N
(alveolar dead space)			N	N
Regional decreased $\dot{V}/\dot{Q}$	↓	(↑)	↓	↓
(venous admixture)			↓	N

Based on data from Comroe et al. (117) and Cherniack et al. (153).

$^a P_{aO_2}$, arterial P_{O_2}; P_{aCO_2}, arterial P_{CO_2}; $\dot{V}/\dot{Q}$, ventilation-perfusion ration; ↑ increased value; ↓, decreased value; N, normal value.

monary hypertension occurs in high altitude as a rule, but only in a proportion of hypoxic patients with chronic lung disease.

3. The pulmonary stretch receptors have been described as insensitive to hypoxia (42). Only recently their sensitivity toward carbon dioxide has been re-examined and established (154–156). Any analysis of P_{O_2}-P_{CO_2} relationships on the stretch receptor is still missing.

4. There is no evidence of a possible sensitivity of irritant and type J receptors to hypoxia or hypoxia-carbon dioxide interaction.

5. When breathing air with low P_{O_2}, the alveolo-venous gradient for oxygen is decreased. This effect tends to decrease the oscillations of P_{O_2} in arterial blood.

6. Breathing hypoxic mixtures is accompanied by hypocapnia in healthy subjects; patients with respiratory insufficiency typically have normo- or hypercapnia.

Carbon Dioxide Inhalation Compared to
Arterial Hypercapnia in Respiratory Insufficiency

The conventional methods used to increase P_{CO_2} when testing the ventilatory response to carbon dioxide use the inhalation of mixtures with fixed carbon dioxide concentrations or rebreathing from a closed system. Both methods can be performed in hyper-, normo-, or hypoxia.

It was pointed out by Fenn and Craig (110) that such methods do not allow the control system of the organism to maintain isocapnia easily with lower cencentrations of inhaled carbon dioxide and not at all with higher concentrations.

There are several points of theoretical difference between carbon dioxide retention or increased carbon dioxide production and carbon dioxide inhalation:

1. Normally—and also during increased carbon dioxide production—the carbon dioxide concentration in the airways during inspiration is negligible. This fact is especially interesting in view of the recent observations on the possible existence of carbon dioxide-sensitive structures in the lungs or airways (157) and on the carbon dioxide sensitivity of the pulmonary stretch receptors (154–156).

2. When the venous load of carbon dioxide increases as the result of carbon dioxide retention or increased carbon dioxide production, and when tidal volume increases as the result of stimulation of breathing, the P_{CO_2} oscillations in arterial blood will normally increase; this is not true for carbon dioxide inhalation.

3. Normally, the arterial P_{CO_2} is regulated within rather narrow limits. Carbon dioxide inhalations, especially in higher concentrations, establish, therefore, a breakdown of the control system. (Fenn and Craig (110) suggested the term of carbon dioxide "tolerance" rather than "sensitivity" curve.)

4. Increased carbon dioxide production is usually accompanied by an increased cardiac output (158).

5. In lung disease, hypercapnia of any degree is matched by a correlated degree

of hypoxemia. Although hypoxia can be produced at will together with inhaling carbon dioxide mixtures, the changes in gas tensions will rarely resemble those in the natural conditions.

It thus seems that adding an extra dead space (see under "Ventilatory Response to Carbon Dioxide") will best simulate the situation of respiratory insufficiency (in which alveolar dead space often is actually present).

INCREASED FUNCTIONAL RESIDUAL CAPACITY

Mechanics of Increased Functional Residual Capacity

FRC is the volume of air contained in the lungs at the end of a spontaneous expiration (159). We speak, therefore, of an increased FRC when the volume of lungs at end expiration exceeds that in the control period or that in comparable subjects under control conditions.

Under physiological conditions, the end-expiratory volume is realized under good muscular relaxation. Otherwise, the following inspiration starts "from a more or less relaxed state at end expiration, i.e., from the FRC" (159). In this chapter, when speaking of the FRC, the end-expiratory volume is meant, including the possibility of incomplete muscular relaxation.

There are two basic mechanisms leading to an increased FRC (Figure 2): dynamic and static.

Dynamic increase of FRC implies the presence of the dynamic component, i.e., lung ventilation. The increase of FRC depends on the act of air filling and

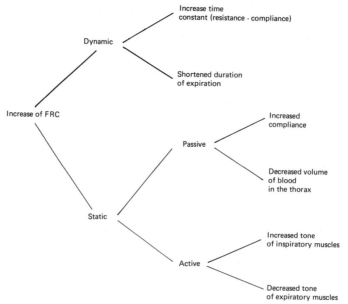

Figure 2. Mechanics of increased functional residual capacity.

leaving the lungs and occurs only when ventilation goes on. In a paralyzed subject during an apneic period, therefore, normalization of a dynamically increased FRC would be expected.

The concept of a dynamic increase of FRC assumes a disproportion between the time available for expiration and the forces responsible for expiration. The frequency of breathing is thus the first determinant; with slow frequencies, the dynamically increased FRC would be expected to be smaller.

Under physiological conditions, there is a neat balance between the forces providing for expiration and lung resistance opposing the air flow. Increased lung resistance, *ceteris paribus*, slows expiratory air flow, resulting in a greater lung volume for the next inspiration, until the expiratory forces balance the resistance within the time available. Lung resistance can be divided into several components of which only some are under clear control (Figure 3).

Static increase of FRC implies that the increase of FRC can be observed also in static conditions, i.e., independent of ventilation and the balance of expiratory forces and lung resistance.

Static increase of FRC can be accomplished passively or actively. Passive increase can be due to increased specific lung compliance. Decrease of elastic lung recoil tends to adjust the resting point of equilibrium between the elasticity of lungs and thorax toward higher volumes, approaching the resting volume of the thorax (160). A decrease of FRC, together with a decrease of lung compliance, was described for human subjects during general anesthesia (161).

The blood present in the lungs may have a 2-fold effect on FRC. Lung congestion decreases lung compliance (162) and, at the same time, competes for the intrathoracic volume otherwise occupied by air. In this way an increase of FRC might be expected after withdrawal of part of the blood from the thoracic cage (163, 164).

The active static increase of FRC is the result of the resting tone of respiratory muscles. Increase of resting inspiratory muscle tone or decrease of expiratory muscle tone or both may be the cause of increased FRC. Such an

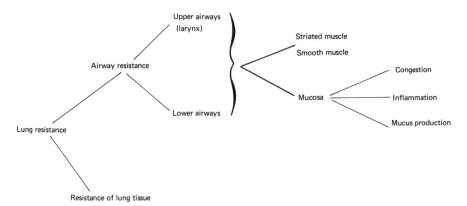

Figure 3. Diagram of factors constituting and influencing lung resistance.

increase of tonic activity in intercostals has been shown, e.g., in chronic obstructive lung disease (165).

Control of Functional Residual Capacity

Increased FRC would be sensed primarily by the pulmonary stretch receptors. When long lasting, adaptation is likely to occur. Adaptation of stretch receptors had been demonstrated with lung inflations (96, 99) and also with increased FRC. To increase FRC experimentally, an "expiratory threshold load" can be used, i.e., submerging the expiratory outflow line in a defined column of water (83, 166). It has been shown that with the expiratory threshold load abdominal expiratory muscles are activated, depending on the integrity of the vagus nerves (83). Adaptation of pulmonary stretch receptors may be responsible for the fact that the duration of inspiration depends only on lung volume changes above end-expiratory level and is independent of the absolute end-expiratory volume. There is, however, another vagal mechanism affecting the duration of expiration that may be functionally inoperative at the control level of FRC and prolongs expiration with increased FRC (93, 166).

It seems to be established today that hypoxia increases FRC via peripheral chemoreceptors (167), whereas the possible role of P_{CO_2} is doubtful.

Pronounced changes in FRC due to changed body position must not be neglected (145).

Consequences

Although increased FRC by itself does not directly affect gas exchange, there are several ways in which it can modify it.

1. With FRC increased by positive pressure breathing (168, 169) or by expiratory threshold loading (83, 170, 171), a decreased ventilatory response to carbon dioxide has been observed.
2. The buffering effect of increased volume of alveolar air tends to decrease the sensitivity of the chemical feedback by damping the oscillations of P_{O_2} and P_{CO_2} in arterial blood.
3. The diffusion area is increased with increased FRC. It was speculated that in hypoxia an increased diffusion area would tend to maintain a higher level of carbon dioxide in the organism, because less alveolar ventilation would be needed for the same amount of oxygen intake, and thus the hypoxic hypocapnia from hyperventilation would be reduced (172).
4. With very high FRC, the pressure-volume curve is shifted toward lower lung compliance. This effect may help to counteract a loss of elasticity and maintain adequate expiration by passive means of elastic recoil of the lungs and thorax rather than by the action of expiratory muscles.
5. Distension of the lungs helps to maintain the small airways open during expiration and to increase the diameter of airways generally. This may be of special importance when increased airway resistance is the primary reason for increased FRC.

6. A linear relationship has been shown between the FRC and breathing frequency (in the absence of breathing movements), increased FRC leading to a slower rate of breathing due to prolongation of the expiratory time (93, 166).

Increased Functional Residual Capacity
in Some Naturally Occurring and Modeled Lung Diseases

Lung emphysema is a typical disease characterized by increased FRC (146). Apart from numerous, largely not very successful attempts to produce emphysema in animals (see review 173), in the last few years papain by aerosol or intrapulmonary injection (174–177) has been widely used. Although papain alone can produce emphysema, the changes become much more pronounced when papain administration is combined with artificially increased airway resistance (177). In rats of conventional breeding, the increase of FRC seems to precede pronounced morphological changes suggestive of emphysema (178). Thus, it can be proposed that an increase in FRC can eventually precede the occurrence of morphologically demonstrable emphysema.

Bronchial asthma is characterized by increased airway resistance. Increased FRC was found in the period between attacks (179); an acute increase in asthmatic children upon exercise could be reversed by bronchodilators (180).

There is no evidence for changes of FRC in bronchitis or pneumonia in man. However a significant increase of FRC was observed in experimental pneumonia in rats after intrapulmonary administration of carragheenin (181) or paraquat (182). The increased FRC decreased after bilateral cervical vagotomy.

Increased FRC is recognized as a clinical feature of lung silicosis, being usually ascribed to the concomitant emphysema (146). In animal experiments, increased FRC was among the prominent and early symptoms of the disease (183, 184).

It thus appears that an increase of FRC may represent a nonspecific reaction to various stimuli. Among them an important role may be ascribed to hypoxia. The decrease of pathologically increased FRC after vagotomy is more difficult to interpret: the slow rate of breathing, changes in lung resistance and/or compliance, and blood volume in the lungs may all indirectly influence the FRC as the result of vagotomy. A direct reflex action on FRC through the vagus nerves is still far from being established.

"NEW INPUTS"

Some lung diseases are accompanied by alveolar hyperventilation and corresponding arterial hypocapnia. When those that are likely to be due to severe hypoxemia are disregarded, there is still a group in which the causes of the changes in gas tensions can be classified as nervous (13).

The nervous inputs that increase ventilation may follow the regular pathways of thoracoabdominal and pulmonary feedbacks (185) as in health, or they may constitute "new inputs" from pulmonary and other receptors, which are not thought to participate in the control of breathing in healthy man at rest. Some pulmonary receptors, namely the irritant and type J receptors, may thus be considered as the source of "new inputs" as opposed to the "regular" feedback inputs.

Clinically, a changed pattern of breathing has been well known in conditions such as pneumonia, lung edema, pulmonary embolism, etc. The changes in the pattern of breathing in lung edema have been ascribed mainly to the stimulation of irritant receptors (186), after microembolism to the type J receptors (187); hyperventilation with pneumothorax (23) was mentioned earlier (see review 9). There are indications that the type J receptors may also be responsible for the major part of hyperventilation in experimental pneumonia of cats and rabbits (188) together with a weakened inflation reflex (189). Dependence of tachypnea due to lung inflammation on intact vagal conduction was further demonstrated in experimental pneumonia due to intrapulmonary injections of carragheenin (181) or paraquat (182) in rats.

The hyperventilation in human diffuse fibrosis of the lungs is not dependent upon hypoxic drive (190, 191). In experimental lung silicosis in rats, apart from tachypnea and increased FRC (183, 184), an increased breathing responsiveness to carbon dioxide has been described, which was present in hyperoxia (192).

In guinea pigs, inhalation of lung irritants and histamine-induced attacks of bronchial asthma are thought to produce hyperventilation by a reflex action, in which the irritant ("collapse") receptors participate (193–196). Similar results have been obtained in experimental asthma in dogs (197).

Occasionally, a distinction is made between "specific' and "nonspecific" inputs (198). Vagi, sinus nerves, and central chemosensitivity were called "specific" and essential for the effects of "nonspecific" inputs, such as noise, touch, and electrical stimulation of dorsal roots or femoral nerves on respiration (199). A reflex increase of ventilation after vibrations applied to the calf muscles of the cat has been described (200). Rhythmical stimuli applied to the femoral nerve in the dog or the carotid sinus nerve in the cat reduced tidal volume when applied in early inspiration, but decreased it when applied in late inspiration or early expiration. Respiratory rate generally increased in either mode of stimulation (201). In vagotomized rabbits, electrical stimulation of the sciatic nerve increased ventilation (202). It was also shown that in vagotomized rats strong rhythmical stimuli applied to the sciatic nerve produce effects similar to those from weak stimuli applied to the central stump of the cut vagus nerve (203). The effects on breathing of afferentation from abdominal viscera via the splanchnic nerves seem to be mainly subservient to functions other than respiratory (204).

FEEDBACK RELATIONSHIPS

Thoracoabdominal and Pulmonary Feedback

Von Euler and Fritts (25) evaluated the relative importance of vagal and thoracic feedbacks. They characterized the regulatory mechanism by its "gain," defined as change in the output per unit change of the input. For output units, they selected the intrapulmonary pressure developed by the inspiratory muscles during tracheal occlusion on various levels of lung volume. Lung volume served as the input. They found that sectioning the dorsal roots of vagotomized cats lowered the pressure changes produced by muscle contraction and, therefore, the α-motoneuron output was facilitated by impulses transmitted through the dorsal root fibers.

Vagotomy alone increased the pressures developed by the inspiratory muscles. Because this increase could be elicited with the dorsal roots sectioned, it seemingly did not depend chiefly on the external loop of γ-motoneurons and muscle spindle afferents. They concluded that the vagi exert an inhibitory influence on inspiratory muscle contraction and that the caudal dorsal root afferents facilitate the contraction. They also concluded that an inhibition of the stretch reflexes in the chest wall is maintained from supraspinal structures.

Gautier (26) presented results qualitatively similar. His experiments on rabbits included dorsal rhizotomy (from T 1–2 to T 12) combined with bilateral cervical vagotomy. The chest wall afferents had a facilitatory influence on tidal volume, slowing down the rate of breathing. The vagi inhibited the inspiratory discharge, decreasing tidal volume and inspiratory duration, and facilitated expiratory duration.

A species difference was observed in experiments on anesthetized and vagotomized dogs and cats. Dogs, like cats, have no extravagal mechanoreceptor information contributing to the control of respiratory frequency during external elastic loading. They do, however, respond to chest compression with an extravagally mediated reflex increase of respiratory frequency (205).

Apart from the dorsal ascending spinal paths, afferent information carried along ventrolateral ascending paths is important for the control of breathing. Transection of these pathways in decerebrated cats resulted in a smaller tidal volume without a change of the breathing rate (33). Carbon dioxide stimulation in this condition also did not change the rate of breathing, and the minute ventilation decreased. Additional vagotomy or midpontine transection changed breathing to an apneustic pattern (33).

Thus, acute elastic loading of the respiratory system is compensated by mechanisms which seem to involve a) intrinsic muscle properties, b) changes of the breathing frequency, and c) vagal feedback (206).

Resistance to Breathing   Work of breathing that increases out of proportion to the amount of oxygen delivered to the body may lead to fatigue of the respiratory muscles. Cherniack and Chodirker (207) deduced from observations on healthy subjects that an individual may breathe less and tolerate hypercapnia with high levels of the work of breathing, but he will tolerate increased work of breathing rather than become more hypoxic. According to mathematical model analysis, the respiratory muscles seem to follow the requirement of least energy expenditure (208–210). Only 50% of the 15-s maximum voluntary ventilation can be maintained "indefinitely" in man (211). The inability to sustain the 15-s maximum voluntary ventilation for longer periods is ascribed to the fatigue of respiratory muscles.

Thus, muscular fatigue exists although it is not well understood. For practical purposes, it may be characterized as an inability of the muscles to respond adequately to neural stimuli as the result of previous contractile activity. The development of fatigue may be influenced by an inadequate supply of substrate (212, 213), oxygen, inadequate circulation, and resting muscle length (214). Muscular fatigue is sensed and, therefore, neural afferents are also involved.

It has been known for a long time that addition of small resistances tends to decrease ventilation at the expense of an elevation of alveolar P_{CO_2} (215). This observation was confirmed by quantitative measurements for resistive and elastic loads and their effects on the ventilatory response to carbon dioxide (216–220) and hypoxia (221). These observations have been further developed into the concept of the ventilatory response to carbon dioxide as dependent on the work of breathing (see review 222). Increased airway resistance can be–at least in some cases–the reason for apneic periods in patients with the Pickwick syndrome (223).

With regard to the suggested opposing role of dorsal root afferents from respiratory muscles and the afferent pulmonary vagus on the pattern of breathing (26), it would be interesting to compare their interaction in the ventilatory response to carbon dioxide. The flattening of the ventilatory response curve to carbon dioxide after bilateral cervical vagotomy (or infiltration vagal anesthesia) is well known (224–229). From Gautier's work (26) on dorsal root rhizotomy (in rabbits), alone or combined with vagotomy, it seems that rhizotomy alone may have somewhat depressed the response to carbon dioxide in his experiments. On the other hand, in the same work, the responses to carbon dioxide after vagotomy and vagotomy combined with dorsal rhizotomy are practically indistinguishable from control responses.

Pulmonary and Chemical Feedback

In 1964 Widdicombe (43) found it difficult to draw a conclusion about the effects of vagal afferentation on the chemical control of breathing. He found among fifteen papers three indicating a decrease of alveolar ventilation, six indicating a stimulation, and six an inconsistent change after vagotomy. Since then, several authors have evaluated the ventilatory response to carbon dioxide and concluded unequivocally that with vagal afferentation blocked or the vagi cut, ventilation is less for a given increase of P_{CO_2} at higher levels of ventilation (224–229).

There are a few indications that the vagus nerves can transmit impulses which limit the breathing performance. The classic experiment in healthy man (226) showed an increased tolerance to high carbon dioxide concentrations and a lower ventilatory response after blocking the glossopharyngeal and vagus nerves. An indication that vagal afferentation may also have a limiting function on ventilation in lung disease is given by the clinical experience with vagal block in patients with various cardiopulmonary diseases; after the block, dyspnea and trachypnea (when present) mostly decreased, and some of the function tests improved (230, 231). A kind of objective measure is given in the experiments of Phillipson et al. (232) on conscious dogs with experimental pneumonitis. They showed that, in two out of the four dogs studied, exercise tolerance was increased after bilateral cervical vagal block (produced by local cooling). These observations may be likened to the experience from sport medicine, where local anesthesia and thus the removal of painful stimuli from a sprained joint enables the sportsman to go on with physical performance. To what extent this analogy may be true for at least a part of vagal afferentation is a matter of conjecture.

A detailed analysis of the phasic vagal feedback effects on the pattern of breathing was performed on paralyzed dogs with constant chemical feedback, due to cardiopulmonary bypass (233). A linear relationship was found between tidal volume and the inspiratory time; with the chemical feedback functioning, the relationship was curvilinear, resembling the Clark and von Euler (118) hyperbola in the cat.

Hypoventilation Syndrome   Cherniack in 1964 (222) enumerated the following possible reasons for chronic alveolar hypoventilation in patients with lung disease: 1) increased buffering capacity of blood and intracellular fluid; 2) decrease of the hypoxic drive with increasing ventilation; 3) disturbances of the mechanism of breathing; 4) the narcotic properties of carbon dioxide; 5) adaptation of the respiratory system to carbon dioxide. He added two other possibilities: a disproportionately great increase of oxygen consumption by the respiratory muscles with increasing ventilation and the size of the physiological dead space. Electromyographic evidence was used (234) to support the view that in patients with lung emphysema the carbon dioxide retention is due to inefficiency of the respiratory system and not to adaptation of the respiratory center.

Flenley et al. (235) showed that the decreased responsiveness to carbon dioxide in chronic obstructive lung disease cannot be accounted for by concomitant hypoxia or increased buffering capacity of the blood or of the cerebrospinal fluid (236). The possible significance of changes in the activity of carbonic anhydrase for the development of respiratory insufficiency was stressed (237).

It was also shown that the work of breathing correlates well with arterial P_{CO_2} and its increase during rebreathing, both in healthy subjects and in patients with chronic obstructive lung disease, with moderate carbon dioxide retention (arterial $P_{CO_2} \leqslant 55$ Torr) (238). On the other hand, such a correlation was not found in a group of eight patients, except for two with resting arterial P_{CO_2} values of 44 and 51 Torr. The rest of the patients, who all had a depression of the response to carbon dioxide in terms of the rate of total inspiratory work, must have had higher resting arterial P_{CO_2} values (239). The lower responsiveness to carbon dioxide of healthy subjects in unloaded breathing correlated well with the greater depression of breathing with flow-resistive loads (240).

In lung diseases that are accompanied by an increased FRC, the control of breathing may be affected by other two factors: increased FRC may lower the ventilatory response through vagal afferents; and, there may be an increased buffering capacity of the FRC with regard to the P_{CO_2}-pH-P_{O_2} oscillations. The interplay between increased FRC and decreased response to carbon dioxide is indicated by experiments on anesthetized dogs. Positive pressure breathing decreased the ventilatory response to carbon dioxide, the effect being dependent upon intact vagi (168). This observation was re-examined on anesthetized, paralyzed dogs with the use of the integrated phrenic output instead of ventilation (170). Qualitatively similar results were obtained. It was shown, however, that the effect of increased FRC is time-limited. In these experimental conditions, inflation with a pressure of 10 cm H_2O decreased the ventilatory response to carbon dioxide to 45% in 1 min, but to only 88% of the control value after 8 min. The ventilatory response to hypoxia was decreased similarly. There is no indication of whether the control level would be reached (as in analogous experiments with decreased FRC).

With regard to the buffering of P_{CO_2} oscillations by increased FRC, it is assumed that the peripheral chemoreceptor role is accentuated in hypoxia (1). In lung disease, hypoxemia is common; it may be causally related to the increased FRC (167, 241), and it may also make the role of peripheral chemoreceptors more important. It is interesting that, in rats with chronic surgical denervation of the sinocarotid region, in 4 weeks the function reappeared (242), presumably by activation of the aortic bodies.

The importance of the dead space concept was further elaborated by theoretical analyses (243, 244) and clinical observations (245). It was found that, during hyperventilation due to exercise or voluntarily induced, the physiological dead space-tidal volume ratio tended to increase, especially in patients who were unable to increase their carbon dioxide output significantly (12, 246). For some time now, patients with chronic obstructive disease have been divided by some clinicians into two basic groups: the emphysematic type and the bronchitic type (247). The patients of the bronchitic type have lower ventilatory responses to both increased P_{CO_2} and to exercise (248). The different responsiveness of patients with chronic obstructive lung disease can be shown for the pulmonary bed with regard to hypoxia and oxygen breathing (249). The "responsive" patients had a remarkable increase in the dead space-tidal volume ratio during oxygen breathing.

It follows that changed responsiveness to chemical stimuli in lung disease should be considered not only with regard to chemical feedback but also as the result of possible interaction with thoracoabdominal and/or pulmonary feedbacks.

There is an unceasing interest in breathing sensations and dyspnea (85, 250–254). In this connection, it is interesting to speculate on dyspnea as the cortical projection of discordance between respiratory feedbacks and/or new inputs.

CONCLUSIONS

1. The control of breathing in lung disease is different from that in health.

2. The basic differences include a) mismatch of afferent inputs through the different feedbacks, as the result of disturbed functions of breathing and uncoupling of respiratory functions, and b) the existence of new inputs.

3. The present trends of research seem to include a) the functions of respiratory feedbacks, b) the quantitative proportions of differing feedback inputs, and c) the relationship of new inputs to feedback control.

ACKNOWLEDGMENT

I am grateful to Mrs. E. Fialová for help in providing the bibliography.

REFERENCES

1. Cunningham, D. J. C. (1974). The control system regulating breathing in man. Q. Rev. Biophys. 6:433.
2. Cunningham, D. J. C. (1974). Integrative aspects of the regulation of breathing: a personal view. *In* A. C. Guyton and J. G. Widdicombe (eds.), MTP International Review of Science, Physiology Series I, Respiratory Physiology I, pp. 303–369. University Park Press, Baltimore.
3. Fillenz, M., and Widdicombe, J. G. (1972). Receptors of the lungs and airways. *In* E. Neil (ed.), Handbook of Sensory Physiology, Enteroceptors, pp. 81–112. Springer-Verlag, New York.
4. Guz, A. (1975). Regulation of respiration in man. Annu. Rev. Physiol. 37:303.
5. Karcsewski, W. A., and Widdicombe, J. G. (eds.) (1973). Neural Control of Breathing. Proceedings of International Symposium. Acta Neurobiol. Exp. No. 1, Vol. 33. Polish Scientific Publishers, Warsaw.
6. Karczewski, W. A. (1974). Organisation of the brain stem respiratory complex. *In* A. C. Guyton and J. G. Widdicombe (eds.), MTP International Review of Science, Physiology Series I, Respiratory Physiology I, pp. 197–219. University Park Press, Baltimore.
7. Mitchell, R. A., and Berger, A. J. (1975). Neural regulation of respiration. Am. Rev. Respir. Dis. 111:206.
8. Nizovtsev, V. P. (ed.). (1973). Giperkapniya-giperoksiya. (Kuibyshev: Kuibyshevskii Medicinskii Institut).
9. Paintal, A. S. (1973). Vagal sensory receptors and their reflex effects. Physiol. Rev. 53:159.
10. Widdicombe, J. G. (1974). Reflexes from the lungs in the control of breathing. *In* R. J. Linden (ed.), Recent Advances in Physiology, pp. 239–278. Churchill Livingston, London.
11. Cunningham, D. J. C. (1975). Can a particular breathing pattern influence development of respiratory insufficiency in man? Presented at the Second International Congress on Pathological Physiology, July 8–11, Praha.
12. Gilbert, R., Keighley, J., and Auchincloss, J. H. (1965). Mechanisms of chronic carbon dioxide retention in patients with obstructive pulmonary disease. Am. J. Med. 38:217.

278   Palaček

13. Auchincloss, J. H., Jr. (1964). Ventilatory disturbances in disease. *In* W. O. Fenn and H. Rahn (eds), Handbook of Physiology, Section 3, Respiration, Vol. II, pp. 1553—1563. American Physiology Society, Washington, D.C.
14. Senior, R. M., and Fishman, A. P. (1967). Disturbances of alveolar ventilation. Med. Clin. North Amer. 51:403.
15. Shick, L. (1975). Respiratory control and respiratory insufficiency. Presented at the Second International Congress on Pathological Physiology, July 8—11, Praha.
16. Pengelly, L. D., Rebuck, A. S., and Campbell, E. J. M. (eds.). (1974). Loaded Breathing. Proceedings of International Symposium on "The effects of mechanical loads on breathing." Longman Canada Limited, Ontario.
17. Bates, D. V., Anthonisen, N. R., Bass, H., Heckscher, T., and Oriol, A. (1968). Recent observations on the measurement of regional $\dot{V}/\dot{Q}$ ratios in chronic lung disease. *In* G. Cumming and L. B. Hunt (eds.), Form and Function in the Human Lung, pp. 125—134. E. & S. Livingston Ltd., London.
18. Bondarev, I. M., Agapov, Y. Y., Zhigalina, L. I., Boikov, A. K., and Volkova, N. V. (1975). Energetic and plastic metabolism and the lung surfactant system. Presented at the Second International Congress on Pathological Physiology, July 8—11, Praha.
19. Mead, J., and Agostoni, E. (1964). Dynamics of breathing. *In* W. O. Fenn and H. Rahn (eds.), Handbook of Physiology, Section 3, Respiration, Vol. I, pp. 411—427. American Physiology Society, Washington, D.C.
20. Huszczuk, A., and Widdicombe, J. G. (1973). Studies on central respiratory activity in artificially ventilated rabbits. Acta Neurobiol. Exp. 33:391.
21. Johansen, S. H., and Osgood, P. (1970). Ventilatory reserve in the dog during partial curarization. Anesthesiology 33:322.
22. Rigg, J. R. A., Engel, L. A., and Ritchie, B. C. (1970). The ventilatory response to carbon dioxide during partial paralysis with tubocurarine. Br. J. Anaesth. 42:105.
23. Kilburn, K. H. (1963). Cardiorespiratory effects of large pneumothorax in conscious and anesthetized dogs. J. Appl. Physiol. 18:279.
24. Defares, J. G. (1964). Principles of feedback control and their application to the respiratory control system. *In* W. O. Fenn and H. Rahn (eds.), Handbook of Physiology, Section 3, Respiration, Vol. I, pp. 649—680. American Physiology Society, Washington, D.C.
25. von Euler, C., and Fritts, H. W., Jr. (1963). Quantitative aspects of respiratory reflexes from the lungs and chest walls of cats. Acta Physiol. Scand. 57:284.
26. Gautier, H. (1973). Respiratory responses of the anesthetized rabbit to vagotomy and thoracic dorsal rhizotomy. Respir. Physiol. 17:238.
27. Fishman, N. H., Phillipson, E. A., and Nadel, J. A. (1973). Effect of differential vagal cold blockade on breathing pattern in conscious dogs. J. Appl. Physiol. 34:754.
28. Phillipson, E. A., Hickey, R. F., Bainton, C. R., and Nadel, J. A. (1970). Effect of vagal blockade on regulation of breathing in conscious dogs. J. Appl. Physiol. 29:475.
29. Phillipson, E. A., Fishman, N. H., Hickey, R. F., and Nadel, J. A. (1973). Effect of differential vagal blockade on ventilatory response to CO_2 in awake dogs. J. Appl. Physiol. 34:759.

30. Sassen, M., and Zimmermann, M. (1973). Differential blocking of myelinated nerve fibres by transient depolarization. Pfluegers Arch. 341:179.
31. Trenchard, D., and Widdicombe, J. G. (1973). Assessment of differential block to conduction by direct current applied to the cervical vagus nerve. Acta Neurobiol. Exp. 33:89.
32. Guz, A., Noble, M., Trenchard, D., Cochrane, H., and Makey, A. (1964). Studies on the vagus nerves in man: their role in respiratory and circulatory control. Clin. Sci. 27:293.
33. Krieger, A. J., Christensen, H. D., Sapru, H. N., and Wang, S. C. (1972). Changes in ventilatory patterns after ablation of various respiratory feedback mechanisms. J. Appl. Physiol. 33:431.
34. Remmers, E. J., and Tsiaras, W. G. (1973). Effect of lateral cervical cord lesions on the respiratory rhythm of anaesthetized, decerebrate cats after vagotomy. J. Physiol. (Lond.) 233:63.
35. Hainsworth, R., Jacobs, L., and Comroe, J. H. (1973). Afferent lung denervation by brief inhalation of steam. J. Appl. Physiol. 34:708.
36. Reichertz, P., and Zipf, H. F. (1957/58). Optische und akustische Darstellung einer zweimal hintereinander herbeigeführten totalen Endoanaesthesie der Lungenreceptoren. Arch. Exp. Pathol. Pharmacol. 232:367.
37. Fallert, M. (1972). Oxyphenonium als Methode zur selektiven afferenten Vagusblockierung in der Atmungsphysiologie. Pfluegers Arch. 333:182.
38. Dain, D. S., Boushey, H. A., and Gold, W. M. (1975). Inhibition of respiratory reflexes by local anesthetic aerosols in dogs and rabbits. J. Appl. Physiol. 38:1045.
39. Jain, S. K., Trenchard, D., Reynolds, F., Noble, M. I. M., and Guz, A. (1973). The effect of local anaesthesia of the airway on respiratory reflexes in the rabbit. Clin. Sci. 44:519.
40. Dixon, M., Callanan, D., and Widdicombe, J. G. (1975). SO_2 and the pattern of breathing. Bull. Physiopathol. Respir. 11:94P.
41. Grunstein, M. M., Younes, M., and Milic-Emili, J. (1973). Control of tidal volume and respiratory frequency in anesthetized cats. J. Appl. Physiol. 35:463.
42. Adrian, E. D. (1933). Afferent impulses in the vagus and their effect on respiration. J. Physiol. (Lond.) 79:332.
43. Widdicombe, J. G. (1964). Respiratory reflexes. In W. O. Fenn and H. Rahn (eds.), Handbook of Physiology, Section 3, Respiration, Vol. I, pp. 585–630. American Physiology Society, Washington, D.C.
44. Kostreva, R. D., Zuperku, E. J., Hess, G. L., Coon, R. L., and Kampine, J. P. (1975). Pulmonary afferent activity recorded from sympathetic nerves. J. Appl. Physiol. 39:37.
45. Widdicombe, J. G. (1954). Respiratory reflexes from trachea and bronchi of the cat. J. Physiol. (Lond.) 123:55.
46. Fitzgerald, R. S., and Parks, D. C. (1971). Effect of hypoxia on carotid chemoreceptor response to carbon dioxide in cats. Respir. Physiol. 12:218.
47. Goodman, N. W., and McCloskey, D. I. (1972). Intracellular potentials in the carotid body. Brain Res. 39:501.
48. Goodman, N. W., Nail, B. S., and Torrance, R. W. (1974). Oscillations in the discharge of single carotid chemoreceptor fibres of the cat. Respir. Physiol. 20:251.
49. Gray, B. A. (1968). Response of the perfused carotid body to changes in pH and P_{CO_2}. Respir. Physiol. 4:229.

50. Paintal, A. S. (1971). The responses of chemoreceptors at reduced temperatures. J. Physiol. (Lond.) 217:1.
51. Sampson, S. R., and Hainsworth, R. (1972). Responses of aortic body chemoreceptors of the cat to physiological stimuli. Am. J. Physiol. 222:953.
52. Bellville, J. W., Fleischli, G., and Defares, J. G. (1969). A new method of studying regulation of respiration—the response to sinusoidally varying CO_2 inhalation. Biomed. Res. 2:329.
53. Wyss, O. A. M. (1964). Die nervöse Steuerung der Atmung, p. 479. Springer-Verlag, Heidelberg.
54. Black, A. M. S., and Torrance, R. W. (1971). Respiratory oscillations in chemoreceptor discharge in the control of breathing. Respir. Physiol. 13:221.
55. Goodman, N. W. (1974). Some observations on the homogeneity of response of single chemoreceptor fibres. Respir. Physiol. 20:271.
56. Baker, A. B., and Hahn, C. E. W. (1974). An analogue of study of controlled ventilation. Respir. Physiol. 22:227.
57. Barrès, G., Santucci, J., and Marchand, B. (1973). Étude expérmentale en boucle ouverte de la régulation chimique de la respiration. Bull. Physiol. Pathol. Resp., 9:1151.
58. Duffin, J. (1972). A mathematical model of the chemoreflex control of ventilation. Respir. Physiol. 15:277.
59. Grodins, F. S., Gray, J. S., Schroeder, K. R., Norins, A. L., and Jones, R. W. (1954). Respiratory responses to CO_2 inhalation: a theoretical study of a nonlinear biological regulator. J. Appl. Physiol. 7:283.
60. Grodins, F. S., and Gordon, J. (1963). Mathematical models of respiratory regulation. Ann. N.Y. Acad. Sci. 109:852.
61. Hill, E. P., Power, G. G., and Longo, L. D. (1973). Mathematical simulation of pulmonary O_2 and CO_2 exchange. Am. J. Physiol. 22:904.
62. Horgan, J. D., and Lange, R. L. (1968). Chemical control in the respiratory system. Trans. Biomed. Eng. 15:119.
63. Longobardo, G. S., Cherniack, N. S., and Fishman, A. P. (1966). Cheyne-Stokes breathing produced by a model of the human respiratory system. J. Appl. Physiol. 21:1839.
64. Matthews, C. M. E., Laszlo, G., Campbell, E. J. M., and Read, D. J. C. (1968/69). A model for the distribution and transport of CO_2 in the body and the ventilatory response to CO_2. Respir. Physiol. 6:45.
65. Milhorn, H. T., and Brown, D. R. (1971). Steady-state simulation of the human respiratory system. Comp. Biomed. Res. 3:604.
66. Milhorn, H. T., Reynolds, W. J., and Holloman, G. H. (1972). Digital simulation of the ventilatory response to CO_2 inhalation and CSF perfusion. Comp. Biomed. Res. 5:301.
67. Scrimshire, D. A., Tomlin, P. J., and Ethridge, R. A. (1973). Computer simulation of gas exchange in human lungs. J. Appl. Physiol. 34:687.
68. Suwa, K., and Bendixen, H. H. (1972). Pulmonary gas exchange in a tidally ventilated single alveolus model. J. Appl. Physiol. 32:834.
69. Trueb, T. J., Cherniack, N. S., D'Souza, A. F., and Fishman, A. P. (1971). A mathematical model of the controlled plant of the respiratory system. Biophys. J. 11:810.
70. Yamamoto, W., and Hori, T. (1971). Phasic air movement model of respiratory regulation of carbon dioxide balance. Comp. Biomed. Res. 3:699.

71. Euler, C. von. (1973). On the role of proprioceptors in perception and execution of motor acts with special reference to breathing. *In* L. D. Pengelly, A. S. Rebuck, and E. J. M. Campbell (eds.), Loaded Breathing, pp. 139–154. Longman Canada Limited, Ontario.

72. Euler, C. von (1973). The role of proprioceptive afferents in the control of respiratory muscles. Acta Neurobiol. Exp. 33:329.

73. Newsom Davis, J. (1974). Control of the muscles of breathing. *In* A. C. Guyton and J. G. Widdicombe (eds.), MTP International Review of Science, Physiology Series I, Respiratory Physiology I, pp. 221–245. University Park Press, Baltimore.

74. Frankshtein, S. I., Sergeeva, L. N., Sergeeva, Z. N., and Ivanova, E. S. (1975). Prinimaet li uchastie afferentaciya s dykhatelnykh myshts v regulatsii eipnicheskogo dykhaniya u cheloveka? (English summary). Sech. Physiol. J. USSR. No. 2. 61:284.

75. Bland, S., Lazerou, L., Dyck, G., and Cherniack, R. M. (1967). The influence of the "chest wall" on respiratory rate and depth. Respir. Physiol. 3:47.

76. Camporesi, E., and Sant'Ambrogio, G. (1971). Influences on the respiratory rhythm originating from the lungs and the chest wall. Pfluegers Arch. 324:311.

77. Remmers, E. J., and Martilla, I. (1975). Action of intercostal muscle afferents on the respiratory rhythm of anesthetized cats. Respir. Physiol. 24:31.

78. Remmers, J. E. (1970). Inhibition of inspiratory activity by intercostal muscle afferents. Respir. Physiol. 10:358.

79. Orthner, H. F., and Yamamoto, W. S. (1974). Transient respiratory response to mechanical loads at fixed blood gas levels in rats. J. Appl. Physiol. 36:280.

80. Younes, M., Arkinstall, W., and Milic-Emili, J. (1973). Mechanism of rapid ventilatory compensation to added elastic loads in cats. J. Appl. Physiol. 35:443.

81. Campbell, E. J. M., Agostoni, E., and Newsom Davis, J. (1970). The Respiratory Muscles. Mechanics and Neural Control. Ed. 2, p. 348. Lloyd-Luke Ltd., London.

82. Bishop, B. (1967). Diaphragm and abdominal muscle responses to elevated airway pressures in the cat. J. Appl. Physiol. 22:959.

83. Bishop, B., and Bachofen, H. (1972). Vagal control of ventilation and respiratory muscles during elevated pressures in the cat. J. Appl. Physiol. 32:103.

84. Bishop, B., and Bachofen, H. (1973). Comparative influence of proprioceptors and chemoreceptors in the control of respiratory muscles. Acta Neurobiol. Exp. 33:381.

85. Porter, R., (ed.), (1970). Breathing: Hering-Breuer Centenary Symposium. J. & A. Churchill, London.

86. Widdicombe, J. G. (1974). Reflex control of breathing. *In* A. C. Guyton and J. G. Widdicombe (eds.), MTP International Review of Science, Physiology Series I, Respiratory Physiology I, pp. 273–301. University Park Press, Baltimore.

87. Düring, M. v., Andres, K. H., and Iravani, J. (1974). The fine structure of the pulmonary stretch receptor in the rat. Z. Anat. Entwicklungsgesch. 143:215.

88. Armstrong, D. J., and Luck, J. C. (1974). Accessibility of pulmonary

stretch receptors from the pulmonary and bronchial circulations. J. Appl. Physiol. 36:706.

89. Miserocchi, G., Mortola, J., and Sant'Ambrogio, G. (1973). Localization of pulmonary stretch receptors in the airways of the dog. J. Physiol. (Lond.) 235:775.

90. Miserocchi, G., and Sant' Ambrogio, G. (1974). Distribution of pulmonary stretch receptors in the intrapulmonary airways of the dog. Respir. Physiol. 21:71.

91. Sant'Ambrogio, G., and Miserocchi, G. (1973). Functional localization of pulmonary stretch receptors in the airways of the cat. Arch. Fisiol. 70:1.

92. Miserocchi, G., and Sant'Ambrogio, G. (1974). Responses of pulmonary stretch receptors to static pressure inflations. Respir. Physiol. 21:77.

93. Bartoli, A., Bystrzycka, E., Guz, A., Jain, S. K., Noble, M. I. M., and Trenchard, D. (1973). Studies of the pulmonary vagal control of central respiratory rhythm in the absence of breathing movements. J. Physiol. (Lond.) 230:449.

94. Younes, M., Iscoe, S., and Milic-Emili, J. (1975). A method for assessment of phasic vagal influence on tidal volume. J. Appl. Physiol. 38:335.

95. Phillipson, E. A. (1974). Vagal control of breathing pattern independent of lung inflation in conscious dogs. J. Appl. Physiol. 37:183.

96. Stanley, N. N., Altose, M. D., Kelsen, S. G., Ward, C. F., and Cherniack, N. S. (1975). Changing effect of lung volume on respiratory drive in man. J. Appl. Physiol. 38:768.

97. Lin, A. C., Lally, D. A., Morre, T. O., and Hong, S. K. (1974). Physiological and conventional breath-hold breaking points. J. Appl. Physiol. 37:291.

98. Younes, M., Vaillancourt, P., and Milic-Emili, J. (1974). Interaction between chemical factors and duration of apnea following lung inflation. J. Appl. Physiol. 36:190.

99. Stanley, N. N., Altose, M. D., Cherniack, N. S., and Fishman, A. P. (1975). Changes in strength of lung inflation reflex during prolonged inflation. J. Appl. Physiol. 38:474.

100. Luck, J. C. (1970). Afferent vagal fibres with an expiratory discharge in the rabbit. J. Physiol. (Lond.) 211:63.

101. Widdicombe, J. G., Dixon, M., and Paleček, F. (1975). Unpublished results.

102. Mortola, J., Sant'Ambrogio, G., and Clement, M. G. (1975). Localization of irritant receptors in the airways of the dog. Respir. Physiol. 24:107.

103. Sampson, S. R., and Vidruk, E. H. (1975). Properties of "irritant" receptors in canine lung. Respir. Physiol. 25:9.

104. Korpáš, J., and Tomori, Z. (1975). Kašel' a iné respiračné reflexy. (English summary). Veda, Bratislava.

105. Dejours, P. (1962). Chemoreflexes in breathing. Physiol. Rev. 42:335.

106. Kellog, R. H. (1964). Central chemical regulation of respiration. In W. O. Fenn and H. Rahn (eds.), Handbook of Physiology, Section 3, Respiration, Vol. I, pp. 507–534. American Physiology Society, Washington, D.C.

107. Torrance, R. W. (ed.). (1968). Arterial Chemoreceptors. Blackwell Scientific Publications, Oxford.

108. Torrance, R. W. (1974). Arterial chemoreceptors. In A. C. Guyton and J. G. Widdicombe (eds.), MTP International Review of Science, Physiology Series I, Respiratory Physiology I, pp. 247–271. University Park Press, Baltimore.

109. Cunningham, D. J. C., Elliott, D. H., Lloyd, B. B., Miller, J. P., and Young, J. M. (1965). A comparison of the effects of oscillating and steady alveolar partial pressures of oxygen and carbon dioxide on the pulmonary ventilation. J. Physiol. (Lond.) 179:498.

110. Fenn, W. O., and Craig, A. B., Jr. (1963). Effect of CO_2 on respiration using a new method of administering CO_2. J. Appl. Physiol. 18:1023.

111. Fenner, A., Jansson, E., and Avery, M. E. (1968). Enhancement of the ventilatory response to carbon dioxide by tube breathing. Respir. Physiol. 4:91.

112. Goode, R. C., Brown, E. B., Jr., Howson, M. G., and Cunningham, D. J. C. (1969). Respiratory effects of breathing down a tube. Respir. Physiol. 6:343.

113. Yamamoto, W. S., and Edwards McIver, W. (1960). Homeostasis of carbon dioxide during intravenous infusion of carbon dioxide. J. Appl. Physiol. 15:807.

114. Kellog, R. H. (1960). Acclimatization to carbon dioxide. Anesthesiology 21:634.

115. Loeschcke, H. H. (1960). Beziehungen zwischen CO_2 und Atmung. Anaesthesist 9:38.

116. Bouhuys, A. (1964). Respiratory dead space. In W. O. Fenn and H. Rahn (eds.), Handbook of Physiology, Section 3, Respiration, Vol. I, pp. 699–714. American Physiology Society, Washington, D.C.

117. Comroe, J. H., Forster, R. E., Dubois, A. B., Briscoe, W. A., and Carlsen, E. (1962). The Lung, Clinical Physiology and Pulmonary Function Tests, Ed. 2, p. 220. The Year Book Publishers, Inc., Chicago.

118. Clark, F. J., and von Euler, C. (1972). On the regulation of depth and rate of breathing. J. Physiol. (Lond.) 222:267.

119. Gautier, H., Remmers, J. E., and Bartlett, D., Jr. (1973). Control of the duration of expiration. Respir. Physiol. 18:205.

120. Hey, E. N., Lloyd, B. B., Cunningham, D. J. C., Jukes, M. G. M., and Bolton, D. P. G. (1966). Effects of various respiratory stimuli on the depth and frequency of breathing in man. Respir. Physiol. 1:193.

121. Patrick, J. M., and Howard, A. (1972). The influence of age, sex, body size and lung size on the control and pattern of breathing during CO_2 inhalation in Caucasians. Respir. Physiol. 16:337.

122. Bartlett, D., Jr., Remmers, J. E., and Gautier, H. (1973). Laryngeal regulation of respiratory airflow. Respir. Physiol. 18:194.

123. Boushey, H. A., Richardson, P. S., and Widdicombe, J. G. (1972). Reflex changes in airways resistance and the pattern of breathing arising from laryngeal stimulation. Bull. Physiol. Pathol. Respir. 8:449.

124. Boushey, H. A., Richardson, P. S., and Widdicombe, J. G. (1972). Reflex effects of laryngeal irritation on the pattern of breathing and total lung resistance. J. Physiol. (Lond.) 224:501.

125. Stransky, A., Szereda-Przestaszewska, M., and Widdicombe, J. G. (1972). Changes in laryngeal calibre due to vagal lung reflexes and peripheral chemoreceptor stimulation. J. Physiol. (Lond.) 224:88.

126. Widdicombe, J. G., and Szereda-Przestaszewska, M. (1973). Effect of pneumothorax on laryngeal calibre. Int. Res. Com. Syst. 73:3.

127. Fenner, A., Heim, K., and Schalk, U. (1972). Dead space rebreathing of air and oxygen in children. Acta Paediatr. Scand. 61:685.

128. Dejours, P. (1964). Control of respiration in muscular exercise. In W. O. Fenn and H. Rahn (eds.), Handbook of Physiology, Section 3, Respira-

tion, Vol. I, pp. 631–648. American Physiology Society, Washington, D.C.

129. Huch, A., Kötter, D., Loerbroks, R., and Piiper, J. (1969). O_2 transport in anesthetized dogs in hypoxia, with O_2 uptake increased by 2:4-dinitrophenol. Respir. Physiol. 6:187.

130. Levine, S., and Huckabee, E. W. (1975). Ventilatory response to drug-induced hypermetabolism. J. Appl. Physiol. 38:827.

131. Lamb, W. T. (1968/69). Ventilatory response to hind limb exercise in anesthetized cats and dogs. Respir. Physiol. 6:88.

132. Edelman, N. H., Santiago, T. V., and Conn, H. L., Jr. (1975). Luft's syndrome: O_2 cost of exercise and chemical control of breathing. J. Appl. Physiol. 39:857.

133. Wasserman, K., Whipp, B. J., Casaburi, R., Huntsman, D. J., Castagna, J., and Lugliani, R. (1975). Regulation of arterial P_{CO_2} during intravenous CO_2 loading. J. Appl. Physiol. 38:651.

134. Lamb, T. W. (1966). Ventilatory responses to intravenous and inspired carbon dioxide in anesthetized cats. Respir. Physiol. 2:99.

135. Lewis, S. M. (1975). Awake baboon's ventilatory response to venous and inhaled CO_2 loading. J. Appl. Physiol. 39:417.

136. Molnar, I., and Refsum, H. E. (1971). Influence of artificially increased dead space on the pulmonary ventilation and the arterial blood gases in unconscious tracheotomized patients, breathing air. Scand. J. Respir. Dis. 52:90.

137. Kelman, G. R., and Watson, A. W. S. (1973). Effect of added dead space on pulmonary ventilation during sub-maximal steady-state exercise. Q. J. Exp. Physiol. 58:305.

138. Barnett, T. B., and Peters, R. M. (1960). Unanesthetized dogs with increased respiratory dead space. J. Appl. Physiol. 15:838.

139. Dejours, P., Puccinelli, R., Armand, J., and Dicharry, M. (1965). Concept and measurement of ventilatory sensitivity to carbon dioxide. J. Appl. Physiol. 20:890.

140. Lambertsen, C. J. (1960). Carbon dioxide and respiration in acid-base homeostasis. Anesthesiology 21:642.

141. Schaefer, K. E. (1963). Respiratory adaptation to chronic hypercapnia. Ann. N. Y. Acad. Sci. 109:772.

142. Sant'Ambrogio, G., Miani, A., Camporesi, E., and Pizzini, G. (1970). Ventilatory response to hypercapnia in phrenicotomized rabbits and cats. Respir. Physiol. 10:236.

143. Ou, L. C., and Tenney, S. M. (1974). Post-prandial rise in alveolar CO_2 and ventilatory response in cats. Respir. Physiol. 22:263.

144. Duda, P., and Pavlásek, J. (1975). Functional differentiation of splanchnic A delta fibres in relation to viscerosomatic reflexes. Physiol. Bohemoslov. 24:137.

145. Agostoni, E., and Mead, J. (1964). Statics of the respiratory system. In W. O. Fenn and H. Rahn (eds.), Handbook of Physiology, Section 3, Respiration Vol. I, pp. 387–409. American Physiology Society, Washington, D.C.

146. Bates, D. V., and Christie, R. V. (1964). Respiratory Function in Disease: an Introduction to the Integrated Study of the Lung. W. B. Saunders Co., Philadelphia.

147. West, J. B. (1964). Topographical distribution of blood flow in the lung. In W. O. Fenn and H. Rahn (eds.), Handbook of Physiology, Section 3,

Respiration, Vol. II, pp. 1437–1451. American Physiology Society, Washington, D.C.

148. Riley, R. L., Permutt, S., Said, S., Godfrey, M., Cheng, T. O., Howell, J. B. L., and Shepard, R. H. (1959). Effect of posture on pulmonary dead space in man. J. Appl. Physiol. 14:339.

149. Zajíc, F., and Janota, M. (1969). Tonic function of respiratory muscles in passive changes of body position. Cor Vasa 11:237.

150. Rigg, J. R. A., Rebuck, A. S., and Campbell, E. J. M. (1974). Effect of posture on the ventilatory response to CO_2. J. Appl. Physiol. 37:487.

151. Paleček, F. (1972). Chemická regulace dýchání. Presented at the Meeting of Czech and Slovak Society for Physiology and Pathology of Breathing, September 14–15, Martin.

152. Chválová, M., and Paleček, F. (1975). Changes of the effective dead space. Presented at the Second International Congress on Pathological Physiology, July 8–11, Praha.

153. Cherniack, R. M., Cherniack, L., and Naimark, A. (1972). Respiration in Health and Disease. W. B. Saunders Co., Philadelphia.

154. Mustafa, M. E. K. Y., and Purves, M. J. (1972). The effect of CO_2 upon discharge from slowly adapting stretch receptors in the lungs of rabbits. Respir. Physiol. 16:197.

155. Sant'Ambrogio, G., Miserocchi, G., and Mortola, J. (1974). Transient responses of pulmonary stretch receptors in the dog to inhalation of carbon dioxide. Respir. Physiol. 22:191.

156. Schoener, E. P., and Frankel, H. M. (1972). Effect of hyperthermia and Pa_{CO_2} on the slowly adapting pulmonary stretch receptor. Am. J. Physiol. 222:68.

157. Bartoli, A., Cross, A. B., Guz, A., Jain, S. K., Noble, M. I. M., and Trenchard, D. (1974). The effect of carbon dioxide in the airways and alveoli on ventilation; a vagal reflex studied in the dog. J. Physiol. (Lond.) 240:91.

158. Kao, F. F., Lahiri, S., Wang, C., and Mei, S. (1967). Ventilation and cardiac output in exercise. Circ. Res. (Suppl.) 20 and 21:179.

159. Agostoni, E., and Mead, J. (1964). Statics of the respiratory system. In W. O. Fenn and H. Rahn (eds.), Handbook of Physiology, Section 3, Respiration, Vol. I, pp. 387–409. American Physiology Society, Washington, D.C.

160. Robinson, N. E., and Gillespie, J. R. (1973). Lung volumes in aging beagle dogs. J. Appl. Physiol. 35:317.

161. Westbrook, P. R., Stubbs, S. E., Sessler, A. D., Rehder, K., and Hyatt, R. E. (1973). Effects of anesthesia and muscle paralysis on respiratory mechanics in normal man. J. Appl. Physiol. 34:81.

162. Radford, E. P., Jr. (1964). Static mechanical properties of mammalian lungs. In W. O. Fenn and H. Rahn (eds.), Handbook of Physiology, Section 3, Respiration, Vol. I, pp. 429–449. American Physiology Society, Washington, D.C.

163. Fishman, A. P. (1963). Dynamics of the pulmonary circulation. In W. F. Hamilton (ed.), Handbook of Physiology, Section 2, Circulation, Vol. II, pp. 1667–1743. American Physiology Society, Washington, D.C.

164. Janota, M., and Zajíc, F. (1973). The tone of respiratory muscles in acute changes of circulation induced by acetylcholine. Acta Neurobiol. Exp. 33:411.

165. Mikulenka, V. (1975). Funkce mezižeberních svalů u zdravých a

nemocných s chronickou obstrukční chorobou plic. (English summary). Stud. Pneumol. Phtiseol. Cechosl. 36:321.

166. Grunstein, M. M., Wyszogrodski, I., and Milic-Emili, J. (1975). Regulation of frequency and depth of breathing during expiratory threshold loading in cats. J. Appl. Physiol. 38:869.

167. Bouverot, P., and Fitzgerald, R. S. (1969). Role of the arterial chemoreceptors in controlling lung volume in the dog. Respir. Physiol. 7:203.

168. Albers, C., Usinger, W., and Pleschka, K. (1966). Der Einfluss des Lungenvolumens auf die Spontanatmung und die ventilatorische CO_2-Reaktion beim Hund. Pfluegers Arch. 291:221.

169. Flenley, D. C., Pengelly, L. D., and Milic-Emili, J. (1971). Immediate effects of positive-pressure breathing on the ventilatory response to CO_2. J. Appl. Physiol. 30:7.

170. Cherniack, N. S., Stanley, N. N., Tuteur, P. G., Altosa, M. D., and Fishman, A. P. (1973). Effects of lung volume changes on respiratory drive during hypoxia and hypercapnia. J. Appl. Physiol. 35:635.

171. Woldring, S. (1965). Interrelation between lung volume, arterial CO_2 tension, and respiratory activity. J. Appl. Physiol. 20:647.

172. Zajíc, F. (1970). Význam změn funkční residuální kapacity. Tčesk Fysiol. 19:79.

173. Paleček, F. (1969). Patogeneze plicního emfyzému ve světle experimentálních prací. (English summary). Cas. Lek. Cesk. 108:905.

174. Goldring, I. P., Greenburg, L., and Ratner, I. M. (1968). On the production of emphysema in Syrian hamsters by aerosal inhalation of papain. Arch. Envir. Health 16:59.

175. Gross, P., Babyak, M. A., Tolker, E., and Kaschak, M. (1964). Enzymatically produced pulmonary emphysema: a preliminary report. J. Occup. Med. 6:481.

176. Marco, V., Meranze, D. R., Yoshida, M., and Kimbel, P. (1972). Papain-induced experimental emphysema in the dog. J. Appl. Physiol. 33:293.

177. Paleček, F., Palečková, M., and Aviado, D. M. (1967). Emphysema in immature rats produced by tracheal constriction and papain. Arch. Environ. Health 15:332.

178. Paleček, F., and Holuša, R. (1971). Spontaneous occurrence of lung emphysema in laboratory rats. Physiol. Bohemoslov. 20:335.

179. Carel, R. S., Poppel, J. W., and Kopetzky, M. T. (1973). Pulmonary diffusing capacity as a function of lung volume in healthy and asthmatic children. Isr. J. Med. Sci. 9:1535.

180. Cropp, G. J. A. (1973). Exercise induced pulmonary hyperinflation in asthmatics and its reduction by isoproterenol and cromoglycate. Pediatr. Res. 7:427/199.

181. Wachtlová, M., Chválová, M., Holuša, R., and Paleček, F. (1975). Carrageenin-induced experimental pneumonia in rats. Physiol. Bohemoslov. 24:263.

182. Vízek, M., Holuša, R., and Paleček, F. (1975). Lung function in acute paraquat poisoning. Physiol. Bohemoslov. 24:559.

183. Kuncová, M., Havránková, J., Holuša, R., and Paleček, F. (1971). Experimental silicosis of the rat: correlation of functional, biochemical and histological changes. Arch. Environ. Health 23:365.

184. Kuncová, M., Havránková, J., Kunc, L., Holuša, R., and Paleček, F. (1972). Experimental lung silicosis: evolution of functional, biochemical and morphological changes in the rat. Arch. Environ. Health 24:281.

185. Dziewanowska-Kunert, Z., Glogowska, M., and Szereda-Przestaszewska, M.

(1971). Changes of respiratory rhythm in experimentally induced pathological conditions of the respiratory system. Bull. Physiol. Pathol. Respir. 7:933.

186. Glogowska, M., and Widdicombe, J. G. (1973). The role of vagal reflexes in experimental lung oedema, bronchoconstriction and inhalation of halothane. Respir. Physiol. 18:116.

187. Guz, A., and Trenchard, D. W. (1971). The role of non-myelinated vagal afferent fibres from the lungs in the genesis of tachypnoea in the rabbit. J. Physiol. (Lond.) 213:345.

188. Trenchard, D., Gardner, D., and Guz, A. (1972). Role of pulmonary vagal afferent nerve fibres in the development of rapid shallow breathing in lung inflammation. Clin. Sci. 42:251.

189. Frankshtein, S. I., and Sergeeva, Z. N. (1966). Tonic activity of lung receptors in normal and pathological states. Nature 210:1054.

190. Lourenco, R. V., Turino, G. M., Davidson, L. A. G., and Fishman, A. P. (1965). The regulation of ventilation in diffuse pulmonary fibrosis. Am. J. Med. 38:199.

191. Mürtz, R., and Begenat, H. (1971). Über die Wirkung niedriger O_2-Partialdrucke auf die Respiration bei Patienten mit Lungenfibrose. Z. Gesamte. Exp. Med. 154:299.

192. Chválová, M., Kuncová, M., Havránková, J., and Paleček, F. (1974). Regulation of respiration in experimental silicosis. Physiol. Bohemoslov. 25:539.

193. Buff, R., and Koller, E. A. (1974). Studies on mechanisms underlying the reflex hyperpnoea induced by inhalation of chemical irritants. Respir. Physiol. 21:371.

194. Koller, E. A. (1971). Über die Bedeutung des Nervensystems für die Atmungsaktivierung im anaphylaktischen Astma bronchiale des Meerschweinchens. Schweiz. Med. Wochenschr. 101:1823.

195. Koller, E. A. (1975). The role of pulmonary irritant/deflation receptors in lung disease. Presented at the Second International Congress on Pathological Physiology, July 8–11, Praha.

196. Mills, J. E., and Widdicombe, J. G. (1970). Role of the vagus nerves in anaphylaxis and histamine-induced bronchoconstriction in guinea-pigs. Br. J. Pharmacol. 39:724.

197. Gold, W. M., Kessler, G. F., and Yu, D. Y. C. (1972). Role of vagus nerves in experimental asthma in allergic dogs. J. Appl. Physiol. 33:719.

198. Schläfke, M. E., See, W. R., Massion, W. H., and Loeschcke, H. H. (1969). Die Rolle "spezifischer" und unspezifischer Afferenzen für den Antrieb der Atmung, untersucht durch Reizung und Blockade von Afferenzen an der decerebrierten Katze. Pfluegers Arch. 312:189.

199. Schlaefke, M. E. (1973). "Specific" and "non-specific" stimuli in the drive of respiration. Acta Neurobiol. Exp. 33:149.

200. Leitner, L. M., and Dejours, P. (1971). Reflex increase in ventilation induced by vibrations applied to the triceps surae muscles in the cat. Respir. Physiol. 12:199.

201. Howard, P., Bromberger-Barnea, B., Fitzgerald, S. R., and Bane, N. H. (1969). Ventilatory responses to peripheral nerve stimulation at different times in the respiratory cycle. Respir. Physiol. 7:389.

202. Wiemer, W., and Kiwull, P. (1965). Die Bedeutung der Nn.Vagi für die chemische Atmungssteuerung des Kaninchens. Pfluegers Arch. 283:R46.

203. Paleček, F., Chválová, M., and Hritzová, M. (1970). Specific and non-

specific afferentation in the regulation of breathing. Physiol. Bohemoslov. 19:339.

204. Siegelová, J. (1974). Splanchnic ventilation reflexes in rabbit and cat. *In* XXVI International Congress of Physiological Sciences, Vol. XI, p. 89. International Union of Physiological Sciences, New Delhi.

205. Shannon, R. (1975). Respiratory frequency control during external elastic loading and chest compression. Respir. Physiol. 23:11.

206. Pengelly, L. D., Greener, J., Bowmer, I., Luterman, A., and Milic-Emili, J. (1975). Effect of added elastances on the first loaded breath in man. J. Appl. Physiol. 38:39.

207. Cherniack, R. M., and Chodirker, W. B. (1972). Hypercapnia with relief of hypoxia in normal individuals with increased work of breathing. J. Appl. Physiol. 33:189.

208. Ruttimann, U. E., and Yamamoto, W. S. (1972). Respiratory airflow patterns that satisfy power and force criteria of optimality. Ann. Biomed. Eng. 1:146.

209. Yamashiro, S. H., and Grodins, F. S. (1973). Respiratory cycle optimization in exercise. J. Appl. Physiol. 35:522.

210. Yamashiro, S. M., Daubenspeck, J. A., Lauritsen, T. N., and Grodins, F. S. (1975). Total work rate of breathing optimization in CO_2 inhalation and exercise. J. Appl. Physiol. 38:702.

211. Freedman, S. (1970). Sustained maximum voluntary ventilation. Respir. Physiol. 8:230.

212. Hermansen, L., Hultman, E., and Saltin, B. (1967). Muscle glycogen during prolonged severe exercise. Acta Physiol. Scand. 71:129.

213. Spande, J. I., and Schottelius, B. A. (1970). Chemical basis of fatigue in isolated mouse soleus muscle. Am. J. Physiol. 219:1490.

214. Aljure, E. F., and Borrero, L. M. (1968). The influence of muscle length on the development of fatigue in toad sartorius. J. Physiol. (Lond.) 199:241.

215. Davies, H. W., Haldane, J. S., and Priestley, J. G. (1919). The response to respiratory resistance. J. Physiol. (Lond.) 53:60.

216. Cherniack, R. M., and Snidal, D. P. (1956). The effect of obstruction to breathing on the ventilatory response to CO_2. J. Clin. Invest. 35:1286.

217. Eldridge, F., and Davis, J. M. (1959). Factors contributing to the diminished ventilatory response to CO_2 of patients with obstructive emphysema. J. Appl. Physiol. 14:721.

218. Freedman, S., Dalton, K. J., Holland, D., and Patton, J. M. S. (1972). The effects of added elastic loads on the respiratory response to CO_2 in man. Respir. Physiol. 14:237.

219. Julich, H., and Kandt, H. (1960). Der Verlauf der Erregungskurven des Atemzentrums sowie das Verhalten einiger Atemgrössen unter der Wirkung schwacher Stenosen. Z. Gesamte. Exp. Med. 133:135.

220. Milic-Emili, J., and Tyler, J. M. (1963). Relationship between Pa_{CO_2} and respiratory work during external resistance breathing in man. Ann. N. Y. Acad. Sci. 109:908.

221. Rebuck, A. S., and Juniper, E. F. (1975). Effect of resistive loading on ventilatory response to hypoxia. J. Appl. Physiol. 38:965.

222. Cherniack, R. M. (1964). Work of breathing and the ventilatory response to CO_2. *In* W. O. Fenn and H. Rahn (eds.), Handbook of Physiology, Section 3, Respiration, Vol. II, pp. 1469–1474. American Physiology Society, Washington, D.C.

223. Duron, B., Quichaud, J., and Fullana, N. (1972). Nouvelles recherches sur le mécanisme des apnées du syndrome de Pickwick. Bull. Physiol. Pathol. Respir. 8:1277.

224. Chválová, M., Hritzová, M., and Paleček, F. (1970). The role of the vagi in the hyperventilation response of the anaesthetized rat. Physiol. Bohemoslov. 19:316.

225. Euler, C. von, Herrero, F., and Wexler, I. (1970). Control mechanisms determining rate and depth of respiratory movements. Respir. Physiol. 10:93.

226. Guz, A., Noble, M. I. M., Widdicombe, J. G., Trenchard, D., and Mushin, W. W. (1966). The effect of bilateral block of vagus and glossopharyngeal nerves on the ventilatory response to CO_2 of conscious man. Respir. Physiol. 1:206.

227. Nadel, J. A., Phillipson, E. A., Fishman, N. H., and Hickey, R. F. (1973). Regulation of respiration by bronchopulmonary receptors in conscious dogs. Acta Neurobiol. Exp. 33:33.

228. Richardson, P. S., and Widdicombe, J. G. (1969). The role of the vagus nerves in the ventilatory responses to hypercapnia and hypoxia in asesthetized and unanesthetized rabbits. Respir. Physiol. 7:122.

229. Bouverot, P. (1973). Vagal afferent fibres from the lung and regulation of breathing in awake dogs. Respir. Physiol. 17:325.

230. Berglund, E., Furhoff, A. K., Löftström, B., and Öquist, L. (1971). A study of the effects of unilateral vagus nerve block in a dyspnoeic patient. Scand. J. Respir. Dis. 52:34.

231. Guz, A., Noble, M. I. M., Eisele, J. H., and Trenchard, D. (1970). Experimental results of vagal block in cardiopulmonary disease. In R. Porter (ed.), Breathing: Hering-Breuer Centenary Symposium, pp. 315–329. J. & A. Churchill, London.

232. Phillipson, E. A., Murphy, E., Kozar, L. F., and Schultze, R. K. (1975). Role of vagal stimuli in exercise ventilation in dogs with experimental pneumonitis. J. Appl. Physiol. 39:76.

233. Bartoli, A., Cross, B. A., Guz, A., Huszczuk, A., and Jefferies, R. (1975). The effect of varying tidal volume on the associated phrenic motoneurone output; studies of vagal and chemical feedback. Respir. Physiol. 25:135.

234. Panchenko, I. A. (1960). Vozbudimost dykhatelnogo tsentra k uglekislote v usloviyakh khronicheskoy giperkapnii. (English summary). Bull. Eksp. Biol. Med. No. 5, 49:25.

235. Flenley, D. C., and Millar, J. S. (1967). Ventilatory response to oxygen and carbon dioxide in chronic ventilatory failure. Clin. Sci. 33:319.

236. Flenley, D. C., Franklin, D. H., and Millar, J. S. (1970). The hypoxic drive to breathing in chronic bronchitis and emphysema. Clin. Sci. 38:503.

237. Koolik, A. M., Kondratyeva, L. N., and Tarakanov, I. A. (1975). Disturbances of regulation of the respiration in the inhibition of activity of the carbonic anhydrase by acetazolamide. Presented at the Second International Congress on Pathological Physiology, July 8–11, Praha.

238. Herberg, D., Krüger, R., Mulch, G., and Utz, G. (1970). Zur Pathophysiologie der CO_2-Retention bei obstruktiven bronchopulmonalen Erkrankungen. Respiration 27:236.

239. Flenley, D. C., and Millar, J. S. (1968). The effects of carbon dioxide inhalation on the inspiratory work of breathing in chronic ventilatory failure. Clin. Sci. 34:385.

240. Clark, T. J. H., and Cochrane, G. M. (1972). Effect of mechanical loading on ventilatory response to CO_2 and CO_2 excretion. Br. Med. J. 1:351.
241. Verzár, F. (1933). Die Regulation des Lungenvolumens. Pfluegers Arch. 232:322.
242. Breslav, I. S., and Konza, E. A. (1975). Vosstanovlenie khemoretseptornoy funktsii posle deafferentatsii sinokarotidnikh zon u krys. (English summary). Sech. Phys. J. USSR, No. 1, 61:84.
243. Ross, B. B., and Farhi, L. E. (1960). Dead-space ventilation as a determinant in the ventilation-perfusion concept. J. Appl. Physiol. 15:363.
244. Suwa, K., and Bendixen, H. H. (1968). A mathematical analysis of physiological dead space in a lung model. J. Appl. Physiol. 24:549.
245. Martin, C. J., Tsunoda, S., and Young, A. C. (1974). Lung emptying patterns in diffuse obstructive pulmonary syndromes. Respir. Physiol. 21:157.
246. Ingram, R. H., Miller, R. B., and Tate, L. A. (1972). Arterial carbon dioxide changes during voluntary hyperventilation in chronic obstructive pulmonary disease. Chest 62:14.
247. Burrows, B., Fletcher, C. M., Heard, B. E., Jones, N. L., and Wootliff, J. S. (1966). The emphysematous and bronchial types of chronic airways obstruction. Lancet i:830.
248. Ingram, R. H., Miller, R. B., and Tate, L. A. (1972). Ventilatory response to carbon dioxide and to exercise in relation to the pathophysiologic type of chronic obstructive pulmonary disease. Am. Rev. Respir. Dis. 105:541.
249. Rebuck, A. S., and Vandenberg, R. A. (1973). The relationship between pulmonary arterial pressure and physiologic dead space in patients with obstructive lung disease. Am. Rev. Respir. Dis. 107:423.
250. Bakers, J. H. C. M., and Tenney, S. M. (1970). The perception of some sensations associated with breathing. Respir. Physiol. 10:85.
251. Breslav, I. S., Zhironkin, A. G., and Shmeleva, A. M. (1975). O vospriyatii chelovekom svoego dykhatelnogo obema. (English summary). Sech. Physiol. J. USSR No. 4, 61:593.
252. Frankshtein, S. I., Ivanova, E. S., and Sergeeva, L. N. (1972). Oshchushchenie nedostatochnosti dykhaniya. Patol. Fiziol. Eksp. Ter. 1:3.
253. Frankshtein, S. I. (1975). The mechanism of sensation of respiratory insufficiency. Presented at the Second International Congress on Pathological Physiology, July 8–11, Praha.
254. Nizovtsev, V. P. (1975). Respiratory insufficiency and dyspnoea. Presented at the Second International Congress on Pathological Physiology, July 8–11, Praha.

International Review of Physiology
Respiratory Physiology II, Volume 14
Edited by John G. Widdicombe
Copyright 1977   University Park Press   Baltimore

9
Defensive Mechanisms
of the Respiratory System

J. G. WIDDICOMBE

St. George's Hospital
Medical School, London, England

PATTERNS OF INVASION OF RESPIRATORY SYSTEM   292
    Irritant Gases   292
    Aerosols   293
        Deposition of Aerosols in Respiratory System   294
           Particle Size   294
           Nature of Particles   294
    Large Objects and Materials   294
    Pattern of Breathing   295

COMPONENTS OF RESPIRATORY DEFENSIVE SYSTEM   295
    Mucociliary Clearance   295
    Immune Responses and Antimicrobial Defenses   296
    Reflex Responses   296

DEFENSIVE MECHANISMS FROM
  PARTICULAR RESPIRATORY SITES   297
    Nose   297
        Absorption and Deposition of Gases and Aerosols   297
        Mucociliary Clearance   297
        Immune Responses and Antimicrobial Defenses   298
        Reflex Responses   298
    Nasopharynx and Pharynx   299
    Larynx   300
    Tracheobronchial Tree   301
        Mucociliary Clearance   302
           Secretory Mechanisms   302
           Mucociliary Transport   303
        Immune Responses and Antimicrobial Defenses   304
        Reflex Responses   305

Alveoli   307
  Antimicrobial Defenses   307
  Reflex Responses   307

The need for the respiratory tract and lungs to be defended against invasion by harmful materials is obvious; successful invasion may lead to pathological changes which could obstruct the respiratory passages, hinder the respiratory functions of the lungs, or allow absorption of toxic substances or organisms into the body. The defensive mechanisms must be active against three types of invader: gases, solid or liquid aerosols, and large objects and materials such as "foreign bodies" and inhaled vomitus. The defensive process may tend to limit the entry of the invader, to expel it, or to lessen the damage which might occur. The pattern of defense will depend not only on the nature of the invader, but on its site of attack. Although the general patterns of the defensive processes are common to most sites in the respiratory tract, there are important differences for each region. In addition, the pattern of response may depend upon the initial health or disease of the respiratory system and on the subsequent pathological changes if the defensive mechanisms are ineffective.

PATTERNS OF INVASION OF RESPIRATORY SYSTEM

Irritant Gases

The list of gases which "irritate" the respiratory tract and lungs is extremely long, and no attempt will be made here to cover it (see 1–3). An adequate definition of a chemical "irritant" is difficult to give, but, in this chapter, the term will refer to substances which when inhaled either cause tissue damage or stimulate nervous afferent end organs in the respiratory tract and lungs, or both. The types of response they cause may also include mucosal hyperemia or edema, stimulation of secretion by goblet cells or submucous glands, depression of ciliary activity, and contraction of airway smooth muscle. The nature of the damage and of the defensive response will depend not only upon the quantity and concentration of the irritant but also upon the site where it acts; the latter in turn is determined by the pattern of breathing (e.g., through the mouth or nose) and on the solubility of the irritant gas. Highly soluble gases such as sulfur dioxide are almost entirely absorbed in the nose, the concentration reaching the larynx being less than 1% of the inhaled concentration in quiet breathing (4–6). The depth of penetration increases if air flow is faster, and if the inhalation is prolonged the mucous membrane may become saturated with the irritant gas so that concentrations increase at sites deeper in the respiratory tract. Many irritant gases may be inhaled either as aerosol solution or absorbed into solid particulate aerosols (smokes), in which case the considerations concerning aerosols described in the next section apply.

Largely because of the application of irritant gases in warfare and crowd-control, there has been extensive research on the chemical processes whereby the gases may act. Most of this research has dealt with the stimulation of pain or "nociceptive" sensory receptors, and it is not possible to say if the same chemical actions underly other harmful actions. In any case, the very great chemical diversity of the irritant gases suggests that they may act chemically in many different ways.

Probably the earliest hypothesis was that of Peters (7), who concluded that many irritant gases acted on nervous receptors by reacting with SH groups in the receptor membrane or by inhibitory "thiol enzymes" associated with the endings (8–10). Irritant chemicals with this property include some halogenated compounds such as esters and amides of iodoacetate and acrylate and dienophiles such as acrolein and organoarsenicals with trivalent arsenic.

Some widely studied irritants, in particular sulfur dioxide and its products sulfite and bisulfite which are formed in tissues, have no action on SH groups in proteins. They do, however, break S–S linkages, and this has been postulated as the basis of their irritant action (1, 11–14). This group of chemicals contains many known irritants, such as chlorine, ammonia, trivalent arsenicals, phosphenes, and hidrides. Some of these compounds also act on SH groups. Full details of the groups are given by Parker and Kharash (13).

Structure-activity relationships for many irritant compounds acting on SH groups or S–S bonds have been determined and are authoritatively reviewed by Alarie (1). He points out that these molecular changes are closely related to the permeability of cell membranes (15). However, some sensory irritants seem to have a different chemical action, and it should not be assumed that the molecular activities of irritants established for nociceptive end organs in cornea or skin need apply to cellular structures such as cilia, goblet cell membranes, and epithelial layers; these may be as important in respiratory reactions to inhaled irritants as are the unpleasant sensations and reflexes set up by stimulation of nerve endings.

Aerosols

Aerosols may be solid or liquid or both and may be mixed with irritant gases. Cigarette smoke is an obvious example of a mixed aerosol. Solid aerosols (smokes) may be chemically inert (e.g., purified carbon dust) but still provoke defensive reactions by their mechanical effect. Distilled water aerosol, seemingly chemically inert, is a powerful inducer of coughing. Apart from chemical and mechanical actions, aerosols may induce defensive responses by immunological (allergic) mechanisms or by viral or bacterial means. These processes will be considered in a later section.

Dead and nonantigenic aerosols are created in nature in many ways, including bonfires, winds acting on dry soil, water sprays, and gas phase reactions. It has been calculated that $985-2,615 \times 10^6$ metric tons of aerosol are formed each year, and that about one-sixth of this is produced by human activity restricted to 1% of the surface of the earth (16, 17). The majority of these aerosols are formed in the troposphere immediately above the earth's surface, and the formation includes gas phase reactions due to sunlight acting on polluted air (e.g., mist, fog, and smog). The aerosols contain many chemical irritants, including nitrogen dioxide and ozone. Although some of these aerosols are restricted to towns and cities, others can be formed in the country—by lightning, for example. In addition, industrial pollution contributes substantially to this pollution.

Antigenic particles can be derived from many sources, but plant spores, pollens, animal debris, insect parts, and home and industrial dusts are the most important. Most of these aerosols are of relatively large size (10–50 μm). Viral and bacterial aerosols are important in social life.

Deposition of Aerosols in Respiratory System

Particle Size The influence of particle size on the site of deposition has been studied experimentally and analyzed theoretically (18, 19). Particles over 10 μm in diameter nearly all settle in the nose or pharynx, but a small proportion may enter the lungs, especially with mouth breathing (20) and hyperpnea. This deep penetration has been shown for large pollen grains (21). Although studies with man have shown that large pollen grains may be largely or totally retained in the nose (22, 23), a few particles in the lungs or the presence of smaller fragments of pollen may be sufficient to induce pulmonary reactions (24). Particles in a middle range, 2–5 μg, show maximum deposition in the lower respiratory tract (18), whereas those less than 0.5 μm in diameter are mainly exhaled and not retained (e.g., cigarette smoke). Few naturally occurring aerosols are of uniform particle size.

Nature of Particles Irregularly shapes particles act as if they were of smaller diameter. The best example is asbestos dust, of which fibres over 50 μm long can penetrate deeply into the lungs (25, 26). Many particles are hydroscopic and expand when they are exposed to the high humidity in the respiratory tract lumen (27). Their site of deposition will, therefore, depend on the size of this effect.

Large Objects and Materials

The respiratory system must be defended against large structures which may block the respiratory tract, cause collapse of part of the lung if allowed to penetrate deeply, and produce local damage to the walls of the respiratory tract. Inhaled materials are one example and include insects, food, vomitus, and a bizarre variety of objects. In addition, the accumulation of intraluminal mucus, blood clots, and tissue debris may provide material in the disease condition which requires removal before health can be restored.

Pattern of Breathing

It has been mentioned already that pattern of breathing may determine the site of deposition of irritant materials. Nose breathing and mouth breathing are an obvious example, the latter allowing deeper penetration of gases (4, 5), and aerosols (20). Increased air flow draws irritant gases and particles deeper into the respiratory system (28, 29). However, the rapid air flow may also lead to more turbulence, and in turn this will cause greater impaction and deposition of particles in the trachea and large bronchi. Thus, bronchoconstriction leads to more proximal deposition of aerosols, in part due to the more rapid air flow and increased turbulence (30). Therefore, the effects of increased air flow depend on a balance between the deeper penetration into the lungs by axial carriage in the air stream and greater impaction proximally in the respiratory tract due to turbulence.

A similar conflict of mechanisms exists in lung disease. On the one hand, heterogeneous obstructions of the airways will lead to deeper penetration of small particles by increasing air flow velocities in the axial stream, opening collateral channels, and preferentially diverting the air stream to unobstructed parts of the lung (31, 32). On the other hand, irregularities of the airway walls and intraluminal mucus will cause greater turbulence and deposition of relatively big particles in the larger airways.

COMPONENTS OF RESPIRATORY DEFENSIVE SYSTEM

This section will introduce in general terms the various ways in which the respiratory system can defend itself. Some will apply more to aerosols than to gases, or vice versa; not all processes will be present at all sites in the respiratory tract and lungs.

Mucociliary Clearance

Respiratory tract mucus has two possible functions in defensive systems of the lung: 1) a physicochemical medium which may act as a barrier to penetration and as a site of chemical and biological reactions; and 2) the structure in which noxious chemicals and microbial agents may be cleared from the respiratory tract by ciliary transport or by defensive reflexes such as coughing or sneezing. Mucus secretion and ciliary transport have separate control systems, and the functional relationship between the two processes is close.

Several different processes related to mucociliary transport can be measured: ciliary beat, mucus velocity or flow rate, mucus secretion, or clearance from a part of the respiratory system. All these mechanisms are related but, because different mechanisms have been studied mainly in the nose or the lower airways and seldom in both, detailed consideration of them will be in the later anatomically-oriented parts of this chapter.

Immune Responses and Antimicrobial Defenses

General antibody production involves lymphocytes, plasma cells, and probably other secretory cells, mainly derived from the thymus gland and from the bone marrow. These cells produce and liberate antibodies even after the body's invasion by an antigen is complete. The cells that release immunoglobulins are found in all parts of the respiratory tract, but not in the lung parenchyma (33). Immunoglobulins are found in secretions from the nose and tracheobronchial tree, and also in the saliva, and their concentrations and ratios are different from those in serum, indicating that active secretory processes may be involved. This conclusion is supported by changes in concentrations of immunoglobulins during immune responses. Mast cells can be extracted from respiratory tissues and have been shown to have fixed IgE. The cells can be degranulated by specific antigen challenge (34, 35). The biochemical mechanisms whereby antigen-antibody reaction on mast and other cells releases chemical mediators have been reviewed (36–38).

The presence of mast cells and plasma cells in the respiratory tract mucosa may account for local hypersensitivity reactions such as allergic rhinitis and bronchial asthma. Similar conditions affecting the alveoli, such as allergic alveolitis, are more difficult to explain on this basis, if it is accepted that the alveolar wall lacks immune system cells (33).

Microorganisms are ingested and killed by macrophages, and those in the alveoli have been chiefly studied by lung lavage. Similar macrophages are seen in the mucosa of the respiratory tract, including the nose, and presumably have similar functions. Defenses against virus infections have been studied mainly for the nasal mucosa and will be considered later.

Reflex Responses

The main functions of these reflexes are either 1) to prevent further entry and penetration of the invading agent, for example, the apnea caused by inhalation of irritant gases into the nose or larynx; 2) to expel the intruder, for example, coughing or sneezing; or 3) to make appropriate physiological adjustments for lessening the action of the stimulus or to prepare the body against the assault, for example, reflex bronchomotor, cardiovascular, and mucus-secreting responses. These reflex responses are highly specific for the particular respiratory site which has been affected and will, therefore, be considered in detail in a later section.

Apart from reflex changes in breathing, reflexes may be elicited which change bronchomotor tone, laryngeal caliber, cardiovascular variables, mucus secretion in the respiratory tract, and skeletal muscular tone.

DEFENSIVE MECHANISMS FROM PARTICULAR RESPIRATORY SITES

Nose

The structure of the nose in relation to its protective function at the entry to the respiratory tract has been authoritatively reviewed (39, 40). Not only does the nose filter out and absorb gases and aerosols (4–6), but it humidifies inspired air and brings it to body temperature by the time the larynx is reached (41).

The cavity of the nose, except for its most anterior part, is lined with pseudostratified columnar cell epithelium, containing many goblet and ciliated cells. Beneath the epithelium is a layer of glands containing both mucous and serous cells (42). The whole mucosa is richly supplied with blood vessels, with a dense capillary network near the epithelial surface and a cavernous venous plexus beneath the mucous membrane (43, 44). This plexus is the basis of the erectile properties of the nasal mucosa, especially the lower two turbinates and the septum. The arterioles and venules are abundantly supplied with adrenergic nerve fibres (45, 46), and parasympathetic cholinergic nerves have also been described (47). Presumably, the function of the innervation is to change vascular volumes and blood flow with respect to the air conditioning role of the nose. There have been many studies of changes in the nasal vascular bed in various conditions (e.g., 43, 48, 49), but little is known about the mechanisms of control of this function and its modifications in disease.

Absorption and Deposition of Gases and Aerosols   The nose acts as a highly efficient filter. Gases which are very soluble in body fluids are well absorbed. Mainly sulfur dioxide has been studied. In man, less than 1% of the inhaled concentration reaches the pharynx (5, 6) even after 6 hr of inhalation. Similar results have been obtained with experimental animals (50, 51). The filtration of liquid and solid aerosols depends, among other factors, on particle size (18). Those with diameters greater than 10 μm are almost 90% retained in the nose, and maximum deposition occurs with diameters of 1.5–3.0 μm. Particles with diameters 0.2–0.5 μm have minimum deposition in the nose; for example, guinea pigs retain only 30% of inhaled cigarette smoke particles in the nose (52). The hydration of aerosol particles in the nose may have an important effect on their size and deposition.

Mucociliary Clearance   The nasal submucosal glands have a cholinergic motor innervation (53, 54), but the reflex control of their activity has been little studied. It is not known whether the nasal goblet cells have an innervation. The total mucus secretion from the nose is fairly easy to collect for chemical analysis. In addition to mucus glycoproteins, lysozyme, immunoglobulins (IgA, IgE, and IgG), and proteins similar to serum portions have been identified. The composition and water content of nasal secretions vary greatly in diseases (55–57). In the anterior part of the nose, where deposition of particles due to impaction is greatest, ciliary beat moves mucus forward, but elsewhere the mucociliary transport is backward toward the pharynx where mucus is swallowed (58, 59). Recent studies on mucociliary clearance in man by Andersen et al.

$(6, 60, 61, 62)$ have shown that flow rates are usually in the range $2-7$ mm min^{-1} and that the total mucus blanket is cleared every $10-15$ min (40). Flow is depressed by $5-25$ ppm of sulfur dioxide (6).

Immune Responses and Antimicrobial Defenses   Recent research on this subject has been reviewed (55). Nasal viruses, such as the influenza virus, penetrate the mucus layer, possibly aided by neuraminidase in the virus which lowers the viscosity of the mucus and allows the virus to reach the cell layer (63). After nasal infection, various changes take place in the composition of nasal mucus secretions. There is increased mucus output and transudation of fluid, and probably serum proteins, across the epithelium. Interferon appears (64), which may be a factor in limiting the virus infection (65). Immunoglobulin A (IgA), but not antibody to the virus, promptly increases in output, whereas virus antibody, probably also an IgA, is secreted $2-3$ weeks after the start of the infection (66). IgG diminishes in output (66).

With bacterial nasal infections, various secreted constituents of mucus have been described; these include lysozyme and lactoferrin and components of the complement system (67, 68). The importance of these constituents in limiting the bacterial infection is controversial.

In allergic nasal conditions, IgE antibodies appear in the secretions (69) and are related to nasal obstruction due to mucosal swelling. Plasma cells containing IgE (and others with IgA) have been identified in the tonsils and adenoids (33), and IgA, IgE, and IgM have been identified in nasal secretions (70).

Reflex Responses   Although the best known reflex response to an invading challenge to the nose is a sneeze, this is only one of many nasal reflexes and one of the least studied, possibly because it is readily depressed by anesthesia in experimental animals.

There are afferent end organs in the nasal mucosa, but these have not been frequently investigated histologically, and most of the studies have been related more to the sense of smell than to defensive mechanisms (71). The trigeminal nerves carry most of the afferent fibers which respond to chemical irritants and odors, both myelinated (72) and nonmyelinated (73) fibers being concerned. End organs in the nasal epithelium can give rise to various forms of sensation, including smell and pain, and to defensive reflexes, both respiratory and nonrespiratory (74, 75). Which receptors are responsible for which responses is not known.

The most obvious respiratory reflex from the nose is the sneeze. Here the expulsive effort is preceded by a deep inspiration; at least on theoretical grounds, this might have the adverse effect of increasing the inhalation of the irritant substance. Presumably this is compensated for by the added mechanical efficiency of the subsequent expulsive effort. Nonexpulsive respiratory reflexes from the nose include sniffing, usually associated with smells, and an apneic reflex, possibly related in mechanism to the diving reflex of aquatic animals (75, 76). It is not known whether the same receptors, but with different discharge frequencies or patterns, are involved in all three reflex patterns of response or what determines which reflex will occur.

Nonrespiratory reflexes from the nose include laryngeal closure. For sneezing, the sudden opening of a previously closed larynx during the expulsive phase may be mechanically important in aerodynamic terms in removing a solid body from the nose; however, this conventional view is based on little experimental evidence. Weaker irritant stimuli to the nose also cause reflex changes in laryngeal caliber in the absence of sneezing. During apneic responses from the nose, the larynx closes during the apnea and subsequent expiratory phases (77); this reflex might prevent access to the lungs of an irritant gas or aerosol or, in the case of the diving reflex, of water.

There are several studies which show that irritation of the nose causes reflex bronchodilatation (78, 79), together with the laryngeal constriction. Early work indicated that nasal irritation causes bronchoconstriction (80); this result might be explained by diffusion of the irritating agent to the larynx, the bronchoconstrictor reflex from the latter site being dominant. However, recent studies in man have shown that 5–25 ppm of sulfur dioxide in the nose, with pharyngeal concentrations less than 1% of the inhaled value, leads to an increase in airways resistance (6). Whether a response is bronchodilator or bronchoconstrictor may depend on the nature of the irritant gas and on the afferent receptors in the nasal mucosa which are stimulated.

Mechanical or chemical irritation of the nose causes reflex hypertension (75, 78). The reflex has been extensively studied in experimental animals because it is an important component of the diving reflex, and includes vasoconstriction in various vascular beds, release of catecholamines from the adrenal medulla, and sympathetic stimulation of the heart (75, 81). Although stimulation of the nose can cause reflex bradycardia related to the diving reflex, the stimuli usually have to be strong, and the involvement of secondary reflexes from arterial baroreceptors due to blood pressure changes has to be considered.

Reflex secretion of mucus from the trachea of the cat is induced by mechanical or chemical irritation of the nasal mucosa (82, 83). It is not known whether an analogous nose-to-nose reflex exists; if it did, it might contribute to the stimulation of nasal mucus output in nasal irritation and disease.

A final nasal reflex response to irritation must be mentioned; this is the reflex inhibition of spinal reflex skeletal muscle tone that follows strong stimulation on the nose (84). This response may be similar to the inhibition of skeletal muscle tone elicited on stimulation of other visceral nociceptive reflexes (85).

A long list of "defensive" reflexes from the nose has been given. Most of the studies of these reflexes have been analytical investigations with experimental animals. Far more must be learned about the possible significance of the reflexes in the response of the organism to nasal invasion or disease, in particular, in man.

Nasopharynx and Pharynx

These parts of the respiratory tract have stratified, squamous cell epithelium, without cilia, so clearance from them is by force due to air flow or by swallowing. Deep under the epithelium are mucous glands, but these have not been studied physiologically; presumably, their function is mainly lubricative in relation to swallowing, at least for the pharynx. The main defensive mechanisms from the nasopharynx and pharynx which have been studied are reflexes initiated from the epithelium. Problems of lymph drainage and of microbial defenses are clearly important, especially bearing in mind the presence of the tonsils and adenoids; however, in terms of physiological mechanisms these structures have been neglected.

The mucosa of the nasopharynx (or epipharynx, the wall of the respiratory tract above and behind the soft palate) contains fine afferent nerve terminals connected to myelinated fibers which run in the glossopharyngeal nerve (86). The receptors have not been well characterized histologically. Endings with nonmyelinated fibers do not seem to have been studied, but it is unlikely that they are absent because pain (presumably from nociceptors) can be evoked from the nasopharynx. The nasopharyngeal receptors are rapidly adapting with an irregular discharge on mechanical stimulation. They seem to be insensitive to chemical stimuli, at least to those tried, ammonia gas and histamine solution (87). Possibly the squamous cell nature of the epithelium has a protective role.

Mechanical stimulation of the nasopharyngeal mucosa sets up a rapid and repetitive series of vigorous inspiratory efforts. The reflex is "snifflike" and has been named the "aspiration reflex" (78, 88). It is very resistant to anesthesia and hypothermia and causes a powerful arousal reaction. It is associated with reflex hypertension, tachycardia, bronchodilatation, and tracheal mucus secretion (78, 89). Presumably, the main function of the respiratory reflex is to draw a foreign body in the back of the nose into the pharynx, where it is either swallowed or coughed up. The reflex could be important in the newborn, in whom the nasal passages must be cleared at the start of breathing. In man, the cardiovascular reflex, including hypertension and venoconstriction, may be powerful (90).

Mechanical stimulation of the pharynx sets up two reflexes which protect the respiratory system: first, swallowing (91), which removes any possible obstruction, and, second, reflex inhibition of breathing (92), which interrupts the inspiratory force which potentially might draw the obstruction into the lungs.

Larynx

The vocal folds are covered with squamous cell stratified epithelium, which could constitute a block in mucociliary transport if air flow did not remove mucus. The fact that the larynx is more constricted in expiration than in inspiration (91) means that the aerodynamic forces on the mucus will be greater in the expulsive direction, even in the absence of coughing. There are mucous glands under the epithelium on the vocal folds, but their physiology has not been studied. As with the nasopharynx and pharynx, the larynx is the source of several reflexes which play a part in defending the respiratory system.

Three main types of receptor have been described on the basis of light microscopy. First, fine nerve branches spread among the epithelial cells and connect to myelinated nerve fibers (74, 86, 93). By analogy with receptors in the lower respiratory tract, these endings are probably responsible for the cough and other defensive reflexes. Second, there are specialized nervous structures, like corpuscles and taste buds, especially in the epiglottis and presumably related to swallowing and taste (74). And third, fine nerve endings are attached to non-myelinated afferent fibers and probably pain or nociceptive endings. Studies of nerve impulse traffic in afferent fibers from laryngeal receptors confirm the complexity of receptor types (74, 94). One group of fibers comes from receptors generally stimulated by irritant gases and smokes or by mechanical contact, but with great variability of response. Another group of endings has a spontaneous regular discharge and is mechanosensitive, but is little affected by most chemical stimulants. Other fibers are nonmyelinated and may be joined to nociceptive endings in the epithelium.

As might be expected from this summary of laryngeal nervous receptors and their discharges, many reflexes have been described arising from the laryngeal mucosa, especially that over the vocal folds. With minimum effective mechanical or chemical stimulation of the epithelium, there is laryngeal closure, both in man and experimental animals (77, 95). Stronger stimulations also inhibit breathing and cause reflex hypertension, bradycardia, bronchoconstriction, and tracheal mucus secretion. The analogy of these responses with diving reflex is clear; the organism is protected until asphyxial blood gas changes become dangerous.

With stronger stimuli, in particular discrete mechanical stimulation with a catheter to the vocal folds, a short expiratory effort without preceding inspiration is elicited (96, 97). This has been studied by Korpas and his colleagues (97), who call it the "expiration reflex," and its function is the vigorous explusion of a potential laryngeal obstruction. This reflex, unlike the cough, is resistant to general anesthesia and is especially powerful in the newborn. It is active in man and is enhanced in inflammatory conditions of the laryngeal mucosa (97). Reflex laryngeal constriction occurs simultaneously.

Even stronger stimuli to the larynx cause coughing, characterized by an initial inspiratory effort before the expulsive expiration against a closed glottis (97, 98).

In view of the diversity of types of receptor, fiber discharge patterns, and reflex responses seen when the laryngeal mucosa is stimulated, it is not surprising that the roles of the different receptor groups in the various reflexes have not yet been worked out. Probably in most forms of laryngeal stimulation, the total reflex and sensory responses are due to the interaction of all the receptor systems.

Tracheobronchial Tree

Physiological responses to inhaled particles and gases depend on the site of deposition. The large airways have a dense cholinergic bronchoconstrictor innervation and receive their blood from the bronchial arteries. Irritation of their mucosa causes constriction of the larger, proximal airways where most of the lower airway resistance resides, and sometimes an increase in functional residual capacity; however, lung compliance does not change. The smaller, peripheral airways have a large total cross-sectional area and little innervation and receive their blood from the pulmonary artery. Irritation of their mucosa causes constriction of the bronchioles and smaller airways, with a decrease in lung compliance. Reflex changes in breathing are different from the trachea compared with the bronchi. In addition, in healthy lung, only the large airways have submucous glands.

Mucociliary Clearance

Secretory Mechanisms   Mucus is produced both from goblet cells and from submucosal glands. Both types of structure are found throughout the upper respiratory tract and in the trachea and larger bronchi, but goblet cells are absent where there is stratified squamous cell epithelium (i.e., in the nasopharynx, pharynx, and vocal folds). The submucosal glands contain both serous and mucous cells and are under parasympathetic cholinergic nervous control (99). Both parasympathetic nerve stimulation and parasympatholytic drugs (such as acetylcholine, pilocarpine, and methacholine) increase volume output of mucus and quantity of glycoprotein secreted, and this effect is blocked by antiacetylcholine drugs such as atropine. There is evidence that lower airway mucus secretion is also promoted by sympathetic activity, β-receptor adrenergic, at least in the cat (83). All these physiological results are based on nerve stimulation and pharmacological experiments. Total output of mucus or its constituents has usually been measured, and it is sometimes difficult to be sure whether the secretion is coming from goblet cells as well as from mucous glands.

Lower airway mucus secretion is enhanced by a number of reflexes, in particular, by irritation of the nose, nasopharynx, larynx, and tracheal bifurcation (82, 89), including the anatomical site of secretion itself. This secretion might help in removing invading substances and structures from the site of invasion or proximal to it (i.e., on the mouth side). Interestingly, irritants inhaled deep into the lungs do not cause reflex secretion of mucus from the trachea unless they cause coughing; similarly, stimulation of alveolar J receptors, which normally respond to pathological changes at the alveolar level, does not promote tracheal mucus secretion (89).

Apart from the nervous control of respiratory tract mucus secretion, mucus output can be promoted directly by a large number of agents brought into contact with the mucosa (99). These include mechanical and many chemical irritations and several drugs, not all of which are cholinergic. The relative parts played by submucous glands and by goblet cells are unclear.

The control of airway goblet cell secretion has been studied by taking advantage of the fact that birds have only goblet cells in their tracheas and no submucosal glands. Recent work by Richardson and Phipps et al. (100) has established that the goblet cells have a parasympathetic cholinergic innervation.

There have been extensive studies both on the chemistry of respiratory tract mucus and on its rheological properties, both in healthy and diseased animals and man (e.g., 101, 102). Some aspects of the chemistry of mucus will be mentioned in later sections. The significance of changes in the chemical and mechanical properties of mucus in the defense of the respiratory system is at present highly speculative, but the research may be providing the background for future understanding of the subject.

Mucociliary Transport   Ciliated cells are found in the epithelium of the nose and of all parts of the lower airways as far as the bronchioles. Their proportion to other epithelial cells varies with site and possibly with species, being greatest in the bronchioles (65%) and least in the upper trachea (17%) (103). The cilia are about 6 μm long and 0.3 μm wide. They have a pendular motion, the forward stroke being 2–3 times faster than the recovery stroke (104). Iravani and Melville (105) have studied the relationships between ciliary amplitude and beat frequency and the localization in the bronchial tree of the isolated rat lung. Beat frequency increases from terminal bronchioles (ca. 400 beats min^{-1}) to trachea (ca. 1,000 beats min^{-1}); beat amplitude increases from 1.2 μm distally to 10.1 μm proximally. Thus, one would expect transport velocity to increase as mucus moves up the tracheobronchial tree, and this has been established; in bronchioles the velocity is 0.6 mm min^{-1} and, in the trachea, 10.1 mm min^{-1}. All these values apply to the healthy rat. They are qualitatively consistent with the fact that total circumferencial length of the airways decreases many hundredfold from bronchioles to trachea, so that any mucus sheet would need a faster transport velocity in the large airways than in the smaller to prevent accumulation (106). Of course, this argument takes no account of the different degrees of activity of secretory tissues at different levels, there being no mucus glands in the smaller bronchi and many in the trachea; nor of the possibility that mucus or its constituents may be absorbed in transit. It may seem surprising that the proportion of ciliated cells is lower in the larger airways compared with the smaller airways. There are many mysteries yet to be solved concerning the history of respiratory tract secretions on their passage from bronchioles to larynx.

The cilia beat in what is thought to be a low viscosity fluid, through which the tips of the cilia project to touch thick mucus. Little is known of the origin and composition of this interciliary liquid, mainly due to difficulties of collection and analysis. Ciliary beat is coordinated so that each row of cilia moves forward a brief time interval out of phase with the next row, so that a wave appears to travel along the epithelial surface. The direction of stroke of the ciliary beat often does not coincide with the direction of the wave (105, 107). In the intact airways, the ciliated cells seem to be divided into irregular "metachronal fields," with coordinated activity of cells in each field largely independent of neighboring fields (108). Although ciliary beat can have different directions in different fields, the total effect in the bronchi is that mucus flows axially except at points of branching. Here the direction of flow becomes oblique to merge with the mainstream at an acute angle.

In the lower airways, mucus forms as plaques or small platelets, and these only become large in the cartilaginous bronchi when the submucous glands are present (109). The particles of mucus may be as small as 4 μm in diameter, but conglomeration takes place to form stable plaques which become large in the proximal airways. At least in the healthy rat airways, there is no such structure as a "mucus blanket," but one can be induced by use of drugs such as pilocarpine which stimulate mucus secretion. The plaques of mucus are transported in rather irregular directions and at various speeds, even in the same part of the airway.

Mucociliary transport is affected by the chemistry of the liquid in the airways. It is not greatly influenced by pH changes in the range 6.5–8.5, but decreases considerably at pH values less than 6.5 (110), a value which can occur in the nose (111). Doubling or halving the normal osmolality of airway fluid depresses or even stops ciliary movement (105). It is not known if these effects of pH or osmolality can be important in disease or in therapy with aerosols. Decreasing air humidity to below 70% can inhibit ciliary movement, and even lower humidities can abolish it. Ciliary beat frequency increases at temperatures of 40–42°C, but decreases or stops if temperatures go above 42°C, at which temperature ultrastructural changes have been seen in the cilia (112). Body temperatures over 42°C can occur in human hyperthermia. Lowering temperature has less marked effects, most studies suggesting that beat frequency is approximately halved at a temperature of 20°C. The relevance of changes in temperature and humidity on respiratory ciliary activity is doubtful, because the nose is such an efficient air conditioner (56). However, quantitative studies on human nasal mucociliary clearance in this context do not seem to have been done.

Inevitably, much research has been done on the effect of tobacco smoke on mucociliary function. Nearly all authors agree that tobacco smoke has considerable inhibitory effects, including depression of ciliary movement, loss of coordination of cilia, reversal of direction of transport, and depression of airway mucus velocity (105, 113, 114). The fact that tobacco smoke also promotes mucus secretion complicates the picture, and at least one study has suggested that total lung clearance is not affected by smoking (115). Possibly, the cough reflex compensates for damage to the mucociliary defenses.

A long list of drugs have been tested on respiratory mucociliary function, and the effect of only a few will be mentioned here (see 99, 105). Ciliary movement of mucus transport is increased by catecholamines (including β receptor stimulants), acetylcholine and nicotine, and depressed α and β receptor blockers, atropinic drugs, and promazine. Both increases and decreases in mucociliary activity have been reported for 5-hydroxytryptamine and histamine. Some of the differences in results may depend upon the use of different methods of study; ciliary beat frequency, mucus flow rates, and respiratory system clearance are all different and important aspects of the complete mucociliary clearance system.

Immune Responses and Antimicrobial Defenses Mast cells can be identified in the epithelium of the bronchi (116), as well as in submucosal tissue (117).

They can be extracted by brush biopsy of human and monkey airways (34, 35) and can be degranulated by appropriate antigen challenge. Similarly, lymphocytes can be washed from the lungs of animals and probably come from the lower respiratory tract rather than from the alveoli, where such cells have not been seen. Lymphocytes from animals sensitized by an aerosol of antigen contain antibodies and a macrophage antimigratory factor. The epithelium of the bronchial mucosa also contains apparently secretory cells for which the function and mediators are unknown; these include Kultschitzky and AFG cells (118). Thus, the mucosa, including the epithelial layer, contain some of the cell types which might underlie an allergen-antibody reaction and release bioactive mediators.

Specific antigens can be shown to release histamine and slow-reacting substance (SRS-A) from isolated lung tissues (119–122), and it has been proposed that these and similar mediators act on airway smooth muscle to cause the constriction seen in allergic bronchial asthma. An alternative possibility is that the mediators act on "irritant" receptors in the epithelium which set up a reflex bronchoconstriction (55, 123–125). Possibly both mechanisms play a part.

Defenses against microbial invasion have been studied for the lungs, but usually it is not easy to say whether the defensive reactions are bronchial or alveolar or both. The alveolar macrophages may be mainly responsible for killing microorganisms, but similar macrophages occur in the tracheobronchial mucosa. The role of macrophages will be considered later in this chapter.

Reflex Responses   Light microscopy shows nerve fibers entering and ramifying in the epithelium of the airways, from trachea to the bronchioles (86). Those in the larger airways are afferent in function; this conclusion is supported by histochemical and electron microscopic studies. Electron microscopy shows afferent nerve fibers on the luminal side of the basement membrane (126, 127). Many appear in cross section about 1 μm from the luminal surface of the epithelium, usually with structures resembling desmosomes or tight junctions just outside. The nerves are concentrated at the hilum of the lungs and at the tracheal bifurcation, which distribution agrees with the physiological evidence that they are afferent and "irritant" receptors. Their inclusions support an afferent function.

The receptors seen microscopically probably correspond to the cough and lung "irritant" receptors studied by single fiber recording. They have the highest concentration in the trachea and the large bronchi near the hilum of the lung (74, 86). The receptors are stimulated by intraluminal irritants, gases, or aerosols, acting chemically or mechanically. These include "inert" carbon dust, cigarette smoke, and a range of chemicals. The susceptibility of the receptors varies greatly between sites, between irritants, and between receptors (128).

Irritant receptors are also stimulated or sensitized by changes in the mechanical properties of the airway wall underlying the receptor site. Thus, those in the lungs and trachea are stimulated by contraction of airway smooth muscle (129) and sensitized by decreases in lung compliance which lead to greater mechanical pull on the airways during the respiratory cycle (130). This behavior may be especially important in acute experimental lung diseases, such as bronchocon-striction, microembolism, anaphylaxis, congestion, and edema, each of which stimulates lung irritant receptors; presumably, the stimulation contributes to or causes reflex changes in breathing and other variables seen in these conditions. In this respect, it is important that tracheobronchial irritant receptors are stim-ulated by anaphylactic reactions in the lungs (130) and by inhalation of histamine aerosols (128, 131, 132).

Stimulation of irritant receptors in the tracheal epithelium (cough receptors) causes coughing, hypertension, laryngeal constriction, bronchoconstriction, and tracheal mucus secretion (74, 92).

Coughing from the trachea is sensitized in experimental inflammation of the respiratory tract, but severe epithelial damage may abolish the cough reflex (97). The action of mucus either in stimulating coughing or in protecting cough receptors from inhaled irritants requires investigation.

Irritant receptors within the lungs do not seem to cause coughing, because those conditions which stimulate them vigorously cause hyperpnea rather than coughing (74, 133). They are probably responsible for the hyperventilation seen on inhalation of irritant gases and aerosols and for the deep augmented breaths which open up collapsed lung (130). However, the isolated respiratory response to activation of lung irritant receptors is still controversial.

The role of laryngeal closure in coughing induced from the tracheobronchial tree is presumably the same as that already described for coughing from the larynx. Tracheostomized patients do not seem to be at a disadvantage through the lack of a laryngeal component in coughing, and some doubt has been thrown on the importance of laryngeal closure in the aerodynamics of coughing (134).

Irritation of the lungs also causes expiratory constrictions of the larynx, together with the hyperpnea (135). The functional significance of this laryngeal reflex has not been established, but it might increase the duration of expiration and functional residual capacity and thereby promote gas exchange in the lungs. The importance of expiratory resistance to air flow in the larynx has recently been emphasized in relation to its effect on the pattern of breathing (136).

Inhalation of dusts, smokes, irritant gases, and aerosols causes reflex bronchoconstriction when the agent is restricted to the lungs and tracheo-bronchial tree (80). The constriction is slow and long lasting in relation to the stimulus and lacks respiratory phase. The advantage of this bronchoconstriction has been debated. It would increase the rigidity of the airways and thus render them less liable to collapse in the vigorous movements of coughing or hyperpnea (137). The constriction might increase the impaction and absorption of aerosols and gases in the lower airway, thus protecting the alveoli (138). In theory, anatomical dead space ventilation should decrease, but this effect is offset by the increase in physiological dead space due to uneven distribution of inspired air (139).

The possibility that stimulation of irritant receptors in the lungs may underlie the bronchoconstriction of allergic asthma has already been mentioned.

The increase in secretion of mucus in the respiratory tract when irritant gases and aerosols are inhaled into the lungs can be shown to be at least in part a reflex, although direct action by the irritant is also important (89).

Alveoli

Antimicrobial Defenses Particles larger than 10 μm in diamter do not usually reach the alveoli, and most particles that are there are less than 2 μm in diameter. These are ingested by alveolar macrophages and eliminated via the trachea, although some particles may enter the lung tissue directly and be taken up into the lymph stream. It is doubtful whether macrophages can re-enter the lung tissue after ingesting material in the alveoli (140, 141). With the use of lung lavage, Brain (140) has calculated that there are 3–15 $\times$ 10^6 macrophages/g of lung tissue in man, or about 16 macrophages per alveolus. The turnover time of alveolar macrophages is about 24 hr, i.e., the same number of macrophages in the lungs at any time appears in the tracheal mucociliary transport each day (142). Nearly all alveolar macrophages come from the bone marrow (143), probably traveling as macrophage precursors (monocytes) and maturing in the alveolar wall (144). Thus, the macrophages which ingest microorganisms in the alveoli come from the alveolar wall and not the blood stream (145). There is a correlation between alveolar macrophage number and both resistance to infection and clearance of particulate matter from the lungs (141). Alveolar macrophage counts increase in response to inhalation of bacteria or inert dusts (146, 147).

Alveolar macrophages kill ingested microorganisms, and this is their main defensive role, rather than removal of live organisms. Labeled, inhaled bacteria in mice are almost entirely killed within 4 hr, but almost all of the label, now presumably on dead bacteria or debris, remains in the lungs after that time (148, 149).

Alveolar macrophages are inhibited by hypoxia, cold, cigarette smoke, and the presence of viruses (150). They are also inhibited by a factor released from lymphocytes in antigen-antibody reactions, but the factor is different from the antimigration factor that acts on macrophages elsewhere (151). This and other results suggest that the alveolar macrophage differs in important respects from macrophages in other tissues.

Reflex Responses Receptors with nonmyelinated afferent nerve fibers have been identified in the alveolar wall (152, 153). They have been studied extensively by Paintal (85, 154), who has shown that they are stimulated by inhalation of irritant gases such as chlorine, ammonia, ethyl ether, and halothane, as well as by alveolar interstitial edema. They are called "juxta-pulmonary capillary receptors" or J receptors. They probably resemble nociceptive endings with nonmyelinated fibers seen in other viscera.

Excitation of J receptors causes apnea and rapid shallow breathing in cat and man, whereas rabbits show also a large increase in functional residual capacity (85, 92). During the apnea, there is laryngeal closure, hypotension, and bradycardia. All these changes are a vagal reflex. Bronchomotor changes are not prominent, but there is a long lasting inhibition of skeletal muscular tone and of the stretch reflex (85).

It is not clear to what extent J receptors play a part in the defensive responses to inhaled irritants, although the overall pattern of reflex responses has similarities to the diving reflex and might be thought to prevent further entry of an irritant into the respiratory system. However, few irritant gases when inhaled set up the particular pattern of reflexes described for J receptors, and presumably most act on respiratory tract receptors before they reach the alveolar level.

REFERENCES

1. Alarie, Y. (1973). Sensory irritation by airborne chemicals. C.R.C. Crit. Rev. Toxicol. 299.
2. Henderson, Y., and Haggard, H. W. (1943). Noxious Gases and The Principles of Respiration Influencing Their Action. Reinhold, New York.
3. Stupfel, M., and Mordelet-Dambrine, M. (1974). Penetration of pollutants in the airways. Bull. Physiopathol. Respir. 10:481.
4. Brain, J. D. (1970). Uptake of inhaled gases by the nose. Ann. Otol. Rhinol. Laryngol. 79:529.
5. Speizer, F. E., and Frank, N. R. (1966). The uptake and release of SO_2 by the human nose. Arch. Environ. Health 12:725.
6. Andersen, I., Lundqvist, G. R., Jensen, P. L., and Proctor, D. F. (1974). Human response to controlled levels of sulfur dioxide. Arch. Environ. Health 28:31.
7. Peters, R. A. (1963). Biochemical Lesions and Lethal Synthesis. Pergamon Press, Oxford.
8. Bacq, Z. M. (1946). Substances thioloprives. Experientia 2:349.
9. Dixon, M. (1948). Reactions of lachrymators with enzymes and proteins. In R. T. Williams (ed.), Symposium on the Biochemical Reactions of Chemical Warfare Agents. Biochemical Society Symposium No. 2, p. 39. University Press, Cambridge.
10. Dixon, M., and Needham, D. M. (1946). Biochemical research on chemical warfare agents. Nature 158:432.
11. Alarie, Y., Wakisaka, I., and Oka, S. (1973). Sensory irritation by sulfur dioxide and chlorobenzylidene malononitrile. Environ. Physiol. Biochem. 3:53.
12. Alarie, Y., Wakisaka, I., and Oka, S. (1973). Sensory irritation by sulfite aerosols. Environ. Physiol. Biochem. 3:
13. Parker, A. J., and Kharasch, N. (1959). The scission of the sulfur-sulfur bond. Chem. Rev. 59:583.
14. Roy, A. B., and Trudinger, P. A. (1970). The Biochemistry of Inorganic Compounds of Sulphur. University Press, Cambridge.
15. Sobrino, J. A., and Del Castillo, G. (1972). Activation of the cholinergic end plate receptors by oxidizing reagents. Int. J. Neurosci. 3:251.
16. First, M. W. (1973). Aerosols in nature. Arch. Intern. Med. 131:24.

17. Study of man's impact on climate (SMIC). (1971). *In* Inadvertent Climate Modification, p. 308. MIT Press, Cambridge, Massachusetts.

18. Stuart, B. O. (1973). Deposition of inhaled aerosols. Arch. Intern. Med. 131:60.

19. Hatch, T., and Gross, P. (1964). Pulmonary Deposition and Retention of Inhaled Aerosols. Academic Press, New York.

20. Hoehne, J. H., and Reed, C. E. (1971). Where is the allergic reaction in ragweed asthma? J. Allergy Clin. Immunol. 48:36.

21. Hobday, J. D., and Townley, R. G. (1971). Deposition of inhaled pollen grains in the lower respiratory tract of the guinea pig. J. Allergy Clin. Immunol. 48:254.

22. VanHouten, P. D., Hashimoto, B., and Wilson, A. F. (1973). A technique for intense radiolabeling of pollen and pollen extract with ^{99}mTc. J. Allergy Clin. Immunol. 52:115.

23. Wilson, A. F., Novey, H. S., Berke, R. A., and Surprenant, E. L. (1973). Deposition of inhaled pollen and pollen extract in human airways. N. Engl. J. Med. 288:1056.

24. Busse, W. W., Reed, C. E., and Hoehne, J. H. (1972). Where is the allergic reaction in ragweed asthma? II. Demonstration of ragweed antigen in airborne particles smaller than pollen. J. Allergy Clin. Immunol. 50:289.

25. Trimbell, V. (1965). The inhalation of fibrous dusts. Ann. N. Y. Acad. Sci. 132:255.

26. Trimbrell, V., Pooley, F., and Wagner, J. C. (1970). Characteristics of respirable asbestos fibres, *In* H. A. Shapiro (ed.), Pneumoconiosis: Proceedings of the International Conference, p. 120. Oxford University Press, Capetown.

27. Wilson, I. B., and LaMer, V. K. (1948). The retension of aerosol particles in the human respiratory tract as a function of particle radius. J. Ind. Hyg. Toxicol. 30:265.

28. Beeckmans, J. M. (1972). Deposition of ellipsoidal particles in the human respiratory tract. *In* T. T. Mercer, P. E. Morrow and W. Stöber (eds.), Assessment of Airborne Particles, p. 361. Thomas, Springfield, Illinois.

29. Denis, W. L. (1971). The effect of breathing rate on the deposition of particles in the human respiratory system. *In* W. Walton (ed.), Inhaled Particles and Vapours, Vol. III, pp. 1, 91. Gresham, Surrey.

30. DuBois, A. B., and Dautrebande, L. (1958). Acute effects of breathing inert dust particles and of carbachol aerosol on the mechanical characteristics of the lungs in man. Changes in response after inhaling sympathomimetic aerosols. J. Clin. Invest. 37:1746.

31. Goldberg, I. S., and Lourenco, R. V. (1973). Deposition of aerosols in pulmonary disease. Arch. Intern. Med. 131:88.

32. Macklem, P. T., Hogg, W. E., and Brunton, J. (1973). Peripheral airway obstruction and particulate deposition in the lung. Arch. Intern. Med. 131:93.

33. Tada, T., and Ishizaka, K. (1970). Distribution of gamma E-forming cells in lymphoid tissues of the human and monkey. J. Immunol. 104:377.

34. Patterson, R., Head, L. R., Suszko, I. M., and Zeiss, C. R., Jr. (1972). Mast cells from human respiratory tissues and their in vitro reactivity. Science 175:1012.

35. Patterson, R., Suszko, I. M., and Zeiss, C. R., Jr. (1972). Reactions of primate respiratory mast cells. J. Allergy Clin. Immunol. 50:7.

36. Austen, K. G. (1973). A review of immunological, biochemical and pharmacological factors in the release of chemical mediators from human

8777887878878787878778787

87878787887878

lung. *In* K. F. Austen and L. M. Lichtenstein (eds.), Asthma: Physiology Immunopharmacology and Treatment, p. 109. Academic Press, New York.

37. McCombs, R. P. (1972). Disease due to immunologic reactions in the lungs. N. Engl. J. Med. 286:1186.

38. Lichtenstein, L. M. (1973). The control of IgE-mediated histamine release: implications for the study of asthma. *In* K. F. Austen and L. M. Lechtenstein (eds.), Asthma: Physiology, Immunopharmacology and treatment, Academic Press, New York.

39. Negus, V. E. (1958). Comparative Anatomy of the Nose and Paranasal Sinuses. E. & S. Livingstone, Edinburgh.

40. Proctor, D. F., Andersen, I., and Lundqvist, G. (1973). Clearance of inhaled particles from the human nose. Arch. Intern. Med. 131:132.

41. Ingelstedt, S. (1956). Studies on the conditioning of air in the respiratory tract. Acta Otorinolaryngol. Belg. Suppl. 131:1.

42. Burton, P. A., and Dizon, M. F. (1969). A comparison of changes in the mucous glands and goblet cells of nasal, sinus, and bronchial mucosa. Thorax 24:180.

43. Drettner, B. (1963). Blood vessel reactions in the nasal mucosa. Int. Rhinol. 1:40.

44. Dawes, J. D. K., and Prichard, M. M. L. (1953). Studies of the vascular arrangements of the nose. J. Anat. 87:311.

45. Dahlstrom, A., and Fuxe, K. (1965). The adrenergic innervation of the nasal mucosa of certain mammals, Acta Otorhinolaryngol. 59:65.

46. Rooker, D. W., and Jackson, R. T. (1969). The effects of certain drugs, cervical sympathetic stimulation and section on nasal patency. Ann. Otol. Rhinol. Laryngol. 78:403.

47. Ishi, T., and Toriyama, M. (1972). Acetylcholinesterase activity in the vasomotor and secretory fibers of the nose. Arch. Klin. Exp. Ohren Nasen Kehlkopfheilkd, 201:1.

48. Davis, D. L., and Hertzman, A. B. (1957). The analysis of vascular reactions in the nasal mucosa with the photoelectric plethysmograph. Ann. Otol. Rhinol. Laryngol. 66:

49. Malcolmson, K. G. (1959). The vasomotor activities of the nasal mucous membranes. J. Laryngol. Otol. 73:73.

50. Balchum, O. J., Dylincki, J., and Meneely, G. R. (1959). Absorption and distribution of $^{35}SO_2$ inhaled through the nose and mouth by dogs. Am. J. Physiol. 197:1317.

51. Frank, N. R., Yodder, R. E., Yokoyama, E., and Speizer, F. E. (1967). The diffusion of $^{35}SO_2$ from tissue fluids into the lungs following exposure of dogs to $^{35}SO_2$. Health Phys. 13:31.

52. Hilding, A. C., and Filipi, A. N. (1966). A method of determining nasal filtration of cigarette smoke: application and results in guinea pigs, anesthetized and soon after death. Ann. Otol. Rhinol. Laryngol. 75:714.

53. Ishii, T. (1970). The cholinergic innervation of the human nasal mucosa. Pract. Otorhinolaryngol. 32:153.

54. Eccles, R., and Wilson, H. (1973). The parasympathetic secretory nerves of the nose of the cat. J. Physiol. 230:213.

55. Cohen, A. B., and Gold, W. M. (1975). Defense mechanisms of the lungs. Ann. Rev. Physiol. 37:325.

56. Proctor, D. F., and Adams, G. K. Physiology and pharmacology of nasal function and mucus secretion. Pharm. Ther. B, in press.

57. Bang, B. G., and Bang, F. B. (1963). Responses of upper respiratory mucosae to deydration and infection. Ann. N. Y. Acad. Sci. 106:625.
58. Proctor, D. F., Andersen, I., Lundqvist, G., and Swift, D. L. (1973). Nasal mucociliary function and the indoor climate. J. Occup. Med. 15:169.
59. Proctor, D. F., Aharonson, E. F., Reasor, M. J., and Bucklen, K. (1973). A method for study of normal respiratory mucus. Bull. Physiopathol. Respir. 9:315.
60. Andersen, I., Lundqvist, G., and Proctor, D. F. (1971). Human nasal mucosal function in a controlled climate. Arch Environ. Health 23:408.
61. Andersen, I., Lundqvist, G. R., and Proctor, D. F. (1972). Human nasal mucosal function under four controlled humidities. Am. Rev. Respir. Dis. 106:438.
62. Andersen, I., Lunqvist, G. R., and Proctor, D. F. (1974). Human response to 78 hours exposure to dry air. Arch. Environ. Health 20:319.
63. Gottschalk, A. (1960). Correlation between composition, structure, shape, and function of a salivary mucoprotein. Nature 186:949.
64. Cate, T. R., Douglas, R. G., Jr., and Couch, R. B. (1969). Interferon and resistance to upper respiratory virus illness. Proc. Soc. Exp. Biol. Med. 131:631.
65. Cate, T. R., Rossen, R. D., Douglas, R. G., Jr., Butler, W. T., and Couch, R. B. (1966). The role of nasal secretion and serum antibody in the rhinovirus common cold. Am. J. Epidemiol. 84:352.
66. Buler, W. T., Waldman, T. A., Rossen, R. D., Douglas, R. G., Jr., and Couch, R. B. (1970). Changes in IgA and IgG concentrations in nasal secretions prior to the appearance of antibody during viral respiratory infection in man. J. Immunol. 105:584.
67. Rossen, R. D., Butler, W. T., Cate, T. R., Szwed, C. F., and Couch, R. B. (1965). Protein composition of nasal secretions during respiratory virus infection. Proc. Soc. Exp. Biol. Med. 119:1169.
68. Rossen, R. D., Schade, A. L., Butler, W. T., and Kasel, J. A. (1966). The proteins in nasal secretions: a longitudinal study of the γ A-globulin, γ G-globulin, albumin, sederophilin, and total protein concentrations in nasal washing from adult male volunteers. J. Clin. Invest. 45:768.
69. Samter, M., and Becker, E. L. (1947). Ragweed reagins in nasal secretion. Proc. Soc. Exp. Biol. Med. 65:140.
70. Tomasi, T. B., and Grey, H. M. (1972). Structure and function of immunoglobulin A. Prog. Allergy 16:81.
71. Graziadei, P. P. C. (1971). The olfactory mucosa of vertebrates. In L. M. Beidler (ed.), Handbook of Sensory Physiology, Vol. IV, Chemical Senses, Part 1, p. 27. Springer-Verlag, Heidelberg.
72. But, V. I., and Klimova-Cherkasova, V. I. (1967). Afferentiation from upper respiratory tract. Bull. Exp. Biol. Med. 64:13.
73. Cauna, N., Hinderer, K. H., and Wentges, R. T. (1969). Sensory receptor organs of the human nasal respiratory mucosa. Am. J. Anat. 14:295.
74. Widdicombe, J. G. Respiratory reflexes and defense. In J. D. Brain, D. F. Proctor, and L. Reid (eds.), Respiratory Defense Mechanisms, Vol. 1. Marcel Dekker, New York. In press.
75. Angell-James, J., and Daly, M. de B. (1969). Nasal reflexes. Proc. R. Soc. Med. 62:1287.
76. Angell-James, J. E., and Daly, M. de B. (1972). Some mechanisms included in the cardiovascular adaptations to diving. Symp. Soc. Exp. Biol. 62:313.
77. Szereda-Przestaszewska, M., and Widdicombe, J. G. (1973). Reflex effects

of chemical irritation on the upper airways on the laryngeal lumen in cats. Respir. Physiol. 18:107.

78. Tomori, Z., and Widdicombe, J. G. (1969). Muscular, bronchomotor and cardiovascular reflexes elicited by mechanical stimulation of the respiratory tract. J. Physiol. 200:25.

79. Allison, J. V., and Powis, D. A. (1971). Adrenal catecholamine secretion during stimulation of the nasal mucous membrane in the rabbit. J. Physiol. 217:327.

80. Widdicombe, J. G. (1963). Regulation of tracheobronchial smooth muscle. Physiol. Rev. 43:1.

81. Daly, M. de Burgh (1972). Interaction of cardiovascular reflexes. Sci. Basis Med. 307.

82. Florey, H., Carleton, H. M., and Wells, A. Q. (1932). Mucus secretion in the trachea. Q. J. Exp. Pathol. 13:269.

83. Gallagher, J. T., Kent, P. W., Passatore, M., Phipps, R. J., and Richardson, P. S. (1975). The composition of tracheal mucus and the nervous control of its secretion in the cat. Proc. R. Soc. Lond. Biol. 192:49.

84. Andersen, P. (1954). Inhibitory reflexes elicited from the trigeminal and olfactory nerves in rabbits. Acta Physiol. Scand. 30:137.

85. Deshpande, S. S., and Devanandan, M. S. (1970). Reflex inhibition of monosynaptic reflexes by stimulation of type-J pulmonary endings. J. Physiol. 206:345.

86. Fillenz, M., and Widdicombe, J. G. (1971). Receptors of the lungs and airways, In E. Neil (ed.), Handbook of Sensory Physiology, Vol. 3, p. 81. Springer-Verlag, Heidelberg.

87. Nail, B. S., Sterling, G. M., and Widdicombe, J. G. (1969). Epipharyngeal receptors responding to mechanical stimulation. J. Physiol. 204:91.

88. Ivanco, I., Korpas, J., and Tomori, Z. (1956). Ein Beitrag zur Interozeption der Luftwege. Physiol. Bohemoslov. 5:84.

89. Phipps, J. J., and Richardson, P. S. The effects of irritation at various levels of the airway upon tracheal mucus secretion in the cat. J. Physiol. 261:563.

90. Corbett, J. L., Kerr, J. A. Prys-Roberts, C., Crampton-Smith, A., and Spalding, J. M. K. (1969). Cardiovascular disturbances in severe tetanus due to overactivity of the sympathetic nervous system. Anaesthesia 24:198.

91. Pressman, J. J., and Kelemen, G. (1955). Physiology of the larynx. Physiol. Rev. 34:506.

92. Widdicombe, J. G. (1964). Respiratory reflexes. In Handbook of Physiology, Section 3, Respiration, Vol. 1, p. 585. American Physiology Society, Washington, D.C.

93. Van Michel, C. (1963). Considerations morphologiques sur les appareils sensoriels de la muqueuse vocale humaine. Acta Anat. 52:188.

94. Boushey, H. A., Richardson, P. S., Widdicombe, J. G., and Wise, J. C. M. (1974). The response of laryngeal afferent fibres to mechanical and chemical stimuli. J. Physiol. 240:153.

95. Hinkle, J. E., and Tantum, K. R. (1971). A technique for measuring reactivity of the glottis. Anesthesiology 35:634.

96. Korpas, J. (1972). Differentiation of the expiration and the cough reflex. Physiol. Bohemoslov. 21:677.

97. Korpas, J., and Tomori, Z. (1975). Cough and other Respiratory Reflexes. Slovakiarn Academy of Science, Bratislava.

98. Boushey, H. A., Richardson, P. S., and Widdicombe, J. G. (1972). Reflex

effects of laryngeal irritation on the pattern of breathing and total lung resistance. J. Physiol. 224:501.

99. Richardson, P. S., and Phipps, R. J. The anatomy, physiology, pharmocology and pathology of tracheobronchial mucus secretion and the use of expectorant drugs in human disease. Pharmacol. Therap. B., in press.

100. Phipps, R. J., Richardson, P. S., Corfield, A., Gallagher, J. T., Jeffery, P. J., Kent, P. W., and Passatore, M. A physiological, biochemical and histological study of goose tracheal mucin and its secretion. Philos. Trans. R. Soc. Lond., in press.

101. Litt, M. (1973). Basic concepts of mucus rheology. Bull. Physiol. Pathol. Respir. 9:33.

102. Keal, E. (1971). Biochemistry and rheology of sputum in asthma. Postgrad. Med. J. 47:171.

103. Jeffery, P. K., and Reid, L. (1975). New observations of rat airway epithelium: a quantitative and electron microscopic study. J. Anat. 120:295.

104. Dalhamn, T. (1956). Mucous flow and ciliary activity in the trachea of healthy rats and rats exposed to respiratory irritant gasses (SO_2, H_3N and HCHO). Acta Physiol. Scand. Suppl. 123, 36:1.

105. Iravani, J., and Melville, G. N. Mucociliary function in the respiratory tract as influenced by physiochemical factors. Pharmacol. Therap. B., in press.

106. Hilding, A. C. (1965). Mucociliary insufficiency and its possible relation to chronic bronchitis and emphysema. Med. Thorac. 22:329.

107. Sleigh, M. A. (1962). The Biology of Cilia and Flagella. Pergamon Press, Oxford.

108. Iravani, J. (1969). Zum Mechanismus der Ortsäbhangigkeit der Flimmeraktivität im Bronchialbaum. Naunyn Schmiedebergs Arch. Exp. Pathol. Pharmakol. 264:248.

109. Iravani, J., and Van As, A. (1972). Mucus transport in the tracheobronchial tree of normal and bronchitic rats. J. Pathol. 106:81.

110. Antweiler, H. (1956). Über die Funktion des Flimmerepithels der Luftwege, insbesondere unter Staubbelastung. Beitr. Silikoseforsch. 2:509.

111. Fabrikant, N. D. (1941). Significance of the pH of nasal secretions in situ. Arch. Otolaryngol. 34:297.

112. Mecklenburg, C., van Mercke, U., Häckansson, C. H., and Toremalm, N. G. (1974). Morphological changes in ciliary cells due to heat exposure. Cell Tissue Res. 148:45.

113. Iravani, J., and Melville, G. N. (1974). Long term effect of cigarette smoking on mucociliary function in animals. Respiration 31:350.

114. Iravani, J., and Melville, G. N. (1974). Mucociliäre Funktion und Inhalation des Zigarettenrauches. Pneumonologie 149:211.

115. Pavia, D., Short, M. D., and Thomson, M. L. (1970). No demonstrable long term effects of cigarette smoking on the ciliary mechanism of the human lung. Nature 226:1228.

116. Salvato, G. (1976). Mechanism of the asthma attack. Br. Med. J. 2:179.

117. Salvato, G. (1961). Mast cells in bronchial connective tissues in man: their modification in asthma and after treatment with histamine liberator. Int. Arch. Appl. Immunol. 18:348.

118. Thurlbeck, W. M., and Wang, N. S. (1974). The structure of the lungs. In J. G. Widdicombe (ed.), MTP International Review of Science, Physiology Series I, Respiratory Physiology I, University Park Press, Baltimore.

119. Brocklehurst, W. E. (1960). The release of histamine and formation of a

slow-reacting substance (SRS-A) during anaphlyactic shock. J. Physiol. (Lond.) 151:416.

120. Lichtenstein, L. M., and Osler, A. G. (1964). Studies on the mechanisms of hypersensitivity phenomena. IX. Histamine release from human leukocytes by ragweed pollen antigen. J. Exp. Med. 120:507.

121. Shield, H. (1963). Histamine release and anaphylactic shock in isolated lungs of guinea pigs. Q. J. Exp. Physiol. 26:165.

122. Schild, H. O., Hawkins, D. F., Monger, J. L., and Herxheimer, H. (1951). Reactions to isolated human asthmatic lung and bronchial tissue to specific antigen-histamine release and muscular contraction. Lancet 2:376.

123. Gold, W. M. (1973). Cholinergic pharmacology in asthma. In K. F. Austen and L. M. Lichtenstein, (eds.), Asthma: Physiology, Immunopharmacology and Treatment, p. 169. Academic Press, New York.

124. Gold, W. M., Kessler, G. F., and Yu, D. Y. C. (1972). Role of vagus nerves in experimental asthma in allergic dogs. J. Appl. Physiol. 33:719.

125. Widdicombe, J. G. (1975). Reflex control of airway smooth muscle. Postgrad. Med. J. 51:36.

126. Lucieano, L., Reale, E., and Ruska, H. (1968). Uber eine 'chemorezeptive' Sinnesxelle in der Trachea der Ratte. Z. Zellforsch. Mikrosk. Anat. 85:350.

127. Jeffery, P., and Reid, L. (1973). Intra-epithelial nerves in normal rat airways: a quantitative electron microscopic study. J. Anat. 114:35.

128. Sampson, S. R., and Vidruk, E. H. (1975). Properties of "irritant" receptors in canine lung. Respir. Physiol. 25:9.

129. Mills, J., Sellick, H., and Widdicombe, J. G. (1969). The role of lung irritant receptors in respiratory responses to multiple pulmonary embolism, anaphylaxis and histamine-induced bronchoconstriction. J. Physiol. 203:337.

130. Sellick, H., and Widdicombe, J. G. (1970). Vagal deflation and inflation reflexes mediated by lung irritant receptors. Q. J. Exp. Physiol. 55:153.

131. Koller, E. A. (1973). Afferent vagal impulses in anaphylactic bronchial asthma. Acta Neurobiol. Exp. 33:51.

132. Sellick, H., and Widdicombe, J. G. (1971). Stimulation of lung irritant receptors by cigarette smoke, carbon dust and histamine aerosol. J. Appl. Physiol. 31:15.

133. Mills, J., Sellick, H., and Widdicombe, J. G. (1970). Epithelial irritant receptors in the lungs. In R. Porter (ed.), Breathing: Hering-Breuer Centenary Symposium, p. 77. Churchill, London.

134. Ross, B. B., Gramiak, R., and Rahn, H. (1955). Physical dynamics of the cough mechanism. J. Appl. Physiol. 8:264.

135. Stransky, A., Szereda-Przestaszewska, M., and Widdicombe, J. G. (1973). The effect of lung reflexes on laryngeal resistance and motoneurone discharge. J. Physiol. 231:417.

136. Bartlett, D., Jr., Remmers, J. E., and Gautier, H. (1973). Laryngeal regulation of respiratory airflow. Respir. Physiol. 18:194.

137. Palombini, B., and Coburn, R. F. (1972). Control of the compressibility of the canine trachea. Respir. Physiol. 15:365.

138. Thomson, M. L., and Short, M. D. (1969). Mucociliary function in health, chronic obstructive airway disease, and asbestosis. J. Appl. Physiol. 26:535.

139. Buff, R., and Koller, E. A. (1974). Studies on mechanisms underlying the

reflex hyperpnoea induced by inhalation of chemical irritants. Respir. Physiol. 21:271.

140. Brain, J. D. (1970). Free cells in the lungs. Some aspects of their roles, quantitation, and regulation. Arch. Intern. Med. 126:477.

141. Bowden, D. H. (1971). The alveolar macrophage. Curr. Top. Pathol. 55:1.

142. Spritzer, A. A., Watson, J. A., Auld, J. A., and Geutthoff, M. A. (1968). Pulmonary macrophage clearance: the hourly rates of transfer of pulmonary macrophages to the oropharynx of the rate. Arch. Environ. Health 17:726.

143. Brunstetter, M. A., Hardie, J. A., Schiff, R., Lewis, J. P., and Cross, C. E. (1971). The origin of pulmonary alveolar macrophages: studies of stem cells using the Es-2 marker of mice. Arch. Intern. Med. 127:1064.

144. Bowden, D. H., and Adamson, Y. R. (1972). The pulmonary interstitial cell as immediate precursor of the alveolar macrophage. Am. J. Pathol. 68:521.

145. Hung, K. S., Hertweck, M. S., and Loosli, C. G. (1972). Electron microscopic evidence for innervation of pneumocytes in mouse lung. Am. Rev. Respir. Dis. 105:1008.

146. Gaurneri, J. J., and Laurenzi, G. A. (1968). Effect of alcohol on the mobilization of alveolar macrophages. J. Lab. Clin. Med. 72:40.

147. LaBelle, C., and Brieger, H. (1961). Patterns and mechanisms in the elimination of dust from the lung. In C. N. Davies (ed.), Inhaled Particles and Vapours II, p. 350. Pergamon Press, Oxford.

148. Green, G. M. (1968). Pulmonary clearance of infectious agent. Ann. Rev. Med. 19:315.

149. Green, G. M., and Kass, E. H. (1964). The role of the alveolar macrophage in the clearance of bacteria from the lung. J. Exp. Med. 119:167.

150. Green, L. H., and Green, G. M. (1968). Differential activity as the mechanism of selection of a pathogen in mixed bacterial infection of the lung. Am. Rev. Respir. Dis. 98:819.

151. Heise, E. R., Han, S., and Weiser, R. S. (1968). In vitro studies on the mechanism of macrophage migration inhibition in tuberculin sensitivity. J. Immunol. 101:1004.

152. Meyrick, B., and Reid, L. (1971). Nerves in rat intra-acinar alveoli: an electron microscopic study. Respir. Physiol. 11:367.

153. Hung, K. S., Hertweck, M. S., Hardy, J. D., and Loosli, C. G. (1973). Electron microscopic observation of nerve endings in the alveolar walls of mouse lungs. Am. Rev. Respir. Dis. 108:328.

154. Paintal, A. S. (1969). Mechanism of stimulation of type J pulmonary receptors. J. Physiol. 203:511.

Index

Aerosols, 293–294
Airway
  expansion of, 27–28
  growth of, 15
  nerves in epithelium, 29–30
  and nonadrenergic inhibitory
    nervous system, 28–29
Altitude, high, hemoglobin function
    at, 124–126
Alveoli
  defensive mechanisms from,
    307–308
  expansion of, 19–20
  nerves in, 29–30
Anatomy, functional, of pulmonary
    vessels, 136–140
Anesthesia, effect on tidal volume,
    194–195
Apneusis, 208

Blood chemistry, complications arising
    from, 247–248
Blood flow
  pulsatile, and pulmonary capillary
    bed, 153–154
  three-zone model of distribution of,
    in pulmonary capillary bed,
    144–146
Blood-gas dissociation curves,
    numerical procedures for, 84–86
Brain stem, complexity of discharge
    patterns within, 209–210
Breathing
  basic functions of, 257–258
  control of, in diseases of the
    respiratory system, 255–290
  feedbacks, 258–265
  uncoupling of central motoneuron
    output and lung movements, 258
Breathing pattern
  adaptive phenomena, 209
  apneusis, 208
  complexity of discharge patterns
    within brain stem, 209–210
  control of, 185–217

cortical influences, 200–201
and exercise, 200
influence of pneumotaxic center,
    196–197
intercostal nerve afferents, 199
mechanisms of alteration of,
    196–201
model of expiratory off-switch,
    206–207
model of inspiratory off-switch,
    201–206
pneumotaxic center, 208–209
pulmonary receptors, 197–199
and temperature, 199

Capillaries, pulmonary, time course of
    P_{CO_2} in, 102
Capillary bed
  effects of lung inflation on, 26–27
  pulmonary, 140–154
    distension, 149–150
    effect of surface tension, 146–148
    lung inflation, 148–149
    model of blood flow distribution,
      144–146
    and pulsatile blood flow, 153–154
    recruitment, 151–153
    vascular waterfall, 140–144
Capillary membranes, alveolar,
    ultrastructure of, 167–170
Carbon dioxide
  control of hemoglobin function,
    114–115
  effect on tidal volume, 191
  ventilatory response to, 263–265
Carbon dioxide dissociation curve, 85
Carbon dioxide tension
  relation to pH, 85–86
  time course of, in pulmonary
    capillaries, 102
Chemoreceptor drive, effect of sudden
    changes in, on tidal volume, 195
Chemoreceptor stimulation,
    alternating, effect on tidal
    volume, 195–196

317

Circulation, pulmonary, 135–183
Clara cell, mystery of, 2–3

Dead space, anatomical, axial
    convection, diffusion, and,
    44–50
Defensive mechanisms of the
    respiratory system, 291–315
Diseases of the respiratory system
    control of breathing in, 255–290
    increased functional residual
    capacity, 268–271

Embryo, structure and function of
    hemoglobin, 117–122
Exercise and breathing pattern, 200
Expiration, off-switch model,
    206–207
Expiratory duration and tidal volume,
    188–196

Fetus, structure and function of
    hemoglobin, 122–124
Fick principle, solution of
    ventilation-perfusion ratio
    equation by, 87
Fluid balance, pulmonary, 135–183
Functional residual capacity,
    increased, 268–271

Gas exchange, 83–106
    additional transfer resistances,
    246–247
    air vs. water as external transport
    medium, 223–229
    blood as internal transport medium,
    223
    external, 220–229
    limitation index, 236–237
    in lung models of ventilation-
    perfusion inequality, 88–90
    in nonhomogeneous lungs, formal
    analysis of, 102–104
    in presence of highly soluble inert
    gases, 98–100
    relative partial pressure differences,
    232–236
    with series inequality, 100–102
    total conductance, 236

Gas exchange organs
    anatomy and models of, 229–231
    application of model analysis to,
    240–241
    complications due to anatomical
    arrangement of, 243–245
    functional analysis of, in vertebrates,
    219–253
    inhomogeneities, 245–246
    real systems vs. models, 243–248
Gas mixing
    axial convection, diffusion, and
    anatomical dead space, 44–50
    cardiogenic, 50–52
    during inspiration, 38–52
    in lung, 37–82
    Taylor-type dispersion, 38–44
Gas washout
    bolus studies, 71–72
    cardiogenic oscillations, 73
    inert, inter- and intraregional
    contributions to, 70–74
    irritant, 292–293
    multiple breath, 73–74
    single breath inert, 65–66, 70–73
    tidal breath studies, 72–73
Growth hormone and lung growth,
    17–18

Hemoglobin
    chemical structure, 108–110
    control of function of by allosteric
    effector molecules, 112–117
    embryonic, structure and function
    of, 117–122
    fetal, structure and function of,
    122–124
    function at high altitude, 124–126
    molecular basis for cooperative
    ligand binding, 110–111
    molecular basis of function of,
    108–112
    ontogenic aspects, 117–124
    oxygen equilibrium of, 111–112
    pathological, 126–127
    respiratory function of, 107–134
    special aspects of function, 117–127
"Hey plot," 187
Hyperoxia and lung growth, 18
Hypobaria and lung growth, 18
Hypoxia
    and local $\dot{V}_A/Q$, 161–164
    and lung growth, 18

Immune responses and antimicrobial defenses, 296
Inspiration
  gas mixing during, 38–52
  off-switch model, 201–206
Inspiratory duration and tidal volume, 188–196

Larynx, defensive mechanisms from, 300–301
Ligand binding, cooperative, molecular basis for, 110–111
Lung
  expansion of, 18–28
  gas exchange in models of ventilation-perfusion inequality, 88–90
  gas mixing and distribution in, 37–82
  growth of
    nature of, 4–15
    postnatal, 4–18
  inflation
    by alveolar enlargement and stretching, 20–23
    by alveolar recruitment or unfolding, 23–26
    effect in zone 4, 157–159
    effects on capillary bed, 26–27
    and pulmonary capillary bed, 148–149
  measurement of water in, 172–175
  and its nerves, 28–30
  resection of tissue, 16–17
  structure of, 1–36
  water balance in, 167–176
Lung volume, diminution of, 17
Lymphatic transport, 171

Molecules, allosteric effector, control of hemoglobin function by, 112–117
Morphometry of pulmonary vessels, 136–138
Mucociliary clearance, 295–296

Nasopharynx, defensive mechanisms from, 299–300
Nerves
  in alveoli and airway epithelium, 29–30
  of lung, 28–30
  vagus, influence on tidal volume and respiratory rate, 188
Nervous system, nonadrenergic inhibitory, and airways, 28–29
Nose, defensive mechanisms from, 297–299

Oxygen dissociation curve, 84–85
Oxygen equilibrium of hemoglobin, 111–112
Oxygen sensitivity of pulmonary vessels, 159–161

Perivascular space, 154–155
pH, relation to P_{CO_2}, 85–86
Pharynx, defensive mechanisms from, 299–300
Phosphates, organic, control of hemoglobin function, 115–116
Pneumotaxic center
  and breathing pattern, 208–209
  influence on breathing pattern, 196–197
Protein transport physiological basis for, 170–171
Protons, control of hemoglobin function, 112–114
Pulmonary capillaries: See Capillaries, pulmonary
Pulmonary gas exchange: See Gas exchange

Recruitment and pulmonary capillary bed, 151–153
Respiration, comparative physiology of, 219–253
Respiratory functions, coupling of, 257–258
Respiratory insufficiency
  basic pathophysiological mechanisms of, 265–268
  CO_2 inhalation compared to arterial hypercapnia, 267–268
  hypoxic hypoxia compared to arterial hypoxemia in, 266–267
Respiratory rate
  effect of temperature, 187–188
  influence of mechanical loads, 188
  influence of vagus nerves, 188
  and tidal volume, 187–188

Respiratory system
  aerosols, 293–294
  defensive mechanisms of, 291–315
    components of, 295–296
    from particular sites, 297–308
  diseases of, control of breathing in,
    255–290
  immune responses and antimicrobial
    defenses, 296
  irritant gases, 292–293
  large objects and materials, 294–295
  patterns of invasion of, 292–295
  reflex responses, 296

Series inequality, gas exchange with,
    100–102
Skin breathing, 237–240
Surface tension, effect of, in
    pulmonary capillary bed,
    146–148

Taylor-type dispersion, 38–44
Temperature
  and breathing pattern, 199
  effect on tidal volume, 191–193
  effect on tidal volume and
    respiratory rate, 187–188
Tidal volume
  changes in T_E with volume inflations
    under isocapnic conditions, 190
  effect of alternating chemoreceptor
    stimulation, 195–196
  effect of anesthesia, 194–195
  effect of carbon dioxide, 191
  effect of sudden changes in
    chemoreceptor drive, 195
  effect of temperature, 187–188,
    191–193
  influence of mechanical loads, 188
  influence of vagus nerves, 188
  and inspiratory and expiratory
    durations, 188–196
  and respiratory rate, 187–188
  V_T, T_I, and T_E in man, 193–194
  V_T and T_I in steady state
    conditions, 188–189
  V_T and T_I with volume inflations
    under isocapnic conditions,
    189–190
Tracheobronchial tree, defensive
  mechanisms from, 301–307

Vascular system, pulmonary, growth
    of, 15–16
Vasoconstriction, hypoxic, 159–167
  possible mechanisms, 164–167
Ventilation distribution
  interregional, 52–62
    dynamic, 57–62
    effect of expiratory flow, 57–59
    effect of inspiratory flow, 57
    quasi-static, 53–56
Ventilation distribution
  intraregional, 62–70
    dynamic factors, 66–67
    experimental evidence of
      nonuniformity, 62–63
    functional and structural basis,
      69–70
    model analyses, 64–65
    sequential filling and emptying, 66
    single breath inert gas washouts,
      65–66
    single breath studies with two
      tracer gases, 67–69
    stratified vs. parallel
      inhomogeneity, 63–64
Ventilation-perfusion inequality, gas
    exchange in lung models of,
    88–90
Ventilation-perfusion ratio
  distributions during air breathing,
    92–95
  distribution during oxygen
    breathing, 95
  low, instability of lung units with,
    95–97
  measurement of continuous
    distributions of, 90–95
Ventilation-perfusion ratio equation,
    86–87
  description, 86
  solution by Fick principle for three
    gases, 87
  solution by R lines, 86–87
Vessels
  alveolar, functional anatomy of, 140
  extra-alveolar, 154–159
    definition, 154
    effect of lung inflation in zone 4,
      157–159
    interstitial pressure, 155–157
    perivascular space, 154–155
  extrapulmonary, functional anatomy
    of, 138

intrapulmonary noncapillary,
     functional anatomy of, 139–140
pulmonary
   functional anatomy of, 136–140
   morphometry, 136–138
   oxygen sensitivity of, 159–161

Water, lung
   distribution of, 175–176
   measurement of, 172–175
Water balance in lung, 167–176
Waterfall, vascular, 140–144